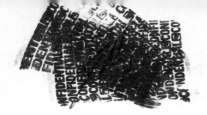

Family Violence and the Caring Professions

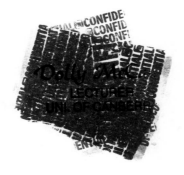

Family Violence and the Caring Professions

Edited by

PAUL KINGSTON

and

BRIDGET PENHALE

Foreword by **Olive Stevenson**

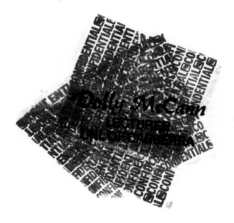

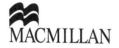

MACMILLAN

First published 1995 by
MACMILLAN PRESS LTD
Houndmills, Basingstoke, Hampshire RG21 2XS
and London
Companies and representatives
throughout the world

ISBN 0-333-60001-0

A catalogue record for this book is available
from the British Library.

10 9 8 7 6 5 4 3 2 1
04 03 02 01 00 99 98 97 96 95

Printed in Malaysia

CONTENTS

v

PART III   ELDER ABUSE

This book is overdue. It offers to British readers for the first time a systematic analysis of abuse to three different categories of people – children, spouses/partners (usually women) and old people – and offers a valuable comparison of the three. Even that bald description hints at the difficulties with which the editors had to grapple. Is it 'ageist' to separate out old people from other adults? What about adults with particular disabilities, especially learning difficulties? And so on. It is a minefield, conceptually and ethically. But all the more credit is due for the decision to grasp the nettle.

The specialist focus on specific groups in nearly all of the literature so far is understandable. Different political and social issues have been on the agenda, different professionals and workers engaged in different ways. However, there was clearly a pressing need for an overview, academically and professionally. The strength of the book is that it does not attempt to 'emulsify' the three groups but tackles each in turn, drawing out in its conclusions, similarities and differences. I have been puzzled in the past by the apparent reluctance to do this. In some quarters, notably governmental, there may be a fear that comparisons of other abuse with child abuse may open a Pandora's Box of trouble and unleash demands for resources. Amongst some academic and professional specialists with elderly people may be a reluctance to get sucked into the world of child abuse which has been so dominant and so voracious. The field of domestic abuse has been less professionalised (an interesting phenomenon in itself) and this has led to a curious split in thought between violence to women and violence to children – so often occurring in the same family and caused by the same man. The 'discourses' have run parallel but have not met in any significant way.

Whatever explanations one advances, the result is unfortunate. It is not a question of stressing similarities; it is a question of using the knowledge and experience gained from one field of study to illuminate another. This book offers rich opportunities to do this and it is particularly useful to have the health and social perspectives presented in turn. Again, rarely do we see these side by side in the same book.

There would seem to be six dimensions in which comparisons are fruitful. These concern: social attitudes to the phenomenon; definitions of it; etiology; the development of a policy response, including law and procedures; assessment processes; and intervention, including evaluation. Each in turn reveals similarities and differences which affect the course of events. For example, it is clear that the plight of abused old people has not raised the same social concern as that of children – which suggests fundamental differences in the value accorded to the two groups. Yet we can also usefully remind ourselves that the level and extent of denial of varying dimensions, including sexual, of child abuse only two or three decades years ago may parallel contemporary reluctance to grapple with this in the field of elder abuse.

Again, in relation to domestic violence, definitions and etiology have been dominated by the feminist paradigm of patriarchal domination, to a far greater extent than the other two groups. Yet this should remind us, first, that a significant number of 'old-age abuse' cases simply carry on a long-standing pattern of marital violence and, secondly, that this way of looking at the phenomenon has a great deal to say to us in relation to child abuse.

When we consider the highly developed law available to us in child protection and the woeful inadequacy of protective law for adults, we have tested legal models to consider (do we want emergency protection orders? for example) but also a responsibility to acknowledge the difference between children and adults in terms of concepts of legal competence with a crucially differing balance between autonomy and protection.

More generally, how can we ensure that assessment of elder abuse takes its proper place within the general framework of community care without excessive prominence, as has happened in child abuse, and that it does not become procedurally driven to the detriment of a sensitive professional response?

These are simply brief examples designed to show how fruitful comparisons are in stimulating high-quality debate among academics and professionals. What is now needed is for specific areas of comparison to be further developed. This book offers numerous such opportunities. It should be warmly welcomed.

Olive Stevenson
Professor of Social Work Studies

ACKNOWLEDGEMENTS

There are a number of people without whom this book would not have been possible. The original concept derives from the earlier American works of Straus, Gelles, and Steinmetz *et al.* to whom we are indebted. Early discussions followed from the initial contact at Action on Elder Abuse, and introduction to each other by Gerry Bennett – our special thanks to him. An initial approach to Kerry Lawrence at Macmillan proved favourable and positive. Our subsequent editor Margaret O'Gorman has proved flexible but committed, for which we are thankful.

Contributors to the book were relatively straightforward to locate: no coercion proved necessary! All have been positive, co-operative and steadfast and produced work of a high quality; our thanks to all. Thanks also to Professor Olive Stevenson for her foreword.

Bridget wishes to thank Dr Shulamith Ramon and Professor Peter Wedge for their initial faith and continuing belief; Ruth and Jenny for their interest and discussions; Dan, Ben and Nick for their unfailing support; and Paul for his commitment to the book/task and his trust and belief that we would complete it.

Paul wishes to thank the friendship and encouragement of Rosalie Wolf and Karl Pillemer and many other American colleagues who continue to keep in contact and consistently stimulate ideas, including Terry Fulmer and Tanya Johnson. Gerry Bennett requires special acknowledgement for his friendship and advice as does Chris Phillipson for his support and provocative ideas that always take the debate forward. Thanks also to all the steering group of Action on Elder Abuse whose ideas continually refresh the family violence debate.

Finally a personal thanks to Ang, Zoe, Lenna and Wookie who continue to tolerate my absences both in England and America.

Paul Kingston
Bridget Penhale

G. C. J. Bennett is Senior Lecturer, London Hospital Medical College, Consultant Physician Health Care of the Elderly CELFACS (City and East London Family and Community Health Services) and Honorary Consultant, Royal Hospital Trust. Chair of Action on Elder Abuse and co-author of *Elder Abuse: Concepts, Theories and Interventions.* Research interests include the epidemiology of abuse and carer perspectives on the issue. Other interests include being co-director of a joint would-care unit with research into all chronic wounds. Other books include *Alzheimer's Disease and Other Confusional States, Essentials of Health Care of the Elderly* and *Wound Care: A Practitioners' Guide.*

Simon Biggs worked as a community psychologist before becoming Programme Co-ordinator to the Central Council for Education and Training in Social Work. He has a wide experience of groupwork with service users, students and professional workers. He is the author of *Understanding Ageing* and co-author of *Understanding Elder Abuse: A Training Manual for Helping Professions.*

Jonathan Dickens and **Jim Ogg** qualified respectively in social work at the Universities of Nottingham and London in 1987. They met as part-time students at the MSc social research course, University of Surrey in 1989, and have both undertaken social work research. Jim Ogg has been a Team Leader with Essex Department of Social Services since March 1994. He has a special interest in the rights of vulnerable older people. Jonathan Dickens has worked as a social worker in an inner London Borough and was a Legal Officer for a London Local Authority until April 1994, acting on behalf of the Social Services Department in court proceedings relating to the care and protection of children.

Christine Hallett is Reader in Social Policy and Head of Department of Applied Social Science at the University of Stirling Scotland. She has researched and published extensively in the field of child protection (with Dr Elizabeth Birchall) and case conferences (with Professor Olive Stevenson). She is currently engaged on a study of decision-making in the Children's Hearings system in Scotland and is Chair of the Child Protection Committee in Central Region, Scotland.

Norman Johnson is Professor of Public Policy at the University of Portsmouth. For four years he was Deputy Director of the Keele research project into marital violence. In 1985 he edited a book entitled *Marital Violence*. He has published several books and numerous papers in the area of social policy.

Paul Kingston is a Research Fellow in the Department of Applied Studies, University of Keele. He is actively involved in research on abuse of elderly people in both England and America. He is Honorary Treasurer of Action on Elder Abuse. Research interests include family violence, falls in the elderly and elderly care in the Accident and Emergency Department. Publications include a co-authored text (with Gerry Bennett) *Elder Abuse: Concepts, Theories and Interventions* and *Elder Abuse: Health and Social Perspectives*.

Siobhan Lloyd is a Lecturer in Sociology/Women's Studies at the University of Aberdeen. She is also Head of the University Counselling Service. Her main research is in the area of violence against women. She has recently completed, with Michele Burman, a study for the Scottish Officer of specialist police units for the investigation of violent crime against women and children.

Jan Pahl is Director of Research at the National Institute for Social Work and an Honorary Reader at the University of Kent. Her research on battered women was funded by the Department of Health and was published in numerous articles and as a book: *Private Violence and Public Policy*. Jan Pahl has worked as a consultant on the topic of violence against women with the United Nations, the World Health Organisation and the Commonwealth Secretariat. She spent six years as a researcher in the health service and is an honorary member of the faculty of Public Health Medicine. Her present job at the National Institute for Social Work involves directing a programme of research on social work and social care, funded by the Department of Health.

Bridget Penhale is currently Team Leader of a team of Hospital Social Workers for the Social Services Department, Norfolk County Council. Prior to this post she held a joint appointment post between the School of Social Work, University of East Anglia, and Norfolk Social Services (1990–2): lecturing part-time and practising as a social worker with older people part-time. With a first degree in psychology, she qualified as a social worker (LSE) in 1981. She has specialised in work with older people since 1984. Her interest in elder abuse arose from practice but was developed through her academic post. She is Vice-Chair of Action on Elder Abuse, Chair of BASW Sub-committee on Community Care (1992–5) and a member of the Executive committee of BASW's Special Interest Group on Ageing. Publications include a number of refereed articles and *Elder Abuse: Health and Social Perspectives*, *Macmillan*.

Chris Phillipson is Professor of Applied Social Studies and Social Gerontology at Keele University and Head of Department. He has published seven books concerned with social, political and health issues arising from an ageing society. His research interests include: the political economy of health and ageing, community care of older people, health education/promotion, drugs and the elderly, old-age abuse and professional training and education. He is a regular consultant to the Health Education Authority, a past executive member of the British Association for Services to the Elderly. He has recently published a study of the future of work and retirement (with Frank Laczko) and a training manual on elder abuse *Understanding Elder Abuse: A Training Manual for Helping Professions* (Simon Biggs).

Stephanie Wheeler is Senior Lecturer at Bournemouth University. Her background has involved general nursing, midwifery and health visiting. In health visiting she spent ten years in the community as a practising health visitor and later a manager. She currently leads the professional studies theme in the Institute of Health and Community Services. She teaches primarily health care ethics and law for nursing and other undergraduate courses and is particularly interested in qualitative research.

Introduction
Family Violence: Framing the Issues

Paul Kingston and Bridget Penhale

Over the past twenty-five years increasing numbers of health and social care professionals have been faced with victims of family violence and abuse, victims from all ages across the life-course. Abuse is suspected, discovered and often proven in a multitude of environments and differing social and institutional circumstances. Abuse may reach the attention of professionals in numerous different ways; sometimes the individual professional suspects abuse and after investigation it is proven. This is probably the case most frequently in the domain of child abuse, and of the three areas considered in this text child abuse clearly has the highest index of suspicion.

Within the domain of adult abuse, health and social care professionals are more frequently approached by the victim after abuse has taken place with requests for advice or help, and an intervention post-abuse is therefore required. Within the sphere of elder abuse, fewer professionals are either knowledgeable about abuse or even suspect that abuse has taken place. However, health and social care professionals are beginning to develop a response to this latest discovery in the field of family violence. The fact is that professionals whenever and wherever they are working are increasingly likely to be caring for victims of abuse.

DEFINING THE CONCEPT

It is perhaps important at this point to mention some of the conceptual difficulties encountered when we sought authors for the text. Firstly the choice of title was relatively easy: we felt that authors would be clear about what would be required in each chapter (particularly because we had talked through the contents of each chapter with authors). It was also apparent that in the USA similar titles had been used to explore the wider issues of abuse and violence within the family, with well-known titles including: *Intimate Violence in families*, Gelles and Cornell (1990); *Current Controversies on Family Violence*, Gelles and Loseke (1993); and *Treatment of Family Violence*, Ammerman and Hersen (1990).

However, it became apparent early on in discussions that family violence was such a complex and multifaceted phenomenon that forms of abuse other than violence would enter into the discourse in all the chapters, and in fact the term 'abuse' is frequently used to encompass violence alongside other pernicious behaviours. Furthermore, differing forms of abuse that are not necessarily physically violent affect the lives of increasing numbers of individuals, for example financial abuse. We make no apologies for this expansion in the types of abuse considered in the text. It is perhaps inevitable and healthy that such developments should occur in an area that is still striving to understand the phenomena in question.

It also became apparent that to subdivide the life-span chronologically was also problematic. When the titles of the chapters were sent out to authors one interesting observation was made about the differentiation between adult abuse and elder abuse. It was suggested that to differentiate between the two phenomena could be construed as ageist, as elders were adults. We sought opinions from all the authors and decided that the consensus was that a differentiation was necessary, although not because of chronology. This was decided on the basis that even though all the victims are adults, the presenting phenomenon and the responses would, in the main, be unique to either elder abuse or adult abuse (Bennett and Kingston, 1993, p. 47). This is a clear example of the delicate task of presenting a precise conceptual framework of the issues under discussion.

DEFINITIONS OF ABUSE

The issue of definitions continues to cause concern and often disagreement amongst researchers, theorists and practitioners; often when practitioners from different professional backgrounds are involved with the same victim. Gelles and Cornell (1990) suggest that students of child maltreatment have identified:

> 'Neglect, emotional abuse, sexual abuse, educational neglect, medical neglect, and failure to thrive as forms of maltreatment.'

It is also apparent that theorists using differing frameworks to conceptualise abuse are in disagreement. For example Gelles and Loseke (1993) offer three differing frameworks for understanding abuse: psychological, sociological and feminist perspectives. Individual authors then proceed to argue their case for using one of the three perspectives. Gelles and Loseke state that this is not just an intellectual debate, that in fact the particular framework used will suggest particular frameworks for policy and intervention. There are also disputes about:

'*Who* is involved? What *behaviours* are of concern? What is the *relationship* between victims and offenders?'

(Gelles and Loseke, 1993)

Debate continues about who is involved in abusive situations and who are the abusers; arguments persist around gender division and whether the abusers are kin or not. Within the field of domestic violence, questions about the likelihood of women abusing men cause heated debate regarding the relative merits of viewing abuse from either a 'family violence' or a 'feminist' perspective (Straus, 1993; Kurz, 1993). In the sphere of elder abuse Pillemer has suggested that:

'Many abusers are not caregivers and many victims are not cared for (at least by their abusers).'

(Pillemer, 1993)

Clearly this view is at odds with the rather simplistic 'stressed caregiver' explanation of elder abuse portrayed by Eastman (1984) and Steinmetz (1988). If the more generic view of elder abuse is to be widely considered then perhaps a more comprehensive definition of elder abuse is required.

The type of behaviours involved in abuse have led feminists to suggest that certain adverts and pornography could be construed as acts of violence towards women (London, 1978). Claims about sexual abuse to older people are beginning to have substance (Holt, 1993; Ramsey-Klawsnik, 1993). Date and acquaintance rape have recently appeared as newly identified phenomena (Koss and Cook, 1993; Murphy, 1988). Within the sphere of learning disability, evidence is accumulating that individuals are the victims of sexual abuse (ARC/NAPSAC, 1993; Brown and Craft, 1989).

In the domain of child abuse, allegations of organised and ritualistic sexual abuse have been investigated (House of Commons, 1992). Current controversies are being fuelled by the debate surrounding corporal punishment by childminders, with confusion over whether a local

3

authority can refuse to register a childminder who refuses to sign an undertaking not to use corporal punishment (see *Sutton London Borough Council* v. *Davis* 1994). The debate about what can be considered violent behaviour within different groups goes on.

Throughout the following chapters issues about the framework and perspectives of abuse will be considered as will the relative merits of definition and intervention. The tensions between differing conceptualisations from professionals from quite different backgrounds will also be explored.

THE EMERGENCE OF DEBATE

Although we have been aware of family violence historically (Radbill, 1980; Dobash and Dobash, 1979; Stearns, 1986), it is only in the last twenty years in the UK that various professional groups, both health and social, have started to advance their expertise to develop a response to various forms of violence. This response has in many ways been congruent with that which appeared in the US where treatment approaches have begun to be implemented in the field of family violence. Ammerman and Hersen (1990) suggest two reasons for these new developments:

- An influx of professionals primarily interested in treatment (e.g., psychologists, psychiatrists, social workers) has occurred on a large scale only during the last decade. It is natural that their research interests should centre on remediation and treatment.
- Research delineating the role of individual and dyadic characteristics, in addition to societal factors as contributors to abuse and neglect, has underscored the utility of psychologically based therapeutic techniques in the treatment and prevention of domestic violence.

It is with the former aspect in mind that the idea of this text developed. Firstly it was felt that with the recently rediscovered phenomenon of elder abuse and neglect, professionals from numerous different agencies are now likely to intervene in cases of abuse throughout the life span. Violence or abuse is truly found from 'cradle to grave'.

These various professional groups have also been expected to work harmoniously together for the benefit of the victims of abuse. Frequently there is professional harmony; sometimes there is friction, with differing perspectives on the most appropriate intervention, if an intervention is even appropriate (see Ogg and Dickens, Chapter 3 in this volume). The aim of this book is therefore to look at family viol-

4

ence from these different professional perspectives in the hope that professionals will gain insight into what drives a particular profession in its aims to offer an intervention in cases of family violence.

The second development in the area of research suggested by Ammerman and Hersen (1990) led us to believe that readers would also need an academic overview of the 'state of the art' knowledge that is available in each area of family violence. If research is to inform the intervention process, then a clear understanding of this research is important. The intention is that the academic overview will show how the knowledge base has been created and how the particular issue has been constructed as a social problem. Because of the development towards a life-span perspective on violence, we also felt it necessary to divide the phenomenon into:

- Child abuse
- Adult abuse
- Elder abuse

Within each area the phenomenon is considered from the perspective of an academic overview, a health perspective and a social perspective. The reasons for this are simple: each area has a unique body of empirical knowledge; each area has a response formulated by health professionals and social professionals. Sometimes the health and social response overlap, often they are separate but complementary.

The following section gives a brief overview of the contents of the chapters that follow.

PART I: CHILD ABUSE

Chapter 1

'Child Abuse: An Academic Overview' by Christine Hallett begins with an analysis of how child abuse has been constructed from a 'claims-making' perspective, suggesting that all social problems need powerful institutions to assist in recognition of the phenomena. Comparisons in the development of the problem with the USA show that the UK is behind in an understanding of the problem and it is noteworthy that this is also found in the area of elder abuse.

A thorough analysis of the definitions of child abuse follow with a particularly valuable perspective on concepts of abuse in other countries, suggesting that abuse may be a fluid concept, ever changing in the face of societal obsessions. The global definition quoted by Gil (1981) is rather more comprehensive, and could be superimposed in the arena of elder abuse. In fact Wolf (1993) has suggested that a way forward in the definitional arena in elder abuse is to 'widen' the definition away from 'carer' abuse. In looking at Gil's definition, by changing the term 'children' to 'elder' we have a definition that encompasses a macro-perspective on elder abuse:

> 'abuse of *elders* is human-originated acts of commission or omission and human-created or tolerated conditions that inhibit or preclude unfolding and development of inherent potential of *elders*.'

> (Gil, 1981, modified by changing 'child' to 'elder')

The definition thus encompasses structural areas that have hitherto been excluded from the arena of elder abuse. This is not the first time that a more generic definition has been suggested for elder abuse; for example, commentators have suggested that the greatest abuse is a failure to 'provide the economic means for a decent life' (Callahan, 1988). Gil also stresses societal abuse, and again, by substituting the term 'elder' for 'child' the congruence of the two forms of abuse can be illuminating:

> 'This definition fits all manifestations of *elder* abuse – individual, institutional and societal. It focuses on human-originated interference with *elder* development whenever, and by whatever means, humans or their institutions and policies interfere with *elder* development, and whether the interference is physical, psychological, social, economic or cultural.'

> (Gil, 1981, modified by changing 'child' to 'elder')

Hallett's chapter then considers how child abuse is also constructed at a micro level with all the inherent dangers of 'subjective professional evaluation' (Hampton and Newberger, 1988). Of particular importance is how the variables of socio-economic status and ethnicity seem to affect the diagnosis of abuse. The prevalence of abuse is also influenced by the difficulties of definition and the fact that abuse is likely to be concealed. The main data sources both in the US and UK consist of sample surveys of the general population considering physical abuse and sexual abuse, sample surveys based on clinical samples and finally register data. The accuracy of each of these data sets is succinctly explored.

The chapter then moves on to consider the nature of abuse and its effect upon the victim. Hallett notes that 'an unknown amount of abuse is thought not to be identified or reported' (again, comparisons with domestic violence and elder abuse can be made); and the wide-ranging degrees of injury are also explored, from soft-tissue injury of a superficial nature, to death itself. There then follows a consideration of neglect with all the difficulties that are encountered when deciding at what threshold neglect should be defined.

Hallett then argues that not only imprecision in terms of definition causes tension amongst professionals, but that tensions are also apparent when causes are considered; that in fact there are competing conceptualisations of aetiology, with both psychological and sociological models being used to described causation.

In conclusion it is suggested that policy has been reactive and not proactive, with concern about identification and less energy spent on intervention. It is hoped that in the arena of elder abuse we can learn from this omission and not replicate the same error.

Chapter 2

'Child Abuse: The Health Perspective' by Stephanie Wheeler opens with definitional issues and epidemiology. The point raised by Hallett of an ever-changing preoccupation with certain elements of child abuse, which affects definitions, is reinforced, suggesting that abuse is influenced by enquiry reports and legislation.

At a micro-definitional level, it is suggested that work with different families can influence professional perceptions of abuse. Wheeler draws on the work of Hallett and Stevenson (1980) who proposed that health visitors might see more 'normal families' than social workers. Wheeler's own work (1992) suggests that tensions between professions makes it difficult to have common inter-professional definitions (this theme is also explored by Ogg and Dickens in Chapter 3). It is argued that to focus on health in terms of child protection using Gil's (1979) definition, linked to Seedhouse's definition of health, allows the health visitor to support parents, rather than view them as potential abusers. Empowerment is then considered within the domain of multi-professional practice. It is noticeable that this concept is a common theme in all areas of family violence.

In the fourth section of her chapter Wheeler produces a case-study from an accident and emergency perspective and focuses on four central themes from child health that she suggests could be utilised in child protection.

- Be an informed flexible practitioner.
- Do not see nursing (and health visiting) as a source of power but accept parents as partners in care.
- Have mature and refined interpersonal skills and awareness.
- Have knowledge related to family and of the processes that influence family functioning.

Firstly it is argued that a clear knowledge base in child abuse is necessary (this is also indispensable in adult and elder abuse). Secondly the nurse views her role in terms of partnership, both with the patient and other professions. Thirdly the nurse has defined and refined her interpersonal skills; this is particularly important when talking to victims of abuse and is clearly influenced by the nurse's value system in the domain of domestic violence (see also Lloyd, Chapter 6). Fourthly the nurse is aware of family dynamics.

The section on ethics and the law reiterates the health professional's position within the frameworks of the Children Act 1989 (DoH, 1989a) and the Code of Conduct (UKCC, 1992). Wheeler poses some awkward dilemmas about confidentiality. The message is clear: concerns must be reported. Nevertheless, for the practitioner the advice may be easier to read than to practise.

In the final section Wheeler considers the legal context of nursing and child protection. The position of health authorities and trusts *vis-a-vis* the Children Act, 1989, and the duty to co-operate on an interagency basis are also explored.

Chapter 3

'Social Perspectives in Child Abuse' by Jim Ogg and Jonathan Dickens starts to develop an understanding of social work intervention strategies in the field of child abuse. In doing so they focus on four distinct areas. Firstly there is an explication of the Children Act. Secondly, by drawing on 'discourse analysis' an exploration of the tensions inherent within practice are focused upon: the areas of 'law' and 'welfare' are specifically examined. Thirdly the practical applications of the Children Act are explored in the 1990s. In the fourth section the growing area of children's rights are considered.

Ogg and Dickens open with an exploration of the recent historical reasons for the 1989 Children Act, including the cases of Jasmine Beckford and Kimberley Carlile and the events in Cleveland in 1987. They then describe some of the main legislative changes found in the Children Act, taking into account how the act has attempted to balance the relative power of social workers, parents and children.

In the second section the conceptual approach of 'discourse analysis' is used to:

'expose the crucial influences which lie behind the way that the Children Act seeks to strike a balance between social workers, parents and children.'

The main discourses considered are 'law', 'welfare', 'the market economy' and 'managerialism' as they apply to practice within the Children Act. Within each discourse the main key signs are explored: for example, in law, 'equality before the law'; in welfare, 'provision of service according to need'; in the market economy, 'independence and state provision', and finally, in managerialism, 'procedures'. The aim in this section is to untangle the inherent tensions that exist between the differing discourses.

In the third section there is an analysis of three crucial developments in practice under the Children Act: care proceedings, case conferences and interviews with children. Within the area of practice tension exists within the differing discourses and Ogg and Dickens offer practical examples of where the tensions originate.

In the final section the issue of children's rights receives attention and again discourse analysis is used as a conceptual framework to deconstruct the inherent difficulties. Ogg and Dickens cite the tension between child-defined choice and adult-defined need as an example of differences in the welfare and legal discourses. This section then debates four issues in the children's rights arena:

• Children's rights to make choices are limited by the range of choices.
• The wishes of a child may not always coincide with legal powers and entitlements.
• Children's choices in matters may have directly harmful consequences.
• Children do not necessarily have the capacity to exercise the responsibilities that follow from their choices.

Clearly these questions and the debates that surround the intrinsic tensions within child protection will continue as an area for debate in future years. Of final note are the analogies that can be drawn in all areas of family violence (adult abuse and elder abuse) between the tensions in the different discourses of 'welfare', 'law', 'market economy' and 'managerialism'.

PART II: ADULT ABUSE

Chapter 4

'Domestic Violence: An Overview' by Norman Johnson opens with the difficulties, described in the child abuse section, of definitions. Johnson discusses the advantages and disadvantages of various terms, including:

- marital violence
- spouse abuse
- battered women
- battered wives
- domestic dispute

eventually settling with the term 'domestic violence'. The chapter then discusses the political dimension of domestic violence. The patriarchal system and the effect of hiding domestic violence is explored, as are the difficulties encountered with social problem construction. Readers will note after reading Chapters 1, 4 and 9 that the theme of 'social problem construction' appears in child, adult and elder abuse. How different types of abuse – child, adult and elder – travelled through Blumer's (1971) taxonomy of social problem construction differs usually because of the professional background of the 'claimsmakers'. It is apparent, for example, that domestic violence is not a major issue for the medical profession (or only in the sense of repairing physical wounds); however, within the spheres of child and elder abuse, the medical profession has taken a lead role.

The chapter then moves on to consider the historical development of the battered-women's movement in the UK. Johnson makes it clear that in terms of trying to make an individual concern a public concern, the women's movement clearly succeeded.

The debate surrounding victims is becoming increasingly heated, with proponents on both sides of the argument. The research quoted in this chapter tries to balance the arguments; however, as new research is constantly being reported, the consensus may change. At present the consensus in the UK suggests that most domestic violence consists of violence by men inflicted upon women. However, in the US the debate has reached new levels of disagreement, with Straus arguing that physical assaults by wives are as frequent as assaults by men (Straus, 1993), and Kurz (1993) arguing the opposite: that women are typically victims.

Johnson moves on to consider the different forms that domestic violence may take, and readers may notice a similarity with the previous chapters on child abuse with classifications of abuse as:

- physical
- sexual
- emotional or psychological

The degree and extensive nature of abuse includes slapping, punching, kicking, choking, butting, biting, burning, hair-pulling and pushing downstairs. Explanations are varied; the first conceptual approach considered by Johnson focuses on the perpetrator as an individual and interprets physiological and psychoanalytical theory. The physiological theory argues that certain genetic and physiological traits predispose all men to violence. From the psycho-pathological perspective, theory suggests the perpetrators are jealous and weak men. Other theorists focus on women as the root cause of violence, suggesting traits in women's personality that provoke violence or even that women are addicted to violence. A further perspective uses social learning theory to try and explain violence. This theory, sometimes called 'the cycle of violence theory', is also referred to as a risk factor in elder abuse, as is the psycho-pathological perspective. In essence it suggests that violence is transmitted generationally.

The final explanation concentrates on socio-structural factors: economic conditions, bad housing, relative poverty, lack of job opportunities. These conditions allied to specific male and female roles are viewed as producing stress with violence as a result. However it is suggested that perpetrators of violence are found in all socio-economic groups and not all men who are close to the above prescribed socio-structural factors abuse.

The chapter concludes with a view of the responses. Firstly there is a synthesis of the criticisms levelled at the police that includes a suggestion that the police are now trying to be more proactive in the area of domestic violence. A resume of the current and potential future legislation follows. Johnson sums up the position by dismissing views that suggest that women are addicted to violence and argues that in many cases it is perhaps too difficult to leave abusive family situations, mainly because of the family social structures.

Chapter 5

'Health Professionals and Violence Against Women' by Jan Pahl opens with an overview of the difficulty in assessing how many victims of violence come into contact with health care professionals. Certainly UK figures are much smaller than US figures, and this in part may be due to the fact that violence to women was discovered earlier in the US.

Other reasons include professional awareness, as research by McLeer and Anwar (1989) clearly indicates. Emergency department staff were subjected to training in the use of a protocol asking direct questions about abuse with positive identifications of female victims increasing from 5.6 per cent to 30 per cent following the use of the protocol. This research suggests that emergency department staff do not identify adult victims of violence. This is also the case for older victims (Kingston and Hopwood, 1994; Kingston and Phillipson, 1994). When McLeer and Anwar's figures are broken down into age, 42 per cent of the victims are 18–20 years old, 35 per cent are 21–30 years old and 18 per cent over 61 years old. It is of interest also that in a recent British survey of the 5 per cent of victims of domestic violence seen in an accident and emergency department, fourteen were male and two female (Smith *et al.*, 1992).

Pahl moves on to consider the effects of abuse. It is disturbing that over two-thirds of women report being subject to abuse for three or more years. The effects on children are also discussed (as seen also in Lloyd's chapter which follows).

The degree of help received from health practitioners clearly varies. Mixed views are reported about general practitioners' responses to women victims, with Binney *et al.*'s (1981) research suggesting 44 per cent finding the contact unhelpful. In Pahl's (1979) study, 56 per cent found the contact helpful and 44 per cent unhelpful. Both these studies are now over a decade old and more recent studies might find attitudinal change amongst general practitioners. This chapter is all the richer for the voices of the women being heard. Health visitors also do not fare well, either because they are seen to be primarily there for the children, or their advice was perceived as inappropriate.

Training for health professionals shows that education can clearly assist in recognising abuse. In a US study of 117 medical schools, over half provided no instruction; the others provided an average of 1.5 sessions of 1.9 hours' duration (McIlwaine, 1989). Smith *et al.* (1992) suggest that medical students in Leicester receive only one session of teaching on family violence given by a psychologist. Pahl in her chapter quotes a study in Detroit that had a profound effect on nurses' attitudes to abuse (Mandt, 1993).

The chapter concludes with recommendations for good practice, including:

- Respecting the woman's account
- Knowing the relevant information
- Keeping careful records
- Giving enough time to the victim

Chapter 6

'Social Work and Domestic Violence' by Siobhan Lloyd develops the now common theme of definition, especially questions about who defines abuse: victims or professionals. Themes then emerge that run through the whole chapter. There is firstly the issue of awareness about domestic violence at both macro and micro levels. Firstly, how aware are politicians and policy-makers of the level of domestic violence in society? Secondly, although social workers and managers are aware of domestic violence, what are their value systems in this area and do they have the prerequisite skills and knowledge to offer the intervention that women (and children) call for?

Lloyd tightens the parameters within which she operates by focusing on women with children who are victims of violence. The justification for this is pragmatic: they have been more thoroughly researched. There are also certain groups who have specific needs because of the unique forms of discrimination they face: black and ethnic minority women; women with disabilities; lesbian women and older women. The particular needs of these groups are sensitively discussed.

It is suggested that social work practice is influenced by two core issues:

- prevalence of domestic violence on case loads
- the way in which domestic violence is understood by social workers

Firstly the extent of the problem may be underestimated by social workers themselves, and secondly the way social workers understand domestic violence will clearly influence their response. The construction of domestic violence as a social problem, not necessarily an individual problem, has also helped women to argue against violence at a political and ideological level.

It is proposed that social workers' understanding of and value systems in domestic violence remain bound to a family systems model (see Straus, 1993, earlier in this chapter). Dobash and Dobash (1992) argue that this is because:

> 'social workers see clients in need of therapy, rather than people in need of alternatives and choices.'

It is particularly important to make this point in a text that is designed to educate those from the 'caring professions' about family violence. This is necessary in order to avoid what Estes (1979) called an 'aging enterprise':

> 'Service strategies in general ... tend to stigmatise their clients as recipients in need, creating an impression that they have somehow failed to assume responsibility for their lives.'

Furthermore, health and social professionals must avoid a 'family violence enterprise': a situation in which service providers extend their service provision, not with the needs of the consumer in mind, but their own vested interests. As Estes perceptively notes:

'particularly in a market economy where profits can be made in human service delivery – the greater the incentives for providers to expand the net of individual needs for which they can provide services.'

(Estes, 1979).

From an historical perspective Lloyd shows how social workers indeed pathologised women (not men) with references to women's supposed faults:

- excessive pressure
- the need to suffer
- rejection of femininity
- sex response

It is also suggested that we have not reached a situation where all social workers challenge the view that women are to blame for the violence. A further concept that has damaged an understanding of domestic violence is 'learned helplessness' (a perspective also discussed by Johnson in Chapter 4). From a service provision perspective, pathologising women or accusing them of suffering from 'learned helplessness', and in need of therapy, should be clearly resisted.

The challenge to the above views comes when the frequency of contact with social workers is considered. Women do approach social workers for help and advice (although it is important to note that some minority ethnic groups were far from happy with the quality of the contact) although they may not find it an easy thing to do. Lloyd outlines some useful suggestions in tabular form to help women disclose domestic violence.

The section on children and domestic violence describes in graphic detail the effect of violence on children, including being used for manipulative purposes, and being forced to watch the abuse. Again the issue of transgenerational violence arises, and the pervasive nature of abuse that affects not only mother but child, often with the social worker not knowing who is most at risk, is explored.

In the section on Women's Aid and social work a familiar issue again arises – the tensions that exist between different agencies, already discussed by Ogg and Dickens, Chapter 3. Multi-agency training is suggested as a way of bringing agencies together to understand each other's intervention philosophy.

The penultimate section considers multi-agency approaches, a theme that arises in all sections of this text (child, adult, elders). The different perspectives of the two agencies are explored: Women's Aid, empowering and autonomous, and social work, paternalistic and patriarchal, with echoes of the 'family violence enterprise'. Lloyd finishes this section with some examples of multi-agency successes, including the recent 'Zero Tolerance' campaign in Edinburgh.

The chapter concludes with a list of measures to help women who are victims. The measures suggested are aimed at both social work agencies and individual social workers.

PART III: ELDER ABUSE

Before considering the three chapters on elder abuse, it is important to note that as far as the editors are aware, this is the first time in the UK that elder abuse has been discussed in a text on family violence alongside child abuse and domestic violence. Despite the existing texts on elder abuse (Eastman, 1984; Pritchard, 1992; Phillipson and Biggs, 1992; DeCalmer and Glendenning, 1993; Bennett and Kingston, 1993), this is the first time that elder abuse has been drawn into a debate that discusses the wider issues of family violence.

Chapter 7

'Elder Abuse: A Critical Overview' by Chris Phillipson and Simon Biggs commences with an analysis of why elder abuse appears to have been rediscovered in the early 1990s, the first reports in the mid-1970s failing to make an impact. Three reasons are given: firstly, professionals were still trying to come to terms with child and spouse abuse; secondly, the status of older people within society; and finally, difficulties of definition. Phillipson and Biggs argue that in the early 1990s the situation is rather different. Professionals in the gerontological arena are more confident of their position and there is a stronger academic framework on which to base practice. There is also a clear debate surrounding community care and the nature of caring, focused on by implementation of the NHS and Community Care Act (DOH, 1989b).

The intrinsic theme of definitions, discussed in the preceding chapters, appears again. A thorough discussion of the relative merits of different definitions follows with the valuable suggestion that consensus

15

and agreement will only be achieved when elders themselves are involved in the debate.

An analysis of the prevalence studies, North American, Canadian and British, clearly indicates that elder abuse exists. These studies under-represent certain groups: frail elders, and disadvantaged and minority ethnic groups – all potentially high-risk victims of abuse. In terms of characteristics, the North American prevalence studies have produced differing profiles for physical/psychological abuse, neglect and financial abuse. Caution is clearly necessary in transferring data from North America to the UK context; on the other hand, it is the only data available at present, so it would be unwise to summarily dismiss the findings. Research in the UK context to replicate such studies for comparative purposes is urgently required.

The next section considers institutional abuse. It is interesting that this phenomenon is not discussed in either of the preceding sections on child and adult abuse. This is to some extent understandable within the adult abuse section, with fewer adults living institutions; however, reports of adults with learning disabilities being subjected to sexual abuse are becoming more frequent (ARC/NAPSAC, 1993; Brown and Craft, 1989). Within the sphere of child protection there is clear evidence of abuse to children living in institutional settings including the Pindown Experience in Staffordshire (Staffordshire County Council, 1991). This is not an issue that can easily be avoided in the arena of ageing studies. Historical and contemporary reports of behaviours inflicted upon elderly people in the 'care' of professionals are available (Bennett and Kingston, 1993). What appears remiss is any concerted effort to tackle the issue of institutional abuse.

Phillipson and Biggs move on to consider theoretical perspectives used to try and understand the dynamics of abuse: the situational model, pathology model, exchange theory, interactionist theory and the social construction of old age. Each theory has its own view of the dynamics involved, either at a macro (societal) level or a micro (individual) level.

The next section considers where elder abuse may fit, if at all, in the wider arena of domestic violence. The similarities with, and differences from, child abuse are clearly explored, with the view being taken that elder abuse is 'similar but also very different to other forms of domestic violence'.

The debate on legislation remains contentious. Phillipson and Biggs take the view that existing legislation is perhaps under-utilised. They further suggest that caution is necessary when new legislation is considered, especially in the absence of any commitment to extra resources.

The chapter concludes with a framework of options that could be utilised to design interventions. These are complemented by four guiding principles in the areas of: vigilance; shared decision-making; empowerment; and policies.

Chapter 8

'Health Perspectives and Elder Abuse' by Dr Gerry Bennett moves straight into the different forms that elder abuse may take, including sexual abuse. Issues of recognition then come to the fore and it is suggested that, in the main, physical abuse is probably the easiest to diagnose, that is, compared with, say, psychological or sexual abuse. Suffice it to say that none of the different forms of abuse are easy to diagnose. One of the reasons suggested is that in the arena of child abuse there are certain development norms and children are in most cases highly visible. Elderly people, on the other hand, have enormously differing health status and can quite often be invisible to health and social care workers. Bennett considers some of the physiological changes due to ageing and how these can affect diagnosis.

Alerting features are then discussed including inappropriate injury and discrepancies between injury and explanation. This is crucial knowledge that all health care professionals should be aware of. Bennett also points out that one of the difficulties of diagnosis is the level of doctors' knowledge of the phenomenon. It has been suggested earlier that family violence is only superficially considered on the medical curriculum; this is also true of nursing curricula (Kingston and Penhale, 1994).

Manifestations of abuse are then examined, from physical indicators to poor hygiene and decubitii. It is important to note that these manifestations do not diagnose abuse, but only lead the professional to ask further questions about their causation.

The section on sexual abuse makes somewhat grim reading. The precise dimensions of the problem are still unknown, this being clearly the most difficult of all the forms of abuse to prove. Bennett draws on the US research to consider the skills necessary to interview potential victims; these guidelines are also useful in the wider arena of abuse. The chapter moves on to consider various myths about victims. Assessment skills are then explored and the necessity for policies and procedures are reiterated. One useful tool, 'The Cost of Care Index' (Kosberg and Cairl, 1986), is also cited as good practice, as is the 'Elder Assessment' instrument (Fulmer, 1984). We believe that this infrastructure of policy and procedure tied to assessment instruments

17

will in retrospect be seen as one of the initial requirements necessary to diagnose elder abuse.

The difficulties encountered when altered mental states are imposed upon older victims of abuse are then explored, followed by a review of legislation, with the final message being one of multi-professional assessment as a crucial first step within the arena of elder abuse.

Chapter 9

'Social Perspectives on Elder Abuse' by Bridget Penhale and Paul Kingston cannot offer the same precise, albeit fluid and developing, response from the social work viewpoint that has been presented by Ogg and Dickens in the child abuse section and Lloyd in the adult abuse section. There are three reasons for this. Firstly, it is only since 1989 that elder abuse has been acknowledged as an issue that needs attention from health and social care professionals (see also Bennett and Kingston, 1993; DeCalmer and Glendenning, 1993; Penhale, 1993; Kingston and Penhale, 1994; Kingston and Phillipson, 1994). Secondly, intervention strategies specifically designed in this area are noticeable by their absence. Thirdly, we are not in a position to evaluate the effectiveness of the superficial work that has developed to date. Studies to evaluate health and social agencies that have responded to the DOH guidelines *No Longer Afraid* (DOH/SSI, 1993) are beginning; however, we are still in the formative stages of responding to abuse. But it is possible to look retrospectively on the recent history of elder abuse and its recognition (or otherwise) as a social problem.

It can be seen that following the early reports in the 1970s, little interest was shown in elder abuse until the late 1980s. This was approximately ten years behind US interest in the area. However, the 1990s have seen a surge in interest in the phenomenon. From a 'social problem perspective' analysis it is possible to compare the development in the US and the UK and this may well aid developments in the future, especially when trying to secure the issue on the political agenda. This chapter uses Blumer's taxonomy of social problem construction to de-construct the developments to date (Blumer, 1971).

In terms of emergence, the 1990s have brought the debate forward, with articles, organisations and research; Phillipson and Biggs in Chapter 7 have also discussed some of the reasons why the debate was delayed. We have suggested that in fact there was not enough room for debate in the arena for elder abuse, child abuse and domestic violence. It would appear that room has had to be somewhat forced by what Best (1989) calls 'claims-makers' and Gusfield (1982) calls 'troubled people professionals'. We further suggest that ageism has helped to keep the issue out of mainstream debate, alongside a late entry for gerontological studies in the UK, arguably 30 years behind the US.

At the level of legitimation it is suggested that elder abuse is accepted by professionals as a serious problem (and perhaps has been for over a decade), but in the wider public and political arena this is clearly not so. If we look at the US experience much media attention was gained through the political hearings in the Senate in 1981. Furthermore, politicians like Claude Pepper invested their personal energies to publicise the debate. There would appear to be a political vacuum outside the Department of Health in the UK.

Mobilisation of action is beginning, reinforced by John Bowis (Junior Minister Of Health) launching Action on Elder Abuse. This, alongside *No Longer Afraid* (DOH/SSI, 1993) is the first official acknowledgement that elder abuse exists in the UK. It is necessary to wait for the last two stages in Blumer's taxonomy: formulation and implementation of the official plan. We are, however, in a position to influence the last two stages, and Action on Elder Abuse alongside other organisations will no doubt be influential in their arguments.

Marginalisation of elderly people is also clearly part of an equation that sees elderly people on the periphery of society. The perceptive views of Townsend (1981) and Walker (1981) although over a decade old are as pertinent as ever, and, it could be argued, there is a continuation and reinforcement of the 'structured dependency' of older people with a protracted reliance on 'care for' older people and not 'care' with the views of elders to the fore.

In conclusion the chapter suggests that a policy response must be unique to elder abuse and that legislation must be clearly thought through before implementation. Empowerment of older people should be the clear goal of any policies. Perhaps the most difficult task will be to educate the wider public, which includes older people themselves; thus far older people's voices have not been heard.

The concluding chapter compares and contrasts the different forms of family violence (child, adult and elder abuse). Some of the common themes within the wider field of family violence, shared by contributors to this text, are then offered by way of synthesis and conclusion to the volume.

This introduction has served to explore the forthcoming chapters. Areas of similarity have been mentioned as have themes that consistently arise. We consider that the reader will begin to have their questions about child, adult and elder abuse answered. However, we also believe that readers will begin to formulate their own questions about family violence, especially many of the moral and ethical issues concerning intervention in what has traditionally been seen as an area that is sacrosanct. We have attempted to offer a beginning to the ongoing debates that we believe are likely for health and social care professionals in the domain of family violence.

PART I

Child Abuse

CHAPTER ONE

Child Abuse: An Academic Overview

Christine Hallett

THE SOCIAL CONSTRUCTION OF CHILD ABUSE

Child abuse, as the term is commonly used in western societies, was discovered, or more properly rediscovered, in the post-war period. The process of rediscovery can usefully be viewed within a sociological framework for analysing the social construction of social problems. This emphasises the complex processes by which behaviours or social conditions, which may have been long experienced as private pains or sorrows, become defined as public ills. It is encapsulated in Manning's observation that social problems 'are not just what people think they are but rather what powerful and influential people think they are' (1985, p.5).

Nelson (1984) explores how and why child abuse claimed a place on the public and political agenda in the United States of America. Underlying her account is the view that governments in western countries are overloaded, given the transformation in the role of the state from a laissez-faire position in the nineteenth century, when relatively little of the nation's wealth was appropriated by the state in taxation for public spending, to contemporary patterns where there is substantial state involvement in many spheres of public policy. In such circumstances, there is more that the state could potentially do than it has power and resources actually to achieve, and so the processes by which some issues successfully claim and maintain a place on the public policy agenda, while others fail to do so, are critical. If, as some assert (Spector and Kitsuse, 1977), social problems are, in essence, the result of groups asserting grievances or making successful claims for attention and resources, the state is a key site for the construction of social problems. A social condition will not be deemed to have been successfully transformed into a social problem if powerful social institutions can, and do, ignore it. Nelson outlines four stages in the policy-agenda-setting process as follows: issue recognition, issue adoption, issue prioritising and issue maintenance. Issue recognition is the point where an issue is noticed and considered to be a potential topic for action. Issue adoption is the decision to respond which involves a perception both of the legitimacy of government responsibility for an issue and of feasibility that an appropriate response could be found if the issue were to be adopted. Issue prioritising involves the reordering of the public policy agenda to make space for the new issue, which may require relegating other topics. Issue maintenance requires sustaining interest in an issue as an addition to the enduring concerns of government.

In the early stages of the social construction of child abuse as a problem in the United States, Nelson highlights the existence of medical interest in the problem, the role of the media in informing political élites of the existence and extensiveness of the problem and in building mass consensus for government action, and the role of prominent politicians championing the cause in the early 1970s. In the United States the emphasis on the physical abuse of children overshadowed the more pervasive problem of child neglect. Physical abuse was the issue on which there was the strongest consensus and the highest emotions, and it represented less of a challenge to the social and economic organisation of society than tackling the problem of child neglect.

The events which occurred in the United States were to have a profound influence on the emergence of child abuse as a social problem in the United Kingdom, which occurred a little later. Parton (1985) has analysed the process, with particular reference to physical abuse, tracing the 'social forces which facilitated, influenced, initiated and reacted' to child abuse. Using, as does Nelson, a 'natural history cycle' approach, Parton suggests that the recognition and response to child abuse did not depend simply on the objective or neutral characteristics of the condition but passed through four stages: discovery, diffusion, consolidation and reification.

Discovery built directly on the work of North American physicians who revealed the problem of child abuse in the post-war years. It should be noted in passing, however, that physical injury, neglect, and emotional and sexual abuse of children had, in fact, been accurately described long before, by a French physician, in the 1850s and 1860s (Tardieu, 1857 and 1860). As Lynch notes, 'much of what was around during his time seems very familiar today' (1992, p. 16). The rediscovery in the post-war years built on the work of Caffey (1946) and Woolley and Evans (1955), paediatric radiologists, who noted a link between fractures of the long bones revealed in X-rays and subdural haematoma (bleeding in the cranium) and postulated trauma as the cause. However, it was the publication in 1962 of an article in the influential *Journal of the American Medical Association*, with the head-line-catching title 'The Battered Child Syndrome' which propelled child abuse into the public arena (Kempe *et al.*, 1962). The article focused on specific injuries (such as broken bones and bruising) inflicted principally on young children. It was a condition which was relatively narrowly defined and which could be diagnosed primarily by doctors. Discovery was professionally led, aided by technological changes which assisted diagnosis. This was important in two respects. First, it established some respectability, credibility and professional legitimacy for the idea that parents or others caring for children could, and did, injure and deliberately harm those in their care. Second, it identified child physical abuse within the medical model. It was identified and publicised by doctors, labelled a syndrome and conceptu-alised as a disease. This was to have important implications for the policy responses to the problem, for child abuse was seen initially as a pathology, with the causes lying in the personality of particular parents, and it was thought to be capable of being diagnosed and treated. As Parton notes, the focus was on dangerous or diseased individuals rather than on the social conditions in which parenting or the care of children took place.

In Britain, as Parton documents, the NSPCC was important in the next phase, diffusion, which took place between 1968 and 1972. Its Battered Child Research Unit was influential in publicising the problem. In campaigning and setting up a demonstration project, the NSPCC forged a new role for itself and began to counteract the financial problems and uncertainly about its function which had stemmed from its duplication of the role of children's departments es-tablished in local government in the 1940s. Thus, as had occurred in the United States of America with respect to paediatric medicine (Pföhl, 1977), organisational and professional interests played a significant part in the emergence of child abuse as a social problem.

Despite the activities of specialist groups such as professions and the NSPCC, there was relatively little public awareness of child abuse in the United Kingdom until the case of Maria Colwell. She was killed in 1973 by her stepfather while under the supervision of the local social services department. A public inquiry was set up following her death. It reported in 1974 (Department of Health and Social Security, 1974) and attracted enormous press and media interest. Parton analyses the role of key politicians and civil servants, particularly the then Secretary of

State for Social Services, Sir Keith Joseph, in deciding to institute a public inquiry, and also locates the developments in a changed political economy of welfare characterised by concern (a 'moral panic') about falling standards in family life, moral degeneracy, the growth of violence and the perceived failure of social workers to remedy the ills. Nonetheless, it remains unclear precisely why this particular case attracted such widespread publicity and why the media took on a crusading and campaigning role. Whatever the reasons, Maria Colwell was front-page news and the effect of this and a succession of later inquiries was to have a profound effect on popular and professional consciousness, and on the policy responses developed to deal with the problem (Department of Health and Social Security, 1982; Hallett, 1989; Hill, 1990; and Department of Health, 1991d). By 1974, child abuse had reached the third of Parton's four stages; it was consolidated as a social problem with public, professional, media and political interest mobilised. The subsequent policy developments reified the problem and affirmed its importance in public policy.

The primary focus of concern in the processes outlined above was physical injury to children. Subsequently, but to a much less significant extent, concerns were raised about children who were neglected or emotionally abused. The second main phase of the rediscovery of child abuse, however, centred on sexual abuse, which entered the public domain in the United Kingdom in the 1980s.

While child physical abuse was identified and publicised by 'experts', a growing recognition of the existence of varied forms of sexual abuse to children resulted in the United Kingdom and in the United States of America (Finkelhor, 1984) from the testimony of adult survivors. As women discussed with each other their childhood experiences, it emerged that what many had thought of as events unique to them were, in fact, shared by others. This feminist analysis which contributed to the discovery and publicity of sexual abuse emphasised not a medical model but a power imbalance in the social structure between adult abusers (principally men) and young people (principally girls and young women) and a process of male socialisation which engendered predatory and exploitative male attitudes and sexual behaviours. In this process the role of professions, particularly medicine, was less dominant (although some clinicians played a prominent role especially in diagnosis) and the activities of self-help groups more prominent (Kelly, 1988; Driver and Droisen, 1989).

A feminist analysis is not, however, the only discourse. Also influential is the family systems model which conceptualises child sexual abuse as a symptom of family dysfunction, emphasising that

26

child sexual abuse within the family arises from disturbances in family relationships (see, for example, Furniss, 1984; CIBA, 1984). In the process, the mother is often portrayed as 'colluding with' or even responsible for the abuse, emphasising the role of women to create and maintain stability within families and underemphasising the power inequalities in family life. The tension and conflict between feminist and family systems approaches remains (Glaser and Forsh, 1988; McLeod and Saraga, 1988).

DEFINITIONS OF CHILD ABUSE

The official definitions of child abuse used in the United Kingdom policy documents have changed and expanded over time in a process described by Dingwall as 'diagnostic inflation' (Dingwall, 1989, p. 29). Initially the focus was relatively narrow, on young children suffering from inflicted physical injuries, epitomised by the term 'battered babies', which was the title of central government circulars of guidance on the topic issued in 1968 and 1970.

Since then the official definitions used when children's names are placed on local child protection registers have widened. These registers are lists maintained by local authority social services departments of 'all children in the area for whom there are unresolved child protection issues and who are currently the subject of an interagency protection plan' (Home Office *et al.*, 1991, p. 48). There are currently four categories in use in England and Wales, defined as follows:

Physical injury:
> Actual or likely physical injury to a child, or failure to prevent physical injury (or suffering) to a child, including deliberate poisoning, suffocating and Munchausen's syndrome by proxy.

Neglect:
> The persistent or severe neglect of a child, or the failure to protect a child from exposure to any kind of danger, including cold or starvation, or extreme failure to carry out important aspects of care, resulting in the significant impairment of the child's health or development, including non-organic failure to thrive.

Sexual abuse:
> Actual or likely sexual exploitation of a child or adolescent. The child may be dependent and/or developmentally immature.

Emotional abuse:
> Actual or likely severe adverse effect on the emotional and behavioural development of a child caused by persistent or severe

emotional ill-treatment or rejection. All abuse involves some emotional ill-treatment. This category should be used where it is the main or sole form of abuse.

(Home Office *et al.*, 1991, p. 48)

Similar categories are in use in Scotland where the official definitions recommended by the Scottish Office for the registration of children are as follows:

Physical injury:

Actual or attempted physical injury to a child, under the age of 16, where there is definite knowledge, or reasonable suspicion, that the injury was inflicted or knowingly not prevented.

Sexual abuse:

Any child below the age of 16 may be deemed to have been sexually abused when any person(s), by design or neglect, exploits the child, directly or indirectly, in any activity intended to lead to the sexual arousal or other forms of gratification of that person, or any other person(s), including organised networks. This definition holds whether or not there has been genital contact and whether or not the child is said to have initiated the behaviour.

Physical neglect:

This occurs when a child's essential needs are not met and this is likely to cause impairment to physical health and development. Such needs include food, clothing, cleanliness, shelter and warmth. A lack of appropriate care results in persistent or severe exposure, through negligence, to circumstances which endanger the child.

Emotional abuse:

Failure to provide for the child's basic emotional needs such as to have a severe effect on the behaviour and development of the child.

Non-organic failure to thrive:

Children who significantly fail to reach normal growth and development milestones (i.e. physical growth, weight, motor, social and intellectual development), where physical and genetic reasons have been medically eliminated and a diagnosis of non-organic failure to thrive have been established.

(Social Work Services Group, 1992)

Two important consequences flow from such definitions. The first is that some forms of harm to children are excluded. The second is that the definitions are phrased in rather general terms and thus require a degree of subjective judgement about the presence or absence of abuse.

THE EXCLUSION OF SOME KINDS OF ABUSE FROM OFFICIAL DEFINITIONS

As was suggested earlier in the chapter, the definition of child abuse is historically and culturally specific. Ideas of what constitutes abuse change over time and vary from place to place, reflecting differing national problems and professional and societal preoccupations. Conceptions of 'abuse' in other countries, for example, include child labour, a prominent issue in the so-called developing countries and in some parts of Europe, e.g. Turkey and Italy (Christopherson, 1989), child prostitution and the harmful consequences for children of war, civil unrest or refugee status, a concern in many parts of the world including Africa, South East Asia and the former republic of Yugoslavia (Garbarino *et al.*, 1991; Ajdukovic, 1993). These issues have been the focus of attention in recent conferences of the International Society for the Study and Prevention of Child Abuse and Neglect (for example, in Hamburg, 1990, Chicago, 1992 and Padua, 1993).

The official definitions in use in the United Kingdom are relatively narrow in their focus on abuse inflicted principally by carers. They implicitly reject the much more radical definition proposed by Gil that

'abuse of children is human-originated acts of commission or omission and human-created or tolerated conditions that inhibit or preclude unfolding and development of inherent potential of children.'

(1981, p. 295)

Gil suggests that

'This definition fits all manifestations of child abuse – individual, institutional and societal. It focuses on human-originated interference with child development whenever, and by whatever means, humans or their institutions and policies interfere with child development, and whether the interference is physical, psychological, social, economic, political or cultural.'

(1981, p. 294)

He stresses, in particular, that societal abuse of children is frequently overlooked. He argues that

'children are abused and their development tends to be stunted as a result of a broad range of perfectly legitimate social policies and public practices which cause, permit and perpetuate poverty, inadequate nutrition, physical and mental ill-health, unemployment, substandard housing and neighbourhoods, polluted and dangerous environments, schooling devoid of meaningful education, widespread lack of opportunities and despair, and similar problems. This massive abuse and destruction of children is a by-product of the normal workings of our established social order and its political, economic and cultural institutions.

This type of abuse, "societal abuse", is usually not addressed by groups or organisations who claim to be committed to the prevention and treatment of child abuse. Preoccupation with child abuse by parents and other individuals, and reluctance to confront institutional and societal abuse, reveal a distorted sense of priorities and tendencies toward scapegoating and victim-blaming; they also create a convenient smokescreen which disguises the nature, scope and dynamics of child abuse.'

(1981, p. 294)

MICRO-LEVEL CONSTRUCTIONS OF CHILD ABUSE

As Hampton and Newberger suggest, since 'child abuse is neither theoretically nor clinically well-defined ... this definitional ambiguity increases the likelihood of subjective professional evaluation' (1988, p. 218). This can be illustrated with reference to the official definitions outlined above. Neglect, for example, has to be persistent or severe but the thresholds are not defined. Sexual abuse involves sexual exploitation of a child or adolescent, but the question remains open (in the official definition) as to whether or not all sexual activity involving a child or adolescent is, *ipso facto*, exploitative since they cannot be presumed to give informed consent.

Since determining such matters involves making value judgements, the construction of child abuse at the case level is dependent upon the decisions made by varied professionals as they operationalise definitions in the course of their practice. Several studies have highlighted the variation evident in these micro-level constructions. Some of these have used standardised material presented in the form of case vignettes to different groups. Perhaps the most famous study is that by Giovannoni and Becerra (1979) *Defining Child Abuse*. They presented brief case vignettes to a group of 263 professionals (doctors, social workers, lawyers and the police) in the United States of America, and asked them to rate the cases on a severity scale. There were significant differences in the severity ratings among the professional groups, and between the professionals and lay members of the community. Gelles

(1982) also reported variations in definition between professional groups, as did O'Toole *et al.*'s (1983) study which also used an experimental design to explore the influence of socio-economic status, ethnicity and the level of injury on physicians' and nurses' recognition and reporting of child abuse in the United States. They reported that physicians' judgements were affected by all three variables, while nurses' judgements were based on the level of injury alone rather than on socio-economic status or ethnicity. For example, in one case vignette involving a child with a serious injury, 70 per cent of physicians judged abuse to be present when the parent(s) were of low socio-economic status compared with 51 per cent when the parents' socio-economic status was high. In another vignette involving a child with a minor injury, 43 per cent of physicians identified abuse when the parent was black compared with 23 per cent when the parent was white. With reference to child sexual abuse, Jackson and Nuttall (1993) explored clinicians' judgements and identified seven factors, including the ethnic origins of the abuser and the abused, the victim's age, the abuser's relationship to the victim, as important in affecting clinical identification.

Others have explored the operationalisation of definitions, not through hypothetical case vignettes but through an examination of practice to see how cases are defined. One such study is by Hampton and Newberger (1988). In the context of a ten-fold rise in reports of child abuse to state welfare agencies over a decade, following the introduction of mandatory reporting laws in the United States, Hampton and Newberger studied hospital staff, who play a key role in the United States of America in both the identification of abuse and the subsequent reporting to child protection agencies. The study was carried out in 26 countries of the United States in 1979–80 involving 805 cases of child abuse and neglect. In the study, child maltreatment was defined as a situation

> 'where, through purposive acts or marked inattention to a child's basic needs, behaviour of a parent/substitute or other adult caretaker caused foreseeable and avoidable injury or impairment to a child, or materially contributed to unreasonable prolongation or worsening of an existing injury or impairment.'

> (1988, p. 214)

The study estimated that approximately 652,000 children per annum in the United States met this operational definition of child abuse and neglect, but only 212,400 of these would have been known to child protection services. Several important differences were found between identified cases which were reported and those which were not. In respect of ethnicity, 60 per cent of identified cases in white families were reported compared with 74 per cent of black and 91 per cent of hispanic families. Hampton and Newberger also found that families who were in the lower income categories had the highest reporting rates: 80 per cent of identified cases in the lowest income categories were reported, while families with high annual incomes (then $25,000 plus) had a better than two-to-one chance of not being reported. There was also a gender differential, with cases in which the alleged perpetrator was not the mother more likely to be reported. Finally, they found that emotional abuse and neglect cases were less likely to be reported than physical injuries. So they conclude:

'disproportionate numbers of unreported cases involved victims of emotional abuse, families of high income, mothers who were alleged to be responsible for the injuries and those who were white.'

and

'for the hospital sample, class and race are the more important factors defining the gradient between reported and unreported cases.'

(1988, p. 217)

The suggest that the greater the social distance between the labeller and the labelled, the more likely is the attribution of the label. Dingwall *et al.* (1983) studied similar processes at work in three local authorities in England. They found that casualty officers' suspicions of child abuse were based on social assessment of the family rather than the specific nature of the child's injuries. They also found a preference for non-intervention (which they termed 'the rule of optimism'), which serves to minimise identifications of child abuse in general. They describe these as essentially moral judgements concerned with the nature of child protection in a liberal democracy and suggested that the processes work 'in such a way as to hold back some upper-middle and "respectable" working-class parents, members of ethnic minorities and "mentally incompetent" parents, while leaving single women and the "rough" indigenous working class as a group proportionately most vulnerable to compulsory measures'. Dingwall *et al.* conclude that

'abuse and neglect are the products of complex processes of identification, confirmation and disposal rather than inherent in the child's presenting condition and, at least in some sense, self-evident.'

(1983, p. 31)

This is important because studies drawing on identified and reported cases are not, therefore, random samples of cases in which child abuse (defined in a particular way) has occurred. Identified cases differ in important but variable ways from a random sample, using a similar definition of abuse. As Gelles observes:

> 'operationally defining "child abuse" as pertaining only to those children publicly labelled "abused" produced a major problem: that is the factors causally associated with abuse became compounded with factors related to susceptibility or vulnerability to having an injury diagnosed as abuse.'

(1980, p. 146)

In the United Kingdom, one of the most important factors which appears to affect the susceptibility to the identification of child abuse is previous contact with the social services department. Whether or not the contact focuses on child-rearing practices, it increases the opportunities for surveillance. In England, two-thirds of a sample of 1,888 families in which there were referrals for abuse had prior contact with the social services department (Gibbons *et al*. 1993) as did 73 per cent in a much smaller sample of 48 registered cases (Hallett, 1993). In a Scottish survey 46 per cent of 199 child abuse referrals were already open cases in the social work department (Taylor and Campbell, 1994).

THE PREVALENCE AND INCIDENCE OF CHILD ABUSE

The definitional ambiguities highlighted above, and the changing definitions used in different times and places, pose considerable problems in estimating both the incidence of child abuse (the number of new cases in a specified time period) and its prevalence (its frequency, usually expressed as a percentage of the child population). The use of non-standard definitions causes difficulty in comparing studies and in documenting changes over time. Another problem stems from the low 'social visibility' of much abuse. Since it is categorised as a crime, it is more likely to be hidden than broadcast, and even if it were decriminalised, it remains a stigmatising activity and one more likely to be concealed than openly espoused.

Three main data sources exist for estimating the incidence and prevalence of abuse. The first, large-scale sample surveys of the general population, have been more prominent in the United States than in the United Kingdom, and are usefully reviewed by Birchall (1989). In 1979, Gil and Noble surveyed a nationwide random sample of adults in the United States about physical injury. Fifty-eight per cent reported that they thought anyone could injure a child. Three per cent reported that they personally knew of a physical injury case to a child in the preceding year and 0.4 per cent admitted abusing a child. From the 3 per cent figure, they derived a figure of 2.5 to 4 million physical injuries to children per annum, an incidence rate of 13–21 per cent of children.

Perhaps the most well-known United States study is that by Straus and his colleagues (1980). In 1979, a nationally representative sample of American parents, with at least one child aged between 1 year and 17 years living at home, was asked about the number of parental attacks on children in the home in the preceding year. Attack was defined to include punching, kicking, biting, hitting with an object, 'beating up' or using a knife or a gun. Straus estimated that 14 per cent of American children aged between 3 and 17 years were subjected to family violence each year. The survey was repeated by Gelles and Straus in 1985 and a lower rate of 10.7 per cent was revealed. Gelles and Straus (1987) suggest that national campaigns in the intervening period had drawn attention to the unacceptability of family violence which led to the reduced incidence, although they acknowledge that it is also possible that the changed climate of public and political opinion led to an increased reluctance to admit to abusive behaviour.

There is little comparable work in the United Kingdom. The Newsons' longitudinal studies of child rearing practices of children aged one, four and seven years in Nottingham shed some light on the topic. They report that straps, sticks and slippers were used on 26 per cent of boys and 18 per cent of girls aged seven, with slaps commonplace at age four and seven (Newson and Newson, 1970 and 1978). They also report a class gradient in the data with greater resort to physical punishment among the lower socio-economic groups. Smith *et al.*'s study (forthcoming) of parental control within the family explored the incidence of physical punishment in a sample of families containing children at ages one, four, seven and eleven. The researchers found that only 9 per cent of the children had never been smacked, and that 72 per cent of one-year-old children had been subjected to physical chastisement. They estimated that 16 per cent of the children had been subjected to hitting defined as severe.

The varying definitions of child sexual abuse pose even greater problems in estimating prevalence. Some studies based on social surveys adopt wide definitions including all unwanted childhood sexual experiences, including, for example, meeting a 'flasher', while others are more restricted. Finkelhor (1986), in reviewing North American studies, found wide variation in rates of abuse ranging from 6 to 62 per cent for girls and from 3 to 30 per cent for boys, reflecting, in part, the different definitions adopted in the studies. In reviewing United Kingdom studies, Birchall concludes that 'reported prevalences ranged from 0.3 per cent to 83 per cent and reflect more light on the construction of the studies than on actual prevalences' (1989, p. 25)

Large-scale United Kingdom studies sampling the general population (Baker and Duncan, 1985; Childwatch, 1986) yielded prevalence rates of between 3 and 36 per cent. One of these, a Mori poll of 2,019 adults, with a response rate of 87 per cent, used a definition of 'any activity which the other expects to lead to their sexual arousal' and concluded that 10 per cent of adults had been abused when under the age of sixteen, 12 per cent of girls and 8 per cent of boys. Forty per cent of those abused knew the abuser and 14 per cent of the abuse took place within the family (Baker and Duncan, 1985). La Fontaine (1988) concluded that a 10 per cent prevalence rate for sexual abuse involving physical contact was likely. The comparative data collated by Finkelhor (1991) shown in Table 1.1 reveals the estimated prevalence of the problem in a range of countries.

Table 1.1   *International comparison of prevalence of child sexual abuse*

Country	Sample sizes and types	Rate %	
		Males	Females
Australia	338 M/603 F	9.0	28.0
(Goldman and Goldman, 1988)	College students		
Canada	1002 M/1006 F	13.0	31.0
(Bagley *et al.*, 1984)	National sample		
Holland	1054 F	–	33.0
(Draijer, 1989)	National sample		
New Zealand	2000 F	–	10.0
(Mullen *et al.*, 1988)	National sample		
Sweden	501 M/501 F	1.0	7.0
(Ronstrom, 1985)	National sample		
United Kingdom	2019 M and F	8.0	12.0
(Baker and Duncan, 1985)	National sample		
United States of America	1252 M/1374 F	16.0	27.0
(Lewis, 1985)	National sample		

Source: Finkelhor, 1991.

Alongside sample surveys, a second data source is estimates of prevalence based on clinical samples. These are problematic partly because of the dangers of extrapolating from small numbers (Hall, 1975; Oliver et al., 1974).

REGISTER DATA

A third important data source comes from child protection registers. By definition, these include only children who have come to the notice of health and welfare agencies and, latterly, only those for whom, in addition, an inter-agency child protection plan is required. They are thus subject to the reporting biases discussed above and also reflect the differing local practices concerning thresholds for registration (Gibbons et al., 1993). Until 1988, the largest source of register data was derived from the NSPCC. Since 1973, they collected data from areas where registers were managed by the NSPCC covering approximately 10 per cent of the child population in England and Wales. The survey, covering some 26,300 children, constitutes 'the largest continuous survey of reported cases of child abuse in the United Kingdom' (Creighton, 1992, p. 7). Reports on the data were published throughout the period (NSPCC, 1975; Creighton and Owtram, 1977; Creighton, 1980; Creighton, 1984; Creighton and Noyes, 1989; Creighton, 1992). The NSPCC survey yielded prevalence rates per 1,000 children of 2.3 in 1988, 3.2 in 1989 and 3.0 in 1990, and estimated incidence rates of 27,000 in 1988, 36,300 in 1989 and 34,700 in 1990.

This survey was ended in 1990, since, by then, the Department of Health was gathering and publishing register data collected from each

Table 1.2   *Categories of abuse*

	Percentage[1]
Neglect	20.0
Physical injury	28.0
Sexual abuse	17.0
Emotional abuse	7.0
Grave concern	34.0

[1]Mixed categories are incorporated with each relevant main category. Totals, therefore, exceed 100.
Source: Department of Health, 1993, p. 8.

local authority in England. The national figures show a steady increase for numbers on the register, new registrations and deregistrations from 1989 to 1991 and a decline in 1992. Numbers on the register increased from 41,200 in 1989 to 45,300 in 1991. In 1992, the number was 38,600 children and the breakdown between categories of abuse was as shown in Table 1.2. (In 1991, government guidance withdrew the registration category of 'grave concern'.) The prevalence rate for all forms of registered child abuse was 3.54 per 1,000 population aged under 18 in England in 1992 (Department of Health, 1993b, p. 6).

National registration criteria were not recommended in Scotland until 1992. In 1991 there was a prevalence rate of registered cases of 3.43 per 1,000 population under 16 (Gough, 1992).

THE NATURE OF THE ABUSE

Some of the difficulties of estimating incidence and prevalence rates are also faced in attempting to determine what is known about the nature of abuse suffered by children. Some forms of abuse are excluded by the official definitions and an unknown amount of abuse is thought not to be identified or reported. It is possible, however, to determine something about the nature of the abuse perpetrated on children from the official records and research studies.

With respect to physical injury to children, the NSPCC register data categorises physical injury to children as follows:

Fatal: all cases which resulted in death
Serious: all fractures, head injuries, internal injuries, severe burns and ingestion of toxic substances
Moderate: all soft tissue injuries of a superficial nature

(Creighton, 1992, p. 5)

The vast majority of abuse (88 per cent in the years 1988–90) is included in the category 'moderate', 43 per cent of cases involving bruising to the body and limbs and 41 per cent to the head and face. The details are provided in Table 1.3.

It is, however, clear that deaths from child abuse are relatively rare. Creighton estimated that such deaths probably numbered about 150 per annum in 1985, although the number decreased between 1988 and 1989. As Birchall (1989) notes, this contrasts with a total of 8,602 children who died in 1987, of whom 358 were killed on the roads. It is, therefore, of interest that child deaths from abuse which featured in many of the key inquiries into child abuse, such as Colwell

Table 1.3   *Nature of abuse sustained (1988–90 combined)*

Injuries	(n = 2786)
Skull fracture	61 (2)*
Subdural haematoma	20 (1)
Retinal haemorrhage	8
Other brain damage	12
Fracture – long bone	91 (3)
Fracture – other	56 (2)
Bruising (head/face)	1150 (41)
Bruising (body/limbs)	1206 (43)
Cut (head/face)	132 (5)
Cut (body/limbs)	85 (3)
Burn, scald	107 (4)
Attempted suffocation/strangulation/drowning	23 (1)
Ingestion	34 (1)
Concussion/convulsions	2
Other	115 (4)

*Bracketed figures show percentage of cases with this abuse. As several cases have more than one type of abuse, the total of these figures exceeds 100 for the injured children.
Source: Creighton, 1992, p. 17.

(Department of Health and Social Security, 1974), Jasmine Beckford (London Borough of Brent, 1985), Kimberley Carlile (London Borough of Greenwich, 1987 and many others, are only a tiny proportion of the cases known to official agencies.

Much more common are injuries categorised as 'moderate'. This category appears to need closer specification since so many are subsumed within it. In a much smaller-scale study, conducted by the author (Hallett, 1993), the proportion of cases in the moderate category was similar (at 85 per cent) to the rates reported by the NSPCC. However, the cases involved those in which implements (e.g. a shoe and a belt) were used to inflict injuries, those in which there was bruising on multiple sites, and others in which one blow, resulting in single bruise, was said to have been inflicted with the hand. In this study, none of the children in the moderate category needed or received *treatment* from their general practitioners or from paediatricians, and their contact with the latter was determined by the need to seek a paediatric opinion about the nature and cause of the injuries. It is clear that the injuries inflicted on children are not, in the main, severe or life-threatening. This is not to condone them. It may be argued that no child should be subjected to inflicted physical injury and that all children have a right to live free from the threat of physical violence (although the United Kingdom has been reluctant to reflect this right in legislation, in contrast to Sweden, for example). It is, however, to acknowledge that, given the apparently widespread recourse to physical chastisement in British child-rearing practices, the children who are registered for physical abuse may not be readily distinguished in terms of their injuries from others in the same age groups from similar backgrounds.

In respect of sexual abuse, the NSPCC register survey required NSPCC team members to assess severity on the basis of their assessment

Table 1.4 *Nature of abuse sustained (1988–90 combined)*

Sexual abuse	(n = 1732)	
Vaginal intercourse	143	(8)*
Anal intercourse	89	(5)
Attempted vaginal/anal intercourse	105	(6)
Vaginal penetration	194	(11)
Anal penetration	109	(6)
Oral penetration	97	(6)
Masturbation of child by perpetrator	97	(6)
Lick/suck/spit on child	30	(2)
Fondle child	370	(21)
Sexually transmitted disease – child	14	(1)
Masturbation of perpetrator by child	103	(6)
Exploitation	15	(1)
Exposure	32	(2)
Indecent assault/gross indecency	169	(10)
Other	117	(7)

*Bracketed figures show percentage of cases with this abuse. As several cases have more than one type of abuse, total of these figures exceeds 100 for the injured children.
Source: Creighton, 1992, p. 17.

of the physical and emotional damage sustained by the child (this method was also used for the categorisation of emotional abuse and neglect and non-organic failure to thrive). In 1,732 sexual abuse cases registered between 1988 and 1990, 38 per cent were categorised as serious, 36 per cent as moderate, with no information in 26 per cent of the cases. The type of activity involved is listed in Table 1.4. Thus, in 42 per cent of the cases, some form of penetrative sexual activity took place, with relatively few cases involving no physical contact.

A similar large-scale study was conducted in Northern Ireland (The Research Team, 1990). Drawing on 408 cases notified to professional agencies in 1987 (an incidence rate of 0.9 per 1,000), the study, *inter alia*, described the nature of the abuse which had occurred, using the following definition of abuse: 'a child, anyone under 17 years of age, is sexually abused when one or more persons involved the child in any activity for the purpose of their own sexual arousal' (p. 15). The study sought to classify the abusive acts in terms of the degree of physical contact. This was an attempt to measure the degree of bodily violation. The categories were as shown in Table 1.5. The study found that the incidence of abuse was substantially higher for girls than for boys (in a ratio of 4.5 to 1). The nature of the abuse suffered in the established cases is shown in Table 1.6.

Table 1.6 shows clearly that, in the established cases, most of the abuse involved sexual contact, with penetrative sexual contact in 65 per cent of cases. In relatively few cases (20 per cent) was there no physical contact. Baker and Duncan's (1985) study, based on a nationally representative sample of adults, suggested that physical sexual contact had occurred in 44 per cent of the sample, with a further 5 per cent having experienced penetration. Besides the degree of physical violation involved in sexual abuse, other factors such as the duration of abuse and the number of abusers have been found to be associated with a more severe impact on the child. Baker and Duncan's study found that 63 per cent of respondents reported one incident of abuse, 23 per cent suffered repeated abuse by one person and 14 per cent suffered repeated abuse by multiple abusers. In the Northern Ireland study, over two-thirds of the established cases were subjected to more than one episode of abuse by the same abuser. The median duration of abuse, in cases (78 per cent) where information was available, was 18 months for boys and 12 months for girls. Most children in the study (90 per cent) were abused by a single abuser and in 9 per cent of the cases there was more than one abuser.

While there are formidable difficulties in commenting authoritatively on the nature of sexual abuse in contemporary society, the available

Table 1.5 *Categories of abusive acts*

Degree of physical contact	Types of abuse
Penetrative sexual contact	Digital penetration Oral genital contact Attempted anal intercourse Anal intercourse Attempted sexual intercourse Sexual intercourse Rape–sexual intercourse with violence
Non-penetrative sexual contact	Physical attack with clear sexual intent Inappropriate fondling or caressing Masturbation of child by adult or adult by child Genital to genital contact
No physical contact exhibitionism to child	Exhibitionism to child with suggestions of further sexual activity Inspection of child's genitals Viewing adult sexual activities Child photographed in sexual pose Viewing blue videos
Miscellaneous	Other types

Source: The Research Team, 1990, pp. 25–6.

Table 1.6 *Distribution of children by highest contact and level of abuse, sex of the child in established cases (N = 408)*

Highest contact level	Female (%)		Male (%)		Total (%)	
Penetrative sexual	214	(64.8)	51	(65.4)	265	(65.0)
Non-penetrative sexual	90	(27.3)	22	(28.2)	112	(27.5)
No physical contact	16	(4.8)	4	(5.1)	20	(4.9)
Miscellaneous	7	(2.1)	0	(0.0)	7	(1.7)
Unclassifiable	3	(0.9)	1	(1.3)	4	(1.0)
Total	330	(100.0)	78	(100.0)	408	(100.0)

Source: Adapted from The Research Team, 1990, p. 123.

data confirm that the identified abuse is serious, with estimates of around half to two-thirds suffering abuse involving physical contact.

NEGLECT

Child neglect did not attract the professional, public and political interest associated with child physical and sexual abuse. There was a long tradition in British child welfare of dealing with cases of child neglect from the voluntary associations such as Dr Barnardo's and the NSPCC, and they were an important part of the work of the Children's Departments established in local authorities in 1948. Child neglect appears to be more mundane and less shocking.

In 1992, over 7,000 children (20 per cent of the total registered) were on child protection registers in England on grounds of neglect. Data from the United States suggest that in the mid-1980s almost half of reported cases (46 per cent) involved neglect, compared with 20 per cent of cases of physical abuse, 11 per cent of sexual abuse and 23 per cent combining abuse and neglect (American Association for Protecting Children, 1986, cited in Crittenden, 1988). Despite the high frequency of neglect, remarkably little is known about the harms suffered by this group of children. As Wolock and Horowitz (1984) note, there is a neglect of neglect. Creighton's (1992) study, for example, while containing data on the nature of the abuse experienced by children in cases of physical and sexual abuse, is silent on the harms suffered by those registered for neglect, beyond noting that workers estimated 24 per cent of the 693 cases registered between 1988 and 1990 to be 'serious' and 52 per cent 'moderate' (with no information concerning 23 per cent).

Neglect is a category of abuse which seems to pose particular problems in identification and in defining thresholds for intervention. In Giovannoni and Becerra's (1979) study and in Birchall's (1992) replication of it in England, vignettes concerning child neglect received severity ratings lower than those given for sexual abuse (the highest) or for physical and emotional abuse. In Birchall's study, neglect cases, together with emotional abuse, also caused most dissensus between the professions. This may partly be because of the difficulty of distinguishing between neglect which should be categorised as abusive and thus registered, and the harsh and depriving social, environmental and economic circumstances in which significant numbers of children live. Since the attribution of the label 'neglect' imputes a deficit in parenting to those with the care of children, there may understandably be a reluctance to use it when the circumstances in which parenting takes place would tax the coping skills of many. Gibbons *et al.* (1993) report that only 7 per cent of cases referred to social services departments for neglect reached the child protection register (compared with 15 per cent of all child abuse referrals) and that most neglect cases were screened out of the child protection system at an early stage, usually without the offer of other services. There is, therefore, an urgent need for further research into the nature of child neglect and into effective intervention to prevent and ameliorate it.

In England, the category of non-organic failure to thrive is subsumed within neglect, while in Scotland it is retained as a separate registration category. It is a term used to describe

> 'infants and children whose growth and development are significantly below age-related norms, and in whom no physical causes can be detected.'

(Iwaniec et al., 1988, p. 230)

The condition is frequently associated with emotional deprivation, family disorganisation and, in particular, difficulties over feeding. It is a relatively rare occurrence comprising less than 2 per cent of the total of 5,728 cases registered between 1988 and 1990 in the NSPCC survey (Creighton, 1992).

EMOTIONAL ABUSE

While all forms of child abuse may involve some emotional harm to the child, this registration category is confined to children whose emotional and behavioural development is severely adversely affected by persistent or severe emotional ill-treatment or rejection. Although the numbers registered are small, comprising only 7 per cent of the total in 1992 (Department of Health, 1993b), these cases share with neglect a lack of data about the harms suffered by the children concerned. As with neglect, there are problems of defining the threshold at which to attribute the label but, in addition, the identification of emotional abuse in the United Kingdom is hampered both by the difficulty of demonstrating that the condition exists and of establishing the relationship between cause and effect which is more difficult in this than in some other forms of abuse. As Iwaniec *et al.* note, 'the very private and highly nebulous intangible qualities of emotional abuse make it a difficult concept to define in a useful, operational sense' (1988, p. 231).

They also note that there may be a significant number of children on child protection registers where the main cause for concern is emotional abuse but where the existence of bruising may be a more straightforward route to child protection.

The identification of emotional abuse appears to be less problematic in systems such as those which prevail in Holland, where there is less involvement of the criminal justice system and less preoccupation with establishing who bears responsibility for the abuse. There, emotional abuse comprised 40 per cent of cases reported to the confidential doctor system in 1991 (de Koning, 1992). The paucity of data on emotional abuse is unfortunate since there is evidence to suggest that these persistent and repeated threats to a child's identity, sense of worth and well-being may be particularly damaging in the long term (Crittenden, 1988).

THE NEED FOR DISAGGREGATION OF THE TERM 'CHILD ABUSE'

This review of the various forms of harm suffered by children, and encompassed by the term 'child abuse' as it is operationalised in British child protection practice, reveals the variety and imprecision of the term. In physical injury, for example, it ranges from death (rarely) to minor bruising. The experience of abuse by the children concerned will vary, *inter alia*, with the precise nature of the harms inflicted, their severity, duration, the degree of breach of trust involved in their perpetration, the child's personal coping strengths and strategies and the nature of the response made when the abuse is discovered, in particular whether the child is believed and supported (Roberts and Taylor, 1993; Monck *et al.*, 1992). Not surprisingly, therefore, Lynch concludes that while 'research studies and clinical experience plainly demonstrate that the outlook for many abused children and their families is grim', nonetheless 'not all abused children have long-term difficulties' (1988, pp. 204 and 209). In similar terms, Berliner (1991) concludes, with reference to sexual abuse, that while studies show that sexually abused children as a group are different from children who have not been sexually abused, there is considerable variation and overlap in the extent of the differences. Furthermore, in a study by Conte and Berliner (1988) 'children were assessed on a symptom checklist derived from the clinical literature … [and] 21 per cent of the children known to have been abused did not display any of these symptoms' (Berliner, 1991, p. 146).

To acknowledge that not all children may suffer long-term adverse consequences is not to imply that the abuse is trivial or acceptable. They may suffer severely in the short term. Furthermore, the rights of children to a life free from inflicted violence, sexual exploitation, emotional rejection or persistent neglect (whatever the short or long-term outcome) may be seen as an inalienable human right. There are parallels here with rape. Debates about the societal response to rape are not usually conducted with reference to any potentially damaging consequences to rape survivors in old age. Rather the act is condemned for its intrinsic assault on the rights, freedom and dignity of the individual, regardless of the long-term consequences.

However, the breadth of the term 'child abuse' makes generalisations about the consequences for individual children difficult. This heterogeneity also affects the characteristics of abusers who commit the varied acts subsumed by the term. Some generalisations may be made, for example, that the majority of identified sexual abusers are men, and that for all forms of abuse, cases that are reported have a clear bias towards abusers of lower socio-economic status (Finkelhor, 1991; Creighton, 1992). Nonetheless, the observation made by Gelles in 1979 remains pertinent, namely that in reviewing studies of the personality characteristics of abusers, nineteen were identified of which only four were common to two or more studies. Gelles observe that 'in some of the current essays, I find profiles of my students, my neighbours, my wife, myself, my son' (1979, p. 135).

The need for disaggregation of the term 'child abuse' can also be illustrated with reference to theories of causation. As with much else in the field, this area is highly contested. As Irvine notes, 'much of the research into child abuse resembles a conceptual battlefield of competing ideologies and assumptions' (1988, p. 119). One tension is between those who see child abuse as a syndrome, tightly bounded and easily identified, and those who emphasise that it is a label applied, albeit with some degree of discretion, but with certain biases, to varied behaviours and outcomes. There is also a tension between those who conceive of it principally as a 'crime' or as a 'sickness'.

The search for causes, which carries implications for prevention and intervention, has been an important part of the research endeavour in child abuse, particularly the attempt to identify the personal and social characteristics of abusers which lead to abuse. As long ago as 1975, Richards raised objections to the term 'non-accidental injury syndrome' because

> 'it may suggest ... a uniformity and similarity between cases which is not found in practice. What is common in all cases is that somebody in a professional position has decided that a child has received injuries deliberately. But this situation may have arisen in a multitude of different ways (and from a multitude of causal factors).'

> (1975, p. 5)

This may be applied to other forms of abuse and, as Belsky suggests, 'no single model can adequately explain the cause of child abuse' (1978, p. 38). The main theoretical perspectives can, nonetheless, be distinguished. Belsky (1978) proposes three: a psychiatric model (focusing on the psychodynamics of the abuser); a sociological model with social factors as primary causes; and an interactive model, emphasising the child's role – for example, prematurity, disability or difficult and unrewarding behaviour – in the interactions which lead to abuse (Elmer and Gregg, 1967; Lynch and Roberts, 1977; Roberts, 1988). Sweet and Resick (1979) propose four models: a psychodynamic model emphasising intrapsychic characteristics – for example, unmet dependency needs; social learning theories, emphasising learned behaviours in parenting; a social/psychological model, focusing on the interaction between adults and their environment; and, finally, a sociological model emphasising social factors. The main distinctions between the models are the emphasis placed on individual psychological characteristics as opposed to social circumstances.

Psychological models

The psychological models reflect the theoretical stance that factors causing child maltreatment are located within the individual abuser. Much of the early work derived from clinical samples, although it was not known whether or how these identified abusers differed from undiscovered abusers in the population at large. In the early years of research in child abuse, there was a concentration on identifying the psychological characteristics of abusing parents (Spinetta and Rigler, 1972; Steele and Pollock, 1968). Gelles summarises it as follows:

'After ten years of conducted research and administration of countless psychological tests, the summary evaluation of the psychopathological approach to domestic violence is that the proportion of individuals who batter their family members and suffer from psychological disorders is not greater than the proportion of the population in general with psychological disorders.'

(1983, p. 152)

The sociological model

The sociological model is founded on the premise that it is societal conditions rather than individual attributes which are primarily responsible for child abuse. This approach emphasises the disproportionate representation of people of low socio-economic status, unemployment, social isolation and harsh environmental conditions among identified abusers (Pelton, 1981; Belsky, 1978; Parton, 1985). Creighton's research (1992), shows that marital instability, early parenthood, large families, criminality and unemployment characterised the parents of the abused children.

However, one problem is that characteristics such as unemployment, marital instability and large families which are associated with families in which abuse has been identified, are present in very large numbers of families experiencing a wide range of social difficulties and some with none. Pelton asserts that

'poverty is not merely "associated" with child abuse; there is good reason to believe that the problems of poverty are causative agents in parents' abusive and negligent behaviours and in the resultant harm to children.'

(1981, p. 33)

He suggests that there is a myth of classlessness which suggests that anyone can harm his/her children, but argues that the

'maintenance of the myth permits many professionals to view child abuse and neglect as psychodynamic problems in the context of a medical model of "disease", "treatment" and "cure" rather than as predominantly sociological and poverty-related problems.'

(1981, p. 31).

While undoubtedly the problems of deprivation, hardship and stress facing many parents compound the problem of parenthood for many poor families, this perspective does not explain why, despite the widespread existence of poverty (Millar, 1993), a relatively small proportion are identified as abusing their children.

A second important strand of sociological theorising of relevance to child abuse has been the identification of the family as a conflict-prone social institution with axes of conflict across gender and generation, that is between men and women and adults and children. In 1979 Gelles and Straus observed that

'with the exception of the police and the military, the family is perhaps the most violent social group and the home, the most violent setting in our society.'

(1979, p. 15)

While presented as a 'haven in a heartless world' (Lasch, 1977) in which love and gentleness may be, and often are, experienced, the family is also a site of conflict in which violence is accepted and, to an extent, condoned. More recently, the family has also been seen as an important site for the sexual abuse of children, predominantly by men. This perspective focuses attention on the nature of the family and the power relations and imbalances within it, particularly between those of a different gender, rather than on the individual characteristics of abusers.

More recently, Gelles (1987) and Browne (1988) have proposed integrated models of the causation of family violence which combine psychological, cultural, social and structural explanations. As Browne notes:

'They assume that violence in the family in influenced by (1) situational stressors, such as distorted family relationships, low self-esteem, unwanted or problem children and other dependents, and (2) structural stressors, such as poor housing, overcrowding, unemployment, social isolation, financial and health problems.'

(1988, p. 22)

Browne further suggests that

'the chances of these situational and structural stressors resulting in family violence are mediated by and depend on the interactive relationships within the family. A secure relationship between family members will "buffer" any effects of stress and facilitate coping strategies on behalf of the family. By contrast, insecure or anxious relationships will not "buffer" the family under stress and "episodic overload", such as an argument, may result in a physical or emotional attack. This will have a negative effect on the existing interpersonal relationships and reduce any "buffering" effects.'

(1988, p. 22)

While such a theory goes some way towards explaining episodic violence, it seems less powerful in explaining the sexual abuse of children. Here a sociological approach emphasising male socialisation and exposing the power imbalance between adults (principally men) and children, especially girls and young women, is more powerful. Even here, however, despite the widespread prevalence of child sexual abuse, we still know too little about how and why some men abuse while others do not.

Thus there is an urgent need for the disaggregation of the term 'child abuse'. While it has proved useful in capturing the political and public imagination, it is too broad and imprecise to give clear indications of the multiple and varied harms suffered by children, the characteristics of those who abuse them, the social conditions which lead to abuse, its multiple and complex causes or, indeed, to strategies of prevention or intervention.

Policy responses to the problem of child abuse are discussed in some detail in the two succeeding chapters. Here, in introduction, it is important to note that the response in the United Kingdom has been characterised by a concern with the identification of abuse and abusers and the determination of case status, in particular whether or not to register the child as abused. In this process, the major emphasis has been placed upon inter-agency co-ordination in the early phases of the construction of a case of abuse, that is identification, referral and initial investigation up to and including the intial child protection conference (Birchall, 1992; Hallett, 1993; Farmer and Owen, 1993; Walton, 1993). To date, less energy and resources have been devoted to subsequent intervention. This is unsurprising given the reactions to the succession of highly publicised child abuse inquiries which have had such a powerful impact upon policy and practice. However, there is now a need to move beyond a somewhat defensive concern with case identification and co-ordinated case management, to develop work in two key areas. The first is to ensure that skills and resources are available to meet the needs of children and families in which abuse had been identified. The second is to work on the complex agenda of identifying, implementing and evaluating a range of preventive programmes, to reduce the incidence and prevalence of the varied forms of harm to children subsumed by the term 'child abuse'.

CHAPTER TWO

Child Abuse: The Health Perspective

Stephanie Wheeler

INTRODUCTION

Current trends in nursing are concerned with providing holistic care and promoting health and healing (McMahon, 1991). Holistic care involves a multidimensional understanding of health that is concerned with physical, emotional, social and spiritual aspects of health. It is appropriate therefore to consider child abuse from a health perspective. Nurses and health visitors have a key role in work for health and child protection. This chapter discusses that particular contribution and provides information for nurses and health visitors in specific areas:

- Child abuse: definitional issues and epidemiology
- Health as a focus for child protection
- Empowerment
- A case study in an accident and emergency department illustrating four key points
- The professional framework: ethics and law
- The Children Act 1989 and *Working Together*

In keeping with the personal philosophy of Reid (1991), the use of 'I' will occasionally occur in the chapter. This is advocated by Webb (1992) when particularly the writer has been involved in the data or ideas presented. During the first six months of a ten-year period as a health visitor I became involved in protecting a young child who was later taken into care by the local social services. This case stimulated an interest in child protection work, particularly inter-agency involvement. I later explored health visitor and social work perceptions concerning child abuse (Wheeler, 1992) which has shaped some of this chapter.

CHILD ABUSE: DEFINITIONAL ISSUES AND EPIDEMIOLOGY

Actually defining child abuse is much more complex than any practitioner might initially be aware of. Practitioners from a health background are heavily influenced by a medical model that adheres to the scientific approach. This is characterised by Munhall and Oiler (1986) in terms of different paradigms or world views. The medical model or received world view follows known physical laws, purports to be objective and neutral, is reductionist (treats the part) and is interested in physical symptomatology (Munhall and Oiler, 1986). The emphasis is on quantitative research that incorporates these aspects and aims to control, manipulate and predict certain variables. In the context of this background the practitioner is given to expect a full explanation concerning every phenomenon. It is at this stage that caution concerning definitions of child abuse must be exercised. Reder *et al.* (1993) cite Gelles (1975) 'who pointed out that there is no objective phenomenon which can automatically be recognised as child abuse'. In their compelling book *Beyond Blame*, Reder *et al.* (1993) describe child abuse as an 'evolving phenomenon' which is influenced by social attributes to children and families which are in turn influenced by inquiry reports and legislation. Within this framework professional practice is modified and guided by theories and knowledge.

In terms of theory and knowledge caution again must be exercised in defining child abuse. In 1985 Parton exposed the political implications of child abuse viewed within a dominant disease model. Parton (1985) argued that this approach ignored the wider legal and socially deviant aspects. Whilst in 1990 Parton pointed out some inadequacies of his earlier work, the dominant disease model is still very relevant. Howitt (1992) gives the history of modern child protection with the underlying medicalisation of child abuse and the medical profession's 'allegiance to science'. He warns of the consequences of this approach, exemplified in the Cleveland Child Sexual Abuse controversy. Howitt (1992) highlights that in the Cleveland inquiry the theory of the anal reflex test (Hobbs and Wynne, 1986) was found to be fundamentally flawed. Further, Howitt (1992) argues that there is evidence that whilst in most cases theory leads to practice, in some circumstances theory may be sought to justify practice, which has other very profound implications.

Lyon and de Cruz (1990), in discussing child abuse and the law, make visible the definitional debate. They argue that research findings are misleading in the absence of a standardised definition. They favour Alan Gilmour's (Director of NSPCC in 1988) working definition:

'Child abuse occurs when any unavoidable act or avoidable failure to act adversely affects the physical, mental or emotional well-being of a child.' An avoidable act is explained by Gilmour as something that has occurred which need not have occurred but would not necessarily be deliberate. This might be, for example, causing a brain haemorrhage unintentionally when shaking a child. Lyon and de Cruz (1990) argue that avoidable harm is a notion familiar to both lawyers and social workers in terms of grounds for care orders, particularly with respect to the Children's and Young Persons' Acts of 1933 and 1969.

Child abuse definitions are influenced by epidemiological evidence. Epidemiology is also an important part of work for health, and according to Farmer and Miller (1991), involves two main areas: first, finding out about disease and its causes, to prevent illness and promote health; second, measuring health care needs and evaluating clinical practice in order to improve health care provision in terms of efficiency and effectiveness. These two areas of concern have obvious implications in the study of child abuse. Nurses and health visitors need to know what child abuse is, how it presents and how often it occurs, in order to try and prevent it happening and manage it effectively and efficiently when it does. The primary focus should be to protect children from child abuse.

What exactly is the incidence (number of cases) of child abuse within the United Kingdom? Christine Hallett answers this question in the preceding chapter when she reviews three main sources of data. Taylor (1992) makes the point that ever since the 1960s, when child abuse emerged as a social problem, practitioners, politicians and the media have wanted reliable evidence concerning the incidence and prevalence. Yet Taylor warns that the validity and reliability of the statistics cannot be taken for granted. As with every type of evidence, numerical data concerning numbers and types of child abuse must be examined critically. Cooper (1993) argues that measuring child abuse is extraordinarily difficult, as the very terms used to describe suffering have changed, from 'child battering' to 'non-accidental injury' and currently 'child abuse'. He further suggests that questions such as, is there more abuse than there used to be? are parents more or less cruel than they used to be? and, are we successfully tackling child abuse? are only solvable in the broadest sense. That is, in western societies there is evidence that children have better health than ever before, they are not working in mines or factories and they are educated in schools.

An area of growing concern, controversy and possible moral panic has been that of child sexual abuse. Again the whole field is beset with definitional problems, as discussed by Blagg *et al.* (1989). They cite

Kempe and Kempe's (1978) definition as the one most commonly used: 'Sexual abuse is defined as the involvement of dependent developmentally immature children and adolescents in sexual activity they do not truly comprehend to which they are unable to give informed consent or that violate the social taboos of family roles.' However, Blagg *et al.* criticise this definition as being too abstract. Yet they consider the Cleveland measurement, centering largely on incest and anal abuse, as far too narrow. Large (1992) investigated health visitor attitudes to child sexual abuse. A total of 103 health visitors in two health districts took part in the study. Significantly 46 per cent of the health visitors reported professional contact with child sexual abuse in the two years prior to the study. Graham (1991), in discussing the incidence and prevalence of child sexual abuse, again points out that the preferred definition of child sexual abuse, together with the techniques used to gather the data, influences the emerging picture which cannot be seen as a true prevalence rate.

Whilst nurses and health visitors need to be aware of the incidence and prevalence of cases of child abuse, the epidemiological evidence must be examined critically. It is important to discover which definition of child abuse was used in the study, and for this to be made clear when reporting research. What appears to be important are the cultural factors which affect decisions about what is defined as child abuse, and the moral judgements used in such processes (see Hallett, Chapter 1).

Each social service area department must maintain a central child protection register. This should list all the children who are considered to be suffering from or likely to suffer significant harm. There must also be a child protection plan for each child. Categories of abuse for registration are listed by Hallett in the preceding chapter, and can be found in the Department of Health (1992a) *Child Protection: Guidance for Senior Nurses, Health Visitors and Midwives*.

Lyon and de Cruz (1990) very clearly discuss each of these categories and set them within the literature and the wider debate. They argue that whilst they provide a working guide to the forms of child abuse currently recognised by professionals, there must be research into definitional issues. My own research findings showed that the assumption that agencies' definitions of child abuse are similar is in fact erroneous (Wheeler, 1992). Some of this can be accounted for in terms of tension between health visitors and social workers. This tension, according to Taylor and Tilley (1990), arises from the different agencies' experience of parenting skills. Ten years earlier, Hallett and Stevenson (1980) suggested that this may be due to the fact that Health Visitors see more 'normal' families than social workers, and consequently definitions of acceptable standards of child care would invariably differ between the two agencies. Taylor and Tilley (1990) argue that health visiting is a preventative service whilst social work is primarily reactive. Health visitors seek to intervene before more serious problems occur and social workers are involved once a crisis has occurred. Knowledge from research such as this is very important, particularly in understanding and preventing communication breakdowns between agencies, an area still criticised in inquiry reports (DoH, 1991d). Yet, returning to definitions of child abuse, Loney (1992) is in favour of David Gil (an American expert) because he views child abuse in the context of the child's potential. So a child is being abused if her or his circumstances do not allow for her or his optimal development. This is most helpful as a link towards the next part of this section, in which (amongst others) David Seedhouse's examination of health in terms of potential is reviewed.

HEALTH AS A FOCUS FOR CHILD PROTECTION

The word 'health' again may appear quite straightforward to define but this is far from the case when individual lives and experiences are shared and examined. An excellent example of these can be found in the works of Oliver Sacks (a neurophysiologist), particularly in his 1985 book in which he presents the cases of individuals with neurological loss.

Ewles and Simnett (1992) make the point that lay people assess their health subjectively, which poses a problem in measuring health as opposed to illness. Also lay and professional views differ, with professionals usually perceiving health as an absence of medically defined disease, illness and disability. Aggleton (1990), in his pathway through health, describes two main types of definition, negative and positive. The negative definitions view health as an absence of disease and illness whilst the positive incorporates certain qualities into the approach to health. Five positive approaches view health as: an ideal state; physical and mental fitness; a commodity; a personal strength or ability; or a basis for personal potential. The latter approach is something David Seedhouse propounds. Seedhouse (1986) makes clear his assumptions concerning human potential that are mainly optimistic. He believes people have a number of potentials that can be fulfilled depending on their circumstances. Further, he considers people want to and can change themselves. Yet in the case of children, parents and care-givers have the main responsibility for the circumstances of their charges. However, Seedhouse argues that health workers have a role in helping people to widen and increase their possibilities for achievement. Health visitors traditionally undertake health status assessments which take account of demographic data, family history, medical history, environmental data, cultural/sociological data, psychological and sociological variables and clients' perceptions of their health and needs (Orr, 1985).

Why Loney (1992) is impressed with David Gil's work concerning child abuse is that it emphasises the importance of the broader social policy in improving or making worse children's potential. Seedhouse (1986) also argues forcefully that a number of factors influence health, such as gender, culture, class, race, education, environment, relationships, employment, diet, smoking and drinking habits and social policy. In many ways it is clearer, he suggests, to describe what affects health rather than what health is. Yet Seedhouse (1986) uses these influences on health as background conditions for his definition of health, which is:

> 'the state of the various background conditions which can enable the achievement of personal potential. The state of a person's health is equivalent to the state of these conditions.'

This definition of health can be linked with Gil's suggestion that child abuse can be viewed as a lack of care or of circumstances which prevent the child's full and proper development (Gil 1979). This would give even more weight to Seedhouse's definition. Where there is a gap in care and understanding of childhood needs, Barker (1990) advocates that health visitors give intensive support and encouragement to parents with children in their first year or two of life. Where there is social stress, Barker suggests support visiting should increase. He argues that viewing parents as in need of support rather than as potential child abusers fosters improved relationships to empower parents to 'end up doing a great job of rearing their children'. In the words of Seedhouse (1986), health workers 'should aim to counter ignorance, lack of reasoning ability, selfishness, disease, illness and injury'. This can only be achieved in conjunction with parents, care-givers and inter-agency co-operation and communication. Ewles and Simnett (1992) suggest that the concept of empowerment is related to ideas of health as the attainment of potential.

EMPOWERMENT

Empowerment is a current concept in the nursing literature with the emergence of the 'New Nursing' (Salvage, 1990, 1992). In social work practice as well, Braye and Preston-Shoot (1993) point out that empowerment and partnership have become accepted principles.

Gibson (1991) highlights the fact that empowerment is from the Latin 'potere', meaning 'to be able'. It is about permitting enabling and the giving of authority and power. She further shows that interest in the concept arose during the 1980s with the World Health Organisation's definition of health promotion. This identifies the process of enabling people to be in control of their own health. Empowerment involves three primary factors: attributes that relate to the client, attributes that relate to the nurse and attributes that belong to both nurse and client (Gibson, 1991).

In the 'New Nursing', Salvage (1990, 1992) identifies the emphasis on the nurse – patient partnership and partnership between doctors and nurses. There is a belief in meeting patients' needs utilising a holistic framework. Patients are helped to use their own resources for healing which enables them to be in control of their health. Primarily the nurse has a teaching and enabling role. This type of nursing appears to have a therapeutic effect on patient health (Pearson *et al.* 1988, cited in Salvage, 1992). Overall the emphasis in 'New Nursing' is on encouraging patients and clients to realise their own power base. Support, education and nursing care is offered in partnership, in difficult and vulnerable circumstances, but only to enable patients to empower themselves. The partnership principle in child protection work is discussed by Peall (1992). She outlines various examples:

- Walter Barker's child development programme in the 1980s, where the key principle was that health visitors worked alongside parents. A mutual sharing of ideas and expertise directed towards the child's best interests occurred.
- The creation of parent-held child health records from a joint interprofessional working party in 1990 set up by the British Paediatric Association.
- Legislation, particularly The Children Act 1989 which encourages partnership with children, parents and professionals.
- DoH guidelines in *Working Together*, suggesting that parents should be invited to child protection case conferences.
- Consumer groups demanding equal partnership (such as the National Childbirth Trust) with professionals.

Empowerment is not without difficulties, Salvage (1992) discusses the constraints on the nurse – patient partnership. She points out that whilst many patients would wish for this style of nursing, it cannot be assumed that everyone would. More fundamental needs such as alleviation from pain and discomfort might be more important than therapeutic relationships. Whilst many case conferences for child protection now include parents, Peall (1992) highlights some of the tensions for community nursing. Many of these concerns are about full disclosure and confidentiality of information and the possibility of parents challenging professional accounts. Peall suggests that challenges should be encouraged to allow parents to express fully their views. This in fact gives professionals the opportunity to understand the family background in depth, for later supportive work.

Skelton (1994) argues that there has occurred an over-acceptance of the currency value of the word 'empowerment' with little critical analysis. He discusses two approaches – the micro, relating to individual patient control, and the macro, which concerns organisational and management structures in the wider society. Skelton suggests that nurses should shift their focus into the macro level. This would require them to become politically involved and press for rights for others. Cloke and Naish (1992) argue that nurses have a role not only in preventative work in child protection but in campaigning in society at large. They suggest pressing for resources for families and children and urging a change in our attitudes, towards the greater value of the parenting role. Cloke and Naish point out that in Britain children are often excluded from certain areas and not viewed as citizens with equal rights. They argue that nurses have a key role in promoting children's rights and cite the Health Visitors' Association work in supporting the campaign to end physical punishment of children.

Both micro and macro levels of empowerment may be appropriate to use in the prevention of child abuse.

Work for child health, then, must involve parental participation. Nethercott (1993) writes eloquently about family nursing and family-centred care when children are ill. She itemises particular knowledge and skills necessary in family care, four of which are central to the work for health and child protection. These are:

1. Be an informed flexible practitioner.
2. Do not see nursing (and health visiting) as a source of power but accept parents as partners in care.
3. Have mature and refined interpersonal skills and awareness.
4. Have knowledge related to family and of the processes that influence family functioning.

Wynne (1992) argues that nurses working in accident and emergency departments have a major role in recognising child abuse and initiating action to protect the child. In so doing, nurses obviously need particular knowledge and skills. The case study which follows may help to illustrate Nethercott's four principles.

CASE STUDY

Deborah, a thirteen-year-old girl, presents herself to the local accident and emergency department with a painful swollen right wrist. It is 11.30 a.m. on a weekday morning and the spring half-term holiday from school. The department is reasonably quiet, and the triage nurse Sarah, a 27-year-old E-grade staff nurse, suspects that Deborah has a Colles fracture.

As she is assessing her, she recognises that Deborah is very distressed and frightened. With careful questionning, Sarah finds that Deborah's stepfather is at home asleep following a night shift as a security guard. Her mother is apparently out at work at her usual day job (a check-out cashier at the local supermarket store). Sarah tries to get Deborah to explain how she hurt her wrist and she appears vague and mutters something about falling off her bike. At the same time Deborah appears very uncomfortable and asks for the toilet. Sarah accompanies her, and helps her with her jeans, and notices bruising to her upper thighs. On return to the cubicle Sarah arranges priority for Deborah to be seen by the casualty registrar who is on duty that day rather than the house officer. She does this because she is suspicious that this is a non-accidental injury and she wants the more experienced medical officer to examine her. As Wynne (1992) advocates, Sarah checks the child protection register for Deborah's name or any family member. In this A/E department a confidential printout of the child protection register is updated and sent out weekly by the local social service department who are the agents responsible. Sarah does not find Deborah's name there. As well as an up-to-date register the A/E department have a liaison health visitor who regularly visits to check casualty admissions and is available for contact.

Point 1

In order to be an informed flexible practitioner Sarah has recently completed the Department of Health training and study pack concerning The Children Act 1989 (DoH 1992b). She knows that in circumstances of non-accidental injury where an emergency protection order may be necessary, the 'welfare principle' applies. This states that the child's welfare is the court's paramount consideration. There is a presumption of 'no order' unless the court considers that to make an order would be better for the child. In her flexibility as an informed practitioner Sarah shares her suspicions with the casualty registrar, Mark. She recommends continued probing into the circumstances of the injury as well as investigation of the bruises noted previously.

Sarah knows that nurses are often worried about asking patients and clients if they have been sexually abused. This is sometimes due to their own emotions about abuse and the uncertainty of how to handle these situations if the answer is yes (McMahon, 1992). Yet Sarah is also aware that individuals are often inviting help with disclosure, to break the cycle of guilt and isolation (McMahon, 1992). Sarah agrees with Mark that they will work together in examination and assessment and Sarah will take the lead role in empowering Deborah to share what has happened to her.

Point 2

Sarah does not view nursing as a source of power and believes strongly in fostering partnership between patients and herself and the medical team.

Point 3

In order to do this she needs to be aware and requires mature and refined interpersonal skills. Sarah explains to Deborah that the doctor will examine her wrist but also needs to check her body in case of other injury. Sarah quietly and calmly asks Deborah if there is anything else she would like to tell her about how her wrist was hurt. Deborah is frightened and needs lots of gentle reassurance and confirmation that Deborah will be with her throughout. Mark conducts the examination with Sarah in close attendance. As well as confirming the probability of a Colles fracture and the need for an X-ray, he notes bruising to Deborah's upper thighs. Mark is concerned, as is Sarah, that Deborah may have been sexually abused. Deborah does not respond to any of his questions and he leaves to arrange an X-ray. As he goes, Deborah bursts into tears and holds Sarah's hand extremely tightly. Sarah asks Deborah if someone has hurt her. Slowly and painfully with Sarah's encouragement Deborah's story unfolds.

Sarah discovers that Deborah has had her wrist broken by her step-father who came home from his night shift and tried to sexually abuse her. Deborah's mother had left for her day job. For many months whilst her mother has been out of the house Deborah has been subjected to sexual taunts and intimacies by her stepfather, who also threatened to kill her if she told anyone.

Point 4

Sarah has gained knowledge of family processes that influence family functioning in possible child abuse cases. For example, Jehu (1988, cited McMahon, 1992) highlighted risk factors in incestuous sexual relationships:

- High marital conflict, often with physical abuse of the mother.
- A father may select children as sexual objects when sexual and emotional needs are not met in the marriage.
- High mobility, with passing to one relative or another leading to a lack of consistent stable care from the parents.
- Families often lack social skills and are isolated from others.
- Confusion in family roles and responsibilities for tasks at home.

McMahon (1991) also reviews Araji and Finkelor's (1986) four preconditions that are necessary before sexual abuse occurs:

1. The perpetrator needs to desire the child, which may occur as a result of disinhibition due to alcohol or drugs. Yet arousal may be part of having a need to dominate or because of low self-esteem or immaturity.
2. Perpetrators can often make the child feel guilty and responsible for abuse. They are sometimes able to persuade themselves that children desire sex. Within situations of step-parenting, because there are no biological ties the taboo is less strong.
3. Constraints from outside need to be considered by the perpetrator. The abuser has more opportunity when the mother is out and when the child is not supervised. Most abuse occurs when children are alone.
4. The perpetrator needs to deal with the child's resistance, usually by threatening violence. Other adults and peers are kept away from the child to lessen the likelihood of discovery, adding to the child's isolation.

Sarah has to be clear about her management of Deborah's story. More information is needed. Wynne (1992) suggests a number of aspects, such as finding out if the child or family are known to social services, communicating with the child's general practitioner and health visitor, and gaining any third-party information. In order to avoid or at least minimise incorrect diagnosis in A/E departments, Wynne suggests a number of stages to work through. Practitioners should obtain:

- the children's views
- the parents'/care-givers' accounts
- the physical examination
- medical investigations (possibly forensic tests)
- the initial opinion

As well as the above, Wynne (1992) recommends adding the view of the health visitor, school nurse, community medical officer, and the knowledge of the general practitioner concerning the child and family, together with social work assessment and investigations from the police.

Clearly Sarah has used particular knowledge and skills in enabling Deborah to share what has happened to her. She has begun the process of investigation and management in order to protect.

THE PROFESSIONAL FRAMEWORK: ETHICS AND LAW

The Department of Health (1991c), in their book entitled *Working Together under the Children Act* (1989), state, 'All agencies working in the area of child protection need to understand something of the legal and ethical constraints which govern workers in other agencies.'

The nursing and health visiting practitioner (as indeed any professional) works within a professional framework which takes account of the legal requirements and ethical dimensions of practice. The nursing professional has a code of professional conduct, now in its third edition (UKCC, 1992). The United Kingdom Central Council (UKCC) has a requirement in law to set up and improve standards in professional conduct, and the code is in response to that. The code of conduct can be viewed as a statement of professional values (Pyne, 1992). Pyne states that it was also produced for three reasons:

1. To establish more clearly than ever before the extent of the accountability of registered practitioners.
2. To assist practitioners in the exercise of their professional accountability so as to achieve high standards of professional practice.
3. To encourage practitioners to assert themselves so that the primacy of the interests of their patients and clients is respected.

Whilst the main aim of the code is to focus attention primarily on the interests of the patient and client, Pyne (1992) gives three other definitions: that the code is a 'portrait' of the practitioner that the UKCC wish to have in professional practice; that it constitutes for nurses, midwives and health visitors an extended definition of accountability; and that it now provides a 'backcloth' for professional judgement in cases of alleged misconduct. The latter definition has implications for the professional registration of the practitioner if during practice behaviour is proven to transgress any of the clauses of the code. Dimond (1990) points out that both UKCC codes of practice and Department of Health circulars are not legally binding and cannot

61

evoke civil or criminal action, but they may be used as evidence in cases where approved practice has not been followed.

There are, however, some tensions between the expectations concerning the requirements of some of the clauses of the code of conduct and the needs in professional practice. In the case of child protection, health visiting and confidentiality is one example. Clause 10 of the UKCC code of conduct (1992) is quite specific with regard to confidentiality. It requires the practitioner not to disclose information about patients and clients without consent except in the case of a court order or the wider public interest. Taylor and Tilley (1989) conducted research in two health authorities concerning health visitor involvement in child protection. They argue that the increased participation of health visitors in this work actually threatens their ethical base. Taylor and Tilley suggest that health visitors enjoy a trusting relationship with parents, as they view the role as supportive, with information given and held in confidence. Health visitors were found to quite rightly maintain that information is only given in court if a subpoena is served. Taylor and Tilley argue that this only supports the public impression that health visitors are unwilling participants in child protection. Yet in contrast to this, health visitors were found to be very willing participants in case conferences where open disclosure of information occurred. The UKCC advisory paper on confidentiality (1987) states, 'In some circumstances the practitioner can be under pressure to divulge information but it must be emphasised that the responsibilities lies with him or her as an individual. This responsibility cannot be delegated.' Taylor and Tilley point out that health visitors cannot agonise about such decisions because concerns about child safety must be reported. They further state that while the advisory paper justifies disclosure of information in order to discharge the nurse's professional responsibility, this is ambiguous in cases where professionals have responsibilities for both child and carer. One possible solution to this problem, Taylor and Tilley suggest, is to accept publicly that the child is the ultimate focus as patient/client and takes priority over the parent and/or carer. Health visitors together with other agencies have perhaps traditionally had a child-centred approach to family intervention (Orr, 1985). The child-centred model, as Orr describes, emphasises the well-being of the child, whilst other family members are secondary to this. Yet in discussing the health visitor – client relationship, Orr, while stressing the therapeutic nature of this, appears to imply that the client is the adult. This is particularly evident in the focus on motherhood, and the discussion concerning the role of women and the lack of theory and research which adequately describes their experiences. Whilst this is of course an extremely valid argument put forward by Orr, and one which health visitors should concern themselves with, yet ambiguity can arise in cases of child abuse.

This ethical dilemma leads pertinently into the next section in which the ethical dimension is examined.

THE ETHICAL DIMENSION

When considering the ethical dimension it is necessary to define the concept; clearly some kind of explanation for the practitioner is needed. Rumbold (1993) argues that ethics is fundamentally about right, wrong, good, bad, ought and duty, and that it forms the basis of our decisions about actions. Tschudin (1992), however, makes the point that often we do not consider our actions, but to behave ethically requires that we do so. In fact, she argues that caring is the basis for ethics and ultimately the relationship between the nurse and the client.

In general there has been an upsurge of interest in health care ethics. Advances in medical science have produced particular dilemmas with literally life-or-death decisions to be made. The case of Tony Bland, who was in a persistent vegetative state, is but one of these (Friend, 1993). Nursing is challenging the traditional notion that ethical issues are the concern primarily of doctors (Chadwick and Tadd, 1992). This has produced a number of courses, conferences and literature designed to assist the nursing practitioner to act ethically in the health care relationship. What must the practitioner do to practise ethically however? One route is to follow codes of conduct, and this is essential to be a safe and competent practitioner, yet tensions may still occur, as discussed previously concerning 'conflict, contradictions and ethical dilemmas' in child protection (Taylor and Tilley, 1989). Therefore more than information about professional codes is required, and practitioners need to draw upon ethical theories and principles in moral reasoning. Whilst there is much valuable and appropriate nursing ethical literature, Beauchamp and Childress (1989) provide a simple linear model to establish where actions, codes, principles and theories fit into the process of ethical decision-making. They recommend that health care practitioners should understand ethical theories and principles so that they can be applied before actions are initiated. In child protection work some cases call for immediate action to safeguard the child; however, there are always opportunities to incorporate the ethical dimension in practice. Two major ethical theories inform our decision-making – the non-consequentialist and consequentialist. A clue to their differences is in the terms used. Non-consequentialist or deontological theory emphasises the process of the action, whilst consequentialist or utilitarian theory emphasises the consequences or outcomes of actions. In child protection work both are often required: that is, the nurse and health visitor should consider the process and the consequences of her or his actions. These major theories are recommended as further reading by the practitioner.

The next level in Beauchamp and Childress's (1989) model concerns the ethical principles, of which there are four:

- the principle of respect for autonomy
- the principle of non-maleficence (doing no harm)
- the principle of beneficence (doing good)
- the principle of justice

Again the practitioner is recommended to further literature for a more detailed discussion of these. Briefly, however, the principle of respect for autonomy involves allowing an individual to act independently, since autonomy literally means self-rule (Gillon, 1986). Respect for individual autonomy is the major focus for empowerment and the 'New Nursing' (Salvage, 1990, 1992), as described earlier.

Orr (1985) states:

'Within a relationship there is respect for different values and the uniqueness of each individual is observed and respected. If such a relationship exists, the health visitor cannot force anything on the client but must recognise that often the client will have different standards which must be respected and observed.'

This statement largely summarises the ethical stance that health visitors should have in the practice setting in terms of respecting individual autonomy. It must be remembered, however, that this principle can equally apply to the child, and there may be conflict of interest in child protection work. With regard to the autonomy of the child, Harding (1991) describes this as one of four value perspectives in child care policy which she puts under the umbrella of 'children's rights and child liberation'. In this perspective children are viewed as having freedom and rights similar to adults, with the focus on autonomy and self-determination. The more extreme approach suggests liberating children from adult control as they are viewed as essentially no different from adults (Harding, 1991). There are in fact a number of problems with this perspective, and Harding discusses them in some detail. The idea of children's autonomy puts into question the whole idea of state involvement in child policy. Further, the implications of policy changes are so vast they are neither realistic nor possible. Most importantly

Harding suggests that if this perspective were implemented it would lead to exploitation of children; also it would leave them in a vulnerable and dangerous position without any regulation to protect them. It could be argued, then, that work to protect children under these circumstances would be greatly hindered.

Two other principles within the four that the nurse and health visitor may be more familiar with are non-malificence and beneficence. The principle of non-malificence requires that one shall do no harm, and is a duty all practitioners owe to their patients and clients. Work for health is primarily about doing good, and therefore the principle of beneficence is at the forefront of practice. In child protection work, nurses and health visitors aim to prevent harm being done to children; the main emphasis for health visitors is prevention. Yet health care practitioners need to consider any harm they may do in the process of their practice. The medical practitioner often has to conduct a cost – benefit analysis in balancing risks and benefits in terms of treatment to patients (Gillon, 1986). In some cases of child abuse, practitioners may need to assess the degree of benefit of a child remaining at home against the risk of potential harm in abusing households. In terms of beneficence (doing good), Seedhouse (1988) argues that 'work for health is a moral endeavour' because it is bound to require intervention into people's lives, which in turn has ethical implications. He considers that the principle of beneficence in part unifies consequential and non-consequential theory because we have a duty to do good and prevent harm. In child protection work it is clear that all practitioners have a duty to prevent child abuse and a duty to protect children from harm.

The fourth principle to briefly outline is that of justice. As Gillon (1985) argues, this has always been of great concern to philosophers, hence Aristotle's formal principle of justice. In this, Aristotle stated that equals must be treated equally and unequals must be treated unequally (Beauchamp and Childress, 1989). On first sight this appears to be rather obscure and indeed begs the question who is equal and who unequal? Yet the notion of equality is central to our considerations of justice and therefore valid in the different theories of justice. In child protection work an important question for practitioners is how just are their actions in respect of children and caregivers? In medical ethics justice is an extremely prominent principle to guide the allocation of resources in the most fairest and deserving way. Notions of fairness and desert are also important concepts in this principle (Beauchamp and Childress, 1989). In child protection work, resources are diverse, from the provision of nursery and daycare facilities to support families in need, to the speciality services such as child psychology and family therapy centres. The funding distribution and allocation of these resources together with the provision of community staff, health visitors, social workers and other agencies involves the principle of justice.

The third tier in Beauchamp and Childress's (1989) model refers to rules and codes in ethical decision-making. These rules relate to such concepts as truth-telling (veracity), promise-keeping (fidelity), confidentiality and respecting privacy of clients. Some rules are set within one principle while others in several of the principles outlined above. For example, confidentiality is set clearly in respect for autonomy whilst truth-telling is part of all the principles. Codes of conduct should reflect principles and rules, and these are apparent within the nursing code of conduct (UKCC, 1992). For example, clauses five and seven refer to aspects of respect for client autonomy, and clause ten, as previously mentioned, deals specifically with confidentiality. Child protection work should be about engaging in truthful and faithful partnership with clients, and recognising if these rules are compromised but essentially trying to prevent this from happening. Commitment to words and concepts is fairly simple, but it is the adherence to these in practice that can be problematic. In the case of truth-telling (veracity) Beauchamp and Childress (1989) describe some of these difficulties in medical ethics where non-disclosure of information to patients concerning their health may occur. Traditionally doctors have justified this in terms of serving the best interests of the patient: i.e. it may be detrimental to the health of the patient to know the full extent of her/his illness. In child protection work an obvious example for health visiting practice may be that an injury is found on a routine developmental check and suspicion of child abuse causes the health visitor to alert other agencies but not disclose this to the carer. In cases such as this it should be acknowledged that both respect for autonomy and truth-telling have been compromised. The practitioner may be able to justify this by appealing to the principle of beneficence in respect of the child. Yet this is a very real dilemma for the health visiting profession and a major argument put forward by Taylor and Tilley (1989) and outlined above. These are the very kind of judgements and actions (the last tier in Beauchamp and Childress's (1989) model) that the practitioner needs to deliberate over and use the knowledge of theories, principles, rules and codes to try and resolve them.

THE LEGAL FRAMEWORK

For the practitioner, accountability concerns how they can be held in law to account for their actions (Dimond, 1990). An individual nurse, midwife or health visitor is accountable to four main arenas, as Dimond points out:

1. the profession – through the code of professional conduct (UKCC, 1992)
2. the employer – via the contract of employment
3. the patient/client – via civil law and civil courts
4. the public – via criminal law and criminal courts.

Dimond (1990) opens her book with an example of a staff nurse who in making a drug error causes the death of a child. In this illustration the staff nurse is liable in all four arenas, and if proven to be grossly negligent Dimond states: 'then consistent results in all four hearings are likely: she will be found guilty in the criminal courts; liable in the civil court; removed from the register by the professional conduct committee; and dismissed by the employer.' For the nursing practitioner this is the worst-case scenario but the example clearly illustrates the extent of accountability.

In child protection work nurses have a clear duty to report any suspicion of or actual child abuse. Dimond (1990) gives a good example of a health visitor making a routine visit to a family with a child of eighteen months and discovering small burn marks. She makes it clear that the health visitor has a duty to report this and procedures are available to do so.

Local authorities have a statutory duty to investigate any suspicion of child abuse and to assess the needs of the child and family (DoH, 1991c, pp. 9). Investigation of abuse and neglect involves:

Section 37 of the Children Act (1989)
Section 47 (1) of the Children Act (1989)
Section 47 (8) of the Children Act (1989)
Schedule 2, paragraph 4 of the Children Act (1989)

(DoH, 1991c, p. 9)

THE CHILDREN ACT (1989)

As has been suggested in this chapter so far, nurses and health visitors have a significant contribution to make in the protection of children. According to the Department of Health (1989), The Children Act 1989 is the most comprehensive piece of legislation ever enacted concerning children. In an introductory guide to the NHS the DoH (1989a, p. 6) points out that,

'The Act has important implications for district and special health authorities, NHS Trusts and family health service authorities in relation to child health and welfare. Health service staff need therefore to understand the provision and aims of the Act and its implications for professional practice.'

In fact the DoH (1989) goes on to state that each health authority and NHS trust has a duty to co-operate with social services departments and assist them in their responsibilities under the Act. Other major aspects highlighted in the guide are that:

- As well as the need for inter-agency co-operation for both the protection of children and the provision of services, GPs and health service staff are to work much more closely with social services departments.
- In order to meet the health needs of children a much greater collaboration is asked for between social services, health professionals, parents and children.

The Children Act 1989 draws together existing legislation and integrates the law concerning private individuals and public authority responsibility, in particular social service departments. The DoH in the foreword (1989) state, 'The Act strikes a new balance between family autonomy and the protection of children'.

Stainton Rogers and Roche (1992) highlight the fact that the Children Act 1989 is very much in harmony with the 'New Nursing' philosophy of holistic health care. They point out that in terms of changes in child protection a major emphasis in the Act is for courts not to intervene unnecessarily. In order to achieve this, two main foci are recommended:

1. Resources should be given to support families with stress in child care.
2. Practitioners should work in partnership with parents to achieve voluntary agreements in protecting children.

The Children Act 1989 does, however, provide clear orders for protection of children if required. The local authority has a duty to investigate any reports concerning child safety. To further any investigation a new order is identified in the Act (Stainton Rogers and Roche, 1992) known as the Child Assessment Order. This order is important in cases where a child has a problem and a medical examination is necessary but the parents are being unco-operative. The order is further reviewed in the sub-section below entitled 'Review of practice procedures'.

Primarily the Act emphasises the notion that children are best looked after within the family and highlights a new concept of parental responsibility. Parental responsibility refers to the duty of care which the parent has in respect of her/his child in terms of moral, physical and emotional health. So important is parental responsibility that if separation or divorce occurs this responsibility continues. Courts must not be used to lessen the duty of parental responsibility in cases of family breakdown. The notion of 'only positive intervention' in the Act prohibits courts from making 'any order unless it is satisfied that the order will positively contribute to the child's welfare' (DoH, 1989a, p. 3). Clearly practitioners need to learn lessons from both the Cleveland controversy (Campbell, 1988) and the removal of children from Orkney (Clyde, 1992).

In the Children Act (1989) another emphasis concerns 'getting the best for children' where the child's welfare is paramount, making the 'overriding purpose of the Act to promote and safeguard the welfare of children' (DoH, 1989b, pp. 3). So whilst the wishes of parents are considered by the courts, actions are directed to the best interests of the child. A checklist is available for the court when considering whether to make a court order and if so which one. The focus of the checklist is on the needs of the child together with his/her views. The latter is developed as a major aspect of the Act termed 'the child and his views in proceedings'. There are two separate proceedings, private and local authority. In private proceedings the Act recognises the tensions between the child's own views and independence, and the potential for the problem caused by the parents resting with the child. In local authority proceedings involving a care order, the child is generally represented by a guardian *ad litem* (a trained social worker). The duty is with the guardian to represent the child's views and safeguard her/his interests. If disagreement occurs between the guardian and child, the child can direct the solicitor who must take her/his instructions (DoH, 1989b, p. 4).

The welfare balance in protecting children is particularly sensitive when suspicion of harm is aroused. The Children Act (1989) 'seeks to protect children both from the harm which can arise from the failures or abuse within the family and from the harm which can be caused by unwarranted intervention in their family life' (DoH, 1989b, p. 5). The Children Act (1989) sets out specific protective orders which allow courts powers to intervene to protect children at risk of harm.

These are outlined in the review of practice procedures and implications below.

Working together for child protection

Working together for child protection is vitally important. No single agency can either prevent child abuse or protect children within one particular professional framework alone. In recognition of this the DoH (1991c) produced a book entitled *Working Together under the Children Act 1989*. This is a guide to inter-agency co-operation for the protection of children from abuse. Every practitioner involved in child protection should have ready access to a copy of this publication. The DoH (1991c) clearly identifies the role of these agencies in child protection.

In terms of race and culture, Narducci (1992) points out that both The Children Act 1989 and *Working Together* require 'due consideration to the religious persuasion, racial origin and cultural and linguistic background of children with whom we are concerned'. He urges that any assessments undertaken and decisions made are not influenced by stereotypic ideas of race and culture. Narducci (1992) cites Dominelli (1988) who identified certain strategies that white people use, such as omission (not acknowledging racism even exists) and decontextualisation (accepting racism but not its affects in everyday practice). He argues for child protection, 'what is perceived as abusive or neglectful in one culture may not be viewed in the same light in others'. There is clearly a need for education, knowledge and respect for culture which allows a full understanding of the multi-ethnic nature of child abuse.

Trowell (1992) has devised a simple model to depict visually agencies that might affect a particular child (see Figure 2.1). These agencies may be involved with an individual child depending on the health protection need identified. In cases of suspected or actual child abuse, Trowell (1992) identifies that the assessment will probably involve health professionals, social service professionals and the police. Continuing work when abuse has been identified will often involve education and probation as well as health and social service professionals. In court cases the legal system is necessarily brought into action with again social and health care professionals and the police. At this stage, Trowell states, the voluntary sector may be involved. Further, she identifies that, after assessment, working with the child and family will involve health and social service professionals, education, the voluntary sector and may include probation, housing, employment and social security. This number of agencies involved presents a significant concern in terms of communication between professionals with regard to both

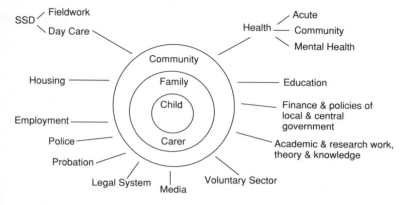

Figure 2.1 *The agencies which may affect a particular child*
Source: Reproduced with kind permission from Trowell (1992).

the protection of the child and the needs of the family or care givers. Trowell (1992) argues that time and again where tragedies have occurred it has been due to a lack of information-sharing between professionals. This communication breakdown is not new. It has been clearly identified in the DHSS (1982) and from professionals themselves (Wheeler, 1992). Yet the most recent inquiry reports, 1980–89 (DoH, 1991a), still uncover problems in inter-agency communication. For example, key words and expressions are identified in this report as having no common meaning, such as 'thriving', 'joint investigation' and 'urgency' (DoH 1991d). This study also highlights difficulties with confidentiality. For example:

'Social worker 2 did not discuss the history of the case with the health visitors because she did not realise that they had been involved with the Gates family for any length of time. Neither did the health visitor realise that social worker 2 and her superiors were not fully conversant with the background. Social worker 2 did not ask her to see their records or to discuss the possible content because in her experience all medical records were regarded as strictly confidential.'   (DoH, 1991d, pp. 100)

So the ethical requirement of confidentiality as outlined above in terms of tension is an issue. This should be addressed in the open more readily, particularly by nurses and health visitors.

71

On-going education and training in child protection for all agencies is necessary. Gilardi's (1991) research concerning the child protection training needs for health visitors in Lewisham and North Southwark significantly found that 97 per cent of a sample of seventy-five health visitors had been involved in at least one case of child protection, and 70 per cent in five cases or more. In terms of shared learning, however, Gilardi reports that only 38 per cent of those educated in the last three years received any form of joint training. Shared learning between agencies is likely to be far more of a feature in future educational programmes. This should enhance communication, as individual professionals from different agencies will have much more understanding of each other's roles and contributions in child protection work. In terms of assessment, apart from Dingwall *et al.*'s (1983) research and Appleton (1993), no study had been undertaken by practitioners to establish how agency workers undertake family assessment (Wheeler, 1992). Following interviews with social workers and health visitors, Wheeler analysed the data phenomenologically and using grounded theory. In the phenomenological data analysis, exhaustive descriptions of both social worker and health visitor family assessments emerged and were compared. When examining these it was shown that the process used by both agencies is very similar. The categories that emerged from the social worker interviews were replicated in the health visitor responses. These were assessing relationships and physical aspects, and in the process using intuition, personal standards and life experience (Wheeler, 1992).

Appleton (1993) conducted a study to explore the procedures and criteria used to define and assess vulnerable families. As well as finding that the concept of vulnerability is highly complex and influenced by multiple factors, indications were that health visitors used their own professional judgements in deciding what constitutes vulnerability. Significantly Appleton (1993) states,

'clearly conflict exists between professional judgements and official guidelines and is displayed in the identification of "other" vulnerable families by the health visitors. Lack of resources and minimal preventative work on the part of social workers means that frequently health visitors are the sole professionals involved with vulnerable families.'

Clearly this study has implications in working together for child protection. It indicates that problems exist in both assessment for so-called vulnerable families in health visiting, and in inter-agency co-operation for prevention in child protection work. Waters (1992) refers to the work of Taylor and Tilley (1989) and suggests that health visitors are constantly examining whether they are agents of social control or educative, supportive and health-promoting practitioners.

Review of practice procedures and implications

In the document *Child Protection: Guidance for Senior Nurses, Health Visitors and Midwives* (DoH, 1992a), the responsibilities of health service staff and the involvement with local authorities is clearly outlined. In cases of suspected or actual child abuse the practitioner needs to use this guidance with the document *Working Together under the Children Act* (DoH 1991c), as previously mentioned. This document comprehensively outlines the investigation of abuse and neglect within the legal framework and professional practice. The practitioner is taken through the stages step by step in the sections 'Working together in individual cases' and 'The child protection conference and the child protection register'. It is pointed out in this document that agencies can only be effective if there is a shared agreement concerning the management of individual cases. The stages necessary are:

1. Referral and recognition
2. Immediate protection and planning the investigation
3. Investigation and initial assessment
4. Child protection conference and decision-making about the need for registration
5. Comprehensive assessment and planning
6. Implementation, review, and where appropriate de-registration.

(DoH 1991c, pp. 26)

The above stages may well overlap and would not necessarily stand separately or be within a time sequence. What is absolutely certain is that

> 'The starting point of the process is that any person who has knowledge of or suspicion that the child is suffering significant harm, or is at risk of significant harm should refer their concern to one or more of the agencies with statutory duties and/or powers to investigate and intervene – the social services department, the police or the NSPCC.'

(DoH, 1991c, pp. 27)

Emergency protection order

In cases where there is risk of serious injury or even death of the child these agencies with child protection powers must secure immediate safety. This can be undertaken by removal of the child on a voluntary basis (parental consent) or by obtaining an emergency protection order. 'An emergency protection order is a short term order which enables a child to be made safe when he might otherwise suffer harm' (DoH, 1989b, p. 62). Application for this is to the court, and the court must be satisfied that there is reasonable cause to believe the child is likely to suffer significant harm or has suffered this (DoH, 1989b, p. 62). The duration of an emergency protection order 'will have effect for as long as the court specifies subject to a maximum of eight days' (DoH, 1989b, p. 65).

In all cases of suspicion of suffering or likelihood of suffering significant harm, investigation must take place. 'In accordance with the Area Child Protection Committee procedures all investigations need to be planned. The prime tasks are:

- to establish the facts about the circumstances giving rise to the concern;
- to decide if there are grounds for concern;
- to identify sources and level of risk; and
- to decide protective or other action in relation to the child and any others.'

(DoH, 1991b, p. 29)

Child assessment orders

In cases where an emergency has not occurred but parents are frustrating the investigation, an application for a child assessment order (CAO) can be considered. The order granted by the court lasts seven days and a full assessment of the child should take place at that time (DoH, 1991c).

The child protection conference

The child protection conference is the key forum for both professionals and the family to share information. In so doing, concerns and risks can be analysed and recommendations for plans of action can be made. A decision as to whether or not to register the child is made and if registration is agreed the key worker must be allocated. The key worker is a social worker from either the social service department or the NSPCC.

The child protection conference is not a forum to decide 'that a person has abused a child which is a criminal offence' (DoH, 1991c, p. 31).

If the child is registered, a comprehensive assessment and plan is required. In the assessment the DoH (1991c, p. 31) outlines the questions where decisions have to be made:

- Who will undertake the assessment?
- Where will it be undertaken?
- What is the time-scale?
- How should it be recorded?
- How to involve the family?
- What is the legal status of the child?
- How will it fit in with any court action and have the necessary steps in relation to this been taken?
- How will it fit with other action, e.g. by the police in respect of the offence?
- What is the SSD's position regarding parental responsibility?

Following this assessment a written plan must be made which involves parents and care-givers. Each agency involved must also identify their particular contribution to the child and family. The expectations of the parents need to be made clear. Once the plan is agreed the implementation must be the responsibility of each individual agency with communication to and co-ordination by the key worker. Each plan must consider the wishes of the child and parents. The plan must also have regard for local resources and specialist services which may address particular needs of the child and family. Both children and parents must be given information about the plan which includes understanding the objectives. It is important that they are able to both accept and work with the plan (DoH, 1991c, p. 32).

CONCLUSION

The Children Act 1989 has certain implications for nursing and health visiting practice. Clearly, as Stainton Rogers and Roche (1992) point out, education and information are fundamental. Relationships between professionals, parents and children should be based on partnership. This does, however, bring tensions, which can only be resolved by 'working together'. Finding new ways of working, communicating, sharing and caring are recognised as essential components of nursing and health visiting practice. The Children Act 1989 offers even greater scope for innovative improvements in child protection work and fits with holistic nursing.

The changes in welfare provision and the reorganised health service (NHS and Community Care Act 1990) have made visible impacts in terms of access to services and provision of resources. It would appear that unemployment, homelessness and ill-health in the poorer sections of our society are growing. Work for health and child protection faces many challenges not just in terms of national aspirations and objectives but within the European community which is shifting radically. Moves towards democracy both in Europe and the former Soviet Union have brought many surprises, but as the market struggles to accommodate these changes economic recession bites deep. The allocation of resources in terms of welfare provision are being adjusted particularly in the United Kingdom. Nurses and health visitors need to be vigilant in advocating for children's and family rights as competition for money from the treasury increases. Ethical theories and principles should be examined and used to justly serve the children and families all social and health care professions seek to protect from harm.

CHAPTER THREE

Social Perspectives in Child Abuse

Jim Ogg and Jonathan Dickens

INTRODUCTION

Social work intervention to protect children from harm and abuse in England and Wales is governed by the legal framework of the Children Act 1989. The Act came into operation on 14 October 1991, and made wide-ranging changes to the law relating to the upbringing, care and protection of children. The aims of the new Act, according to the guidance issued by the Department of Health (DH), are 'to strike a new balance between the rights of children to express their views on decisions made about their lives, the rights of parents to exercise their responsibilities towards the child and the duty of the state to intervene when the child's welfare requires it' (DH, 1991a, p. 1). In this chapter we examine the ways that the Act seeks to achieve these balances, and the ways in which these are reflected in the day-to-day practice of social work with children and families.

The chapter is divided into four sections. First, we present an account of the Act itself, summarising its background and its key concepts. In the second section we adopt a 'discourse analysis' approach to draw out the conceptual and political tensions and ambiguities which lie behind the formulation and putting-into-practice of the legislation, paying particular attention to the discourses of 'law' and 'welfare'. In the third section we look more closely at the practical implications of the Act for child protection work in the 1990s, illustrating our discussion with examples of current developments in social work practice. In the fourth section we add an extra dimension by applying the framework to the emerging field of children's rights and some of its implications for child protection.

THE CHILDREN ACT 1989

The impetus for a reform of child care law which led to the Children Act 1989 came from two principal directions. First, there were long-standing concerns from social work professionals, academics and special interest groups about the quality of social work practice and decision-making for children in care, particularly regarding the involvement of natural families and the maintenance of contact between children and parents. These matters were the subjects of a Parliamentary investigation by the Social Services Select Committee between 1982 and 1984, and its report (published in 1984) gave rise to a government inter-departmental review of child care law (DHSS, 1985a). A summary of research findings into aspects of child care practice was published for dissemination throughout Social Services Departments (SSDs) in 1985 (DHSS, 1985b). These initiatives led to the publication of a White Paper on 'The Law on Child Care and Family Services' in 1987 (DHSS, 1987).

The second source of pressure for reform had a much higher public and media profile. This arose from a series of inquiries in the mid-1980s into child abuse deaths, notably the cases of Jasmine Beckford (London Borough of Brent, 1985) and Kimberley Carlile (London Borough of Greenwich, 1987). These two inquiries – both chaired by a leading barrister, Louis Blom-Cooper QC – made heavy criticism of social workers for inadequate knowledge of child abuse risk indicators and child protection law, and for being reluctant to use the legal powers available to them.

The public interest in child protection matters was heightened even further by the events in Cleveland in 1987. Ninety-one children in Cleveland were made subjects of Place of Safety Orders between January and June that year because of suspicions of sexual abuse (Secretary of State for Social Services, 1988, p. 172). In this case, social workers were criticised for acting over-hastily to remove children from their homes, and there was criticism of the legal processes which enabled them to do so (e.g. that Place of Safety Orders allowed the children to be kept away from home for up to 28 days on suspicion of abuse without any right of appeal for the parents: Secretary of State for Social Services, 1988, pp. 172–3, 226–9). The inquiry into the Cleveland affair was chaired by another prominent legal figure, Lord Justice Butler-Sloss, and her report (published in July 1988) gave the final push for the introduction of new child care legislation. The government published its Children Bill in November 1988.

In the context of the diverse and sometimes contradictory criticisms of social workers – for failing to work in co-operative ways with the parents and families of children in care or at risk of coming into care, for failing to act decisively to protect children from harm, and for taking legal action too quickly – the new law sought to strike better 'balances' between the duties and powers of social workers, the autonomy of families, the rights of children and the rights of parents. One outcome of this 'balancing' process was that the old Place of Safety Order was replaced by a new Emergency Protection Order (EPO), which can only last for 8 days, and which parents have the right to challenge after 72 hours (Children Act 1989, s. 44). Another example is that the new law makes provisions for children to apply for court orders (or the discharge of orders) in their own right, recognising that the interests and wishes of children and their parents may not always coincide.

The Act seeks to achieve its balances between the powers of social workers and the rights of parents and children by introducing two important principles for child care law and practice. The first of these is that statutory intervention in family life should only occur when absolutely necessary. As a rule, *partnership* between social workers and parents is to be preferred. This emphasis is reflected in the 'no order' principle in Section 1(5) of the Act, which states that whenever a court is considering making an order under the Act, 'it shall not make the order … unless it considers that doing so would be better for the child than making no order at all' – in other words, there has to be a demonstrable need for a court order rather than voluntary co-operation.

The partnership principle is further reflected in those parts of the Act which deal with local authority services to 'children in need' and their families. Part III of the Act (Sections 17–30), and Schedule 2 in particular, impose a range of duties on local authorities to provide services such as day care, family centres, advice and counselling, home help and cash assistance to such children and their families. The aims of these services are to 'safeguard and promote' the child's welfare and promote the upbringing of the child by his/her own family (s. 17(1)).

The second important principle is the emphasis on *parental responsibility*, which is loosely defined in the Act as 'all the rights, duties, powers, responsibilities and authority which by law a parent of a child has in relation to the child and his property' (s. 3(1)).

The significant points about parental responsibility are that it can be shared by different people, and that a parent who does not actually have the physical care of a child will retain his/her responsibility and thus have an on-going right to be consulted on decisions about the child's upbringing (s. 2(5)–(7)). Even when a child is the subject of a Care Order, the parent(s) retain their responsibility – although in this case the local authority has parental responsibility too, and is given additional power to determine the extent to which the parent(s) may exercise their responsibility (s. 33(3)).

Parental responsibility can only be acquired by someone who is not actually a parent of the child by an order of court. This put an end to the power of local authorities to pass 'Parental Rights Resolutions' on children who were in 'voluntary care' (itself a concept which has been abolished by the new law). 'Parental Rights Resolutions' were an administrative procedure by which a local authority could terminate the rights of a parent and vest them in itself, without reference to a court.

The new EPO gives parental responsibility to the applicant (usually the SSD) for the duration of the Order, but the parents still retain their responsibility. There is a presumption that the applicant will allow 'reasonable contact' between the child and (amongst others) his/her parents (s. 34). Where the child does not want such contact, or it is not considered to be in the best interests of the child, the SSD has to apply to the court for permission to refuse it. The court has the power to make directions about the sort of contact (if any) which should occur, and also about whether the child should undergo any form of examination or assessment, and if so, what this should involve. In the event that there is, or is considered likely to be, any dispute between the SSD and the parents, directions from the court are required to settle the matter.

The partnership and parental responsibility principles have major implications for social work practice. They require workers to make greater efforts than ever before to consult with parents and to facilitate parental participation in decision-making – even when the children are in care or considered to be at risk of harm. One outcome of this is a greater emphasis on parental attendance at child protection case conferences, which is discussed more fully in the third section of this chapter. Another important consequence of the participatory approach is that it requires workers to observe the highest standards of anti-discriminatory practice if it is to be truly effective with parents and children of all racial and cultural backgrounds. The Act explicitly states that SSDs, in reaching decisions about children whom they are looking after or proposing to look after, should give due consideration to 'the child's religious persuasion, racial origin and cultural and linguistic background' (s. 22(5)).

In the following section we use the theoretical approach of discourse analysis to expose the crucial influences which lie behind the way that the Children Act seeks to strike its balances between social workers, parents and children. (For a fuller discussion of the background and provisions of the Children Act 1989, see especially Parton, 1991; Eekelaar and Dingwall, 1990; and Masson, 1992. Additionally, Fox Harding,

1991, provides useful insights into the different value positions reflected in child care legislation.)

LAW, WELFARE AND OTHER DISCOURSES

The Children Act seeks to balance the powers of social workers and the autonomy of families by promoting the two concepts of partnership and parental responsibility. Although presented as the 'building blocks' from which services to families are to be developed, a closer examination of these principles reveals two very different approaches to the way in which the state can properly intervene in family life. The first emphasises that intervention must be justified according to legal criteria and authorised by a court; the second argues that family and child care matters are best dealt with by welfare practitioners, not lawyers and judges. Both approaches can be detected in the Children Act: on the one hand, there is an emphasis on reducing the need for legal intervention (exemplified by the 'no order' principle); on the other, there is an increasing reliance on the courts and the law as safeguards for parents against over-intervention from social workers. Discourse analysis helps to unravel the tensions which lie behind the 'balances' in the Children Act, and in this section we explore the relationship between four key *discourses* in the formulation and subsequent putting-into-practice of the Act –'law', 'welfare', 'the market economy' and 'managerialism'.

Discourse analysis is an approach which regards language as the key to the structures of knowledge and power through which people experience and make sense of the world around them. Words and concepts are treated as 'signs' which derive their meaning from these structures or 'discourses'. The crucial point is that the signs do not derive their meaning from anything 'real' or 'out there' to which they refer; rather, meaning comes from within the discourse itself, from the interrelationships with other signs, and from the aims and internal rules of the discourse.

The key signs in the legal discourse are concepts such as 'equality before the law', 'rights', 'due process', 'just deserts' and 'deterrence'. The key signs in the welfare discourse, on the other hand, are to do with 'assistance', 'treatment', 'expert assessment', 'provision of services according to need', and 'rehabilitation'. From a discourse perspective, the meaning of these sorts of signs (those which apparently refer to very general or abstract concepts) lies in their function – which is to bestow greater weight on what the user is saying, thus reinforcing the status and power of both the user and the discourse itself.

In arguing that the meaning of a 'sign' is not to be found in anything 'real', 'out there', but within the discourse itself, the intention is not to deny that child abuse occurs. Rather, the value of discourse analysis is that it focuses attention on the way that certain forms of harm to children are presented and understood in such a way that they become the subjects of public debate and state intervention, whilst others – for example, bullying in schools, poor quality housing, road traffic accidents – have not received the same treatment, despite the efforts of certain individuals and groups to increase their profile. Discourse analysis emphasises the importance of studying the specific processes of social change (or "lines of transformation' – Donzelot, 1980) by which certain discourses achieve dominance over others. Applying this approach to the history of the Children Act reveals how the tensions between the discourses of law and welfare lie at the heart of the new 'balances' the Act seeks to create. The Act puts its emphasis on welfare services and voluntary co-operation between parents and social workers as the best ways of meeting children's needs and protecting them from harm; but the law also has a role to play in achieving those aims, and there must be adequate powers for compulsory intervention combined with proper processes to ensure fairness.

Despite the tensions between law and welfare, the two discourses are inter-dependent and neither can achieve its own ends without the assistance of the other. For example, welfare does not possess direct sanctions such as fines, imprisonment or the right to remove children from their parents – when its therapeutic and educational approach fails, it has to look to the courts for reinforcement. However, the relationship is not all one-way, because law itself needs the welfare discourse. The law relies on the recommendations of welfare 'experts' to justify its imposition of disciplinary sanctions. In child care matters, the courts look to welfare practitioners such as social workers, paediatricians and child psychiatrists for assessments of the family and recommendations on the best course of action. The legal discourse can restrict the potential intrusiveness of welfare intervention, but it also enforces those interventions when necessary; on the other hand, the treatment-oriented welfare discourse can ameliorate the formally just but inflexible legal system, but it also furnishes reasons to support 'unavoidable' legal action on occasions (Donzelot, 1980, p. 232). (For discourses generally, see also Rojek *et al.* 1988; Carty and Mair, 1990; King, 1991; King and Piper, 1990; and James, 1992.)

In addition to law and welfare, two other significant discourses lie behind the provisions of the Children Act and the ways in which they are being put into practice. The first of these is the discourse of the 'market economy'. Its key signs are a wish to 'reduce the role of the state'; to increase 'consumer choice'; to promote 'independence and self-provision' to meet needs, rather than dependency on the state; to get better 'value for money' from services provided out of central and local government funds; and to increase the 'privatisation' of such services. These signs have been the dominant elements in the political philosophy and programme (or 'discourse') of the Tory government since 1979. Ever decreasing resources and tighter budgetary constraints for local government (and within that, for SSDs) are justified in terms of this market rhetoric – and indeed, the signs are not the exclusive province of Tory politicians. The interaction of discourses is exemplified by the way that Labour-controlled local authorities have also adopted signs such as 'value for money' and 'consumer choice' in campaigns to enhance the relevance and popularity of their services. The signs have meaning in left-wing as well as right-wing political discourse.

Although the market economy discourse did not become an explicit feature of the debates about the Children Act, it nevertheless had a significant underlying influence. This can be detected from the way in which the resource implications of the new legislation were downplayed by the government. Their line was that local authorities would require very little extra funding to implement the Act – the note on the anticipated financial effects of the new law, included in the Bill in November 1988, put the cost of the extra welfare responsibilities (the services to families and children under Part III of the Act) at just £1.7 million, and estimated that this would require an additional 150 local authority employees in England and Wales (i.e. less than $1\frac{1}{2}$ new posts per SSD). Many of the individuals and organisations involved in the Parliamentary debates had grave doubts about the realism of these figures, but their misgivings were not allowed to undermine the progress of the Bill. The estimates are, however, indicative of the wider political atmosphere in which the Children Act was drafted, and it remains a defining feature of the climate in which the Act has since been put into effect (Frost, 1992).

The second additional discourse is 'managerialism'. The aim here is for a much tighter control of social work practice in order to counter the dangers of 'over-intervention' (as in Cleveland) or 'under-intervention' (as in child abuse deaths). This control is to be achieved from three sources – the courts, central government and managers in SSDs. The key signs include 'procedures', 'supervision', 'inspection', 'regulations', and 'guidance'. Another important sign is 'directions', an example of which is the court-given directions to determine what happens to a child under an EPO (see above). The introduction of the Children Act was accompanied by the publication of nine volumes of DH 'Guidance and Regulations', plus a general introduction to the principles of the new Act and a further summary of research findings (DH, 1990, 1991b). It was also marked by the publication of new, expanded procedures for inter-professional and inter-agency working in child protection (Working Together, DH, 1991c), and had been preceded by extremely detailed and prescriptive guidelines on how social workers should conduct comprehensive family assessments (DH, 1988).

In the following section we move on to a closer examination of social work practice under the Children Act in the light of the tensions and interplay of the various discourses, but concentrating particularly on law and welfare.

CHILD PROTECTION UNDER THE CHILDREN ACT 1989

In this section we discuss three of the main developments in child protection work since the implementation of the Children Act 1989. These topics illustrate current social work practice in this field, and further demonstrate the tensions between law and welfare. They also suggest avenues for further research and evaluation. The three features are the reduction in the number of care cases coming before the courts; greater parental participation in child protection case conferences; and the impact of new legislation and guidelines about video-recorded interviews with children.

Care proceedings

The most notable change since the Children Act came into force has been a dramatic fall in the volume of court proceedings about children brought by local authorities. The DH's report on the first year of the Children Act shows that there were just over 2,200 applications for EPOs between 14 October 1991 and 30 September 1992 (i.e. very nearly the first full year). Approximately 1,900 EPOs were made, compared with about 5,000 Place of Safety Orders during the full year ending 31 March 1991 (DH, 1993, pp. 15–16, 19–20). There were slightly over 3,700 applications for care orders, and by 30 September 1992 a total of 1,607 care orders had been made. There were still over 1,800 applications outstanding, and the DH estimated that the final number of care orders resulting from the first year's activity would be between 2,500 and 3,000. Under the previous legislation there were 5,400 care orders in the year ending 31 March 1991 (DH, 1993, pp. 14–15).

It is important not to draw over-hasty conclusions from the number of care orders 'before' and 'after' the introduction of the Children Act, not least because the extent of the legislative changes makes a straightforward comparison impossible. It is also important to note that the rate of applications increased over the year, and so a possible explanation of the initial drop in court activity is that it was attributable to social workers' uncertainty about the new law, and that as they became increasingly familiar with the new Act, so they became more ready to make court applications. To some extent this is borne out by more recent statistics which show that approximately 14,000 care orders were made in the period January–June 1993, which was over 60 per cent more than in the same period in 1992 (Children Act Advisory Committee, 1993, pp. 92, 96).

The same statistics show, however, that the number of care orders made per quarter reached a peak in the period October–December 1992 and has since declined, so there may be other factors behind the overall decrease in court activity which will not simply wear off over time. Most notably these could include a more widespread and enduring commitment to working in partnership with parents and using the court only as a last resort, but others could be dissatisfaction with the provisions of the new Act or with aspects of the court process. These sorts of issues will need to be addressed by longer-term qualitative research, such as interviews with social workers, to explore their attitudes and the factors which shape their decision-making. It is crucially important that this research addresses the issue of whether the drop in court proceedings is for the 'right' reasons, and that children are not being left at risk of harm as a result.

The Social Services Inspectorate (SSI: a branch of the DH) made a start on this research with a study of decision-making about court applications in four local authorities during the period January–June 1992 (SSI, 1992). The study focused on sixteen cases where there were apparently grounds for an application, but none was made. The findings were that the reasons for not seeking an order were very varied – the most frequent ones were that workers felt that their plans and services would ensure sufficient protection for the child without recourse to the court, that the child was already in a safe environment (e.g. an alternative address), and that there was parental agreement to co-operate with the social services plan (SSI, 1992, pp. 5, 69–73). The study comments on the high level of services put into these families, but does not pay any attention to the efforts which workers may have had to make to secure these services, or the effect of resource shortages on the level of services available to families before matters reach the point of possible court action (SSI, 1992, pp. 46–9).

The study also highlighted a 'widespread anxiety' amongst workers that even if the grounds for an order could be demonstrated, the 'no order' principle would mean that the court would not make the order if there was parental co-operation (SSI, 1992, p. 72). The DH report on the first year of the Children Act picks up on this theme, and warns that it was not the intention of the Act that the 'no order' principle should require partnership to have broken down before a court order can be made. It states 'Local authorities should not feel inhibited by the working in partnership provisions of the Children Act from seeking appropriate court orders ... The two processes are not mutually exclusive' (DH, 1993, p. 19).

By the end of the first year, then, the fall in the volume of care proceedings had provoked a re-examination of the aims of the Act, and in particular the implications of the 'partnership' philosophy. Continued monitoring of the court returns will give an indication of how the Act is being put into effect, but further qualitative research is necessary for a deeper insight into the underlying realities of everyday social work practice.

Child protection case conferences

The second relevant feature of social work practice since the introduction of the Children Act is the greater emphasis on parental participation in child protection case conferences. These are meetings of all the professional workers who have knowledge of a particular family, when there are concerns or allegations about child abuse. Those invited will include social workers, teachers, the police, doctors, day-nursery workers, health visitors and – in what has now become routine practice – the parents. The aims are to share and evaluate information about the family; to make decisions about the level of risk to the child; to make plans for future action; and to decide whether or not the child's name should be on the 'Child Protection Register' (DH, 1991c, p. 41).

The involvement of parents is a relatively recent development, although its introduction has not been uniform across the country – some SSDs have been inviting parents for much longer than others, but for many the change has only come about since the Children Act came into force.

In 1986 the DHSS published a draft edition of *Working Together* (the guide for inter-agency co-operation in child protection work) which explicitly stated that parents should not attend case conferences (DHSS, 1986, p. 19). By the 1988 edition the position had changed, and the DHSS advice was that parents 'should be invited where practicable to attend part, or if appropriate the whole, of case conferences unless in the view of the chairman of the conference their presence will preclude a full and proper consideration of the child's interests' (DHSS, 1988, pp. 29–30). However, the attendance of parents only became more widespread very gradually after the publication of that advice, and the 1991 version of *Working Together* strengthens the expectation that parents will be invited. It argues that there will only be 'exceptional occasions' when it will not be appropriate to invite one or other parent to attend all or part of a conference (DH, 1991c, p. 43).

In terms of the tensions between the legal and welfare discourses, it is interesting to note that the 1988 guidance made explicit reference to the fact that the European Court of Human Rights had found the United Kingdom government to be in breach of the European Convention of Human Rights because of failure to involve parents in decision-making about their children (DHSS, 1988, p. 29). It thereby drew attention to the legal reasons for inviting parents to case conferences; in contrast, the 1991 guidance emphasises the welfare reasons, stressing that the welfare of the child is the 'overriding factor' in child protection work. It emphasises that there should be full parental involvement from the outset of the investigation process, and 'as much openness and honesty as possible between families and professionals' (DH, 1991c, p. 43). Attendance at case conferences is seen as a part of this process, and as a practical consequence of 'partnership' and 'parental responsibility'. There have, however, also been calls to enhance the status of the *Working Together* guidelines by giving them statutory force. These have come from the parental rights pressure group Parents Against Injustice (PAIN), which has argued that if local authorities are legally obliged to follow the *Working Together* guidelines, this will ensure that practice 'reflects the rhetoric of policy' (PAIN, 1992, p. 86).

Parental participation raises a range of practical considerations regarding anti-discriminatory practice: at the most obvious level, provision should be made for parents whose first language is not English, both in terms of written information before and after the conference, and interpretation during it (in this respect, it is salutary to note that after the first year of the Act, nearly half the local authorities in England did not have publicity about their services for children in need in any language other than English: DH, 1993, p. 42). Apart from these practical issues, parents of black children will need to be convinced that their own culture and views are being taken seriously in case conferences where the majority of the practitioners may well be white. Again, the challenge to SSDs is to ensure that the rhetoric of the

Children Act – of taking religion, race, language and culture into account – is achieved in practice.

In terms of discourse analysis, another example of the tensions between and within the legal and welfare discourses is that although the attendance of parents at conferences is required from both points of view, it also creates problems from both perspectives. From the legal side, if the local authority's solicitor attends the conference and hears the views of the parents, he/she will thereby be in a position to assess the evidence the parents may give in advance of the court proceedings, and will thus have gained an unfair and improper advantage. Equally, if the parents bring their own legal representative, there is a danger that the conference may be turned into a pre-trial rehearsal of the court hearing, rather than a meeting focused on how best to protect the child from harm (Thomson, 1992, p. 17). The 1991 guidance states that legal representation for the parents is not appropriate (DH, 1991c, p. 44), but many SSDs have formulated policies on parental participation which do make provision for them to bring their own solicitors. It has also been suggested that parental attendance may militate against the welfare aims of the conference, by inhibiting practitioners from a full discussion about the family, and that the risk of an emotional outburst or argument from the parents will also hinder the conference from achieving its purposes (again, Thomson, 1992, p. 17).

Research into parental participation suggests that the reality is not as problematic as often anticipated by practitioners. A pilot study in Lewisham in 1990, for example, found a 94 per cent response rate amongst professionals that the presence of the parents had not prevented them from sharing relevant information about the family; a 97 per cent rate that, in their opinion, it had not impeded the right decision on whether or not to place the child's name on the Child Protection Register; and a 63 per cent rate that it had actually been 'helpful' or 'very helpful' in enabling the conference to reach appropriate decisions (Shemmings, 1991, esp. pp. 31–50; see also Atherton, 1991, for a summary of research findings). Many SSDs have set up schemes to monitor parental participation, whilst the DH has also sponsored research to identify good models of participatory practice. Inspections by the SSI have also looked at the issue of parental participation in case conferences (such inspections can, of course, be understood as manifestations of, and vehicles for, greater central government control of social work). From a discourse perspective, one of the key issues in any future research will be how the legal and welfare imperatives in favour of parental participation balance with the specified aims of conferences and the legal and welfare responsibilities of the various agencies in attendance.

Interviews with children

The third development in child protection work is closely linked with the implementation of another major piece of legislation – the Criminal Justice Act 1991, which came into force on 1 October 1992. Among the main features of this Act are important changes to the law concerning children's evidence in criminal proceedings about cases of sexual abuse or violence. Children are no longer automatically assumed to be incompetent as witnesses, and the Act allows the court the discretion to receive the initial evidence from a child or young person in the form of a video-recording, rather than requiring him/her to repeat the allegations in the courtroom – although the witness must still be available for cross-examination during the hearing (s. 32A of the Criminal Justice Act 1988, as added by the 1991 Act). However, the cross-examination can be done by means of a live television link, so that the child does not have to be in the same room as the alleged perpetrator.

The *Memorandum of Good Practice on Video-Recorded Interviews with Child Witnesses for Criminal Proceedings* was published by the Home Office in conjunction with the Department of Health in May 1992, in preparation for the implementation of the new Act. It offers advice to social workers and police officers on the preparations required before an interview is carried out, the conduct of the interview itself, and the procedures to follow after it has been completed (Home Office, 1992).

The *Memorandum* is the latest development in a lengthy process of debate and experiments in working practices concerning the relationship between the police and social workers in the investigation of child sexual abuse, and the purposes and conduct of what are now called 'diagnostic' or 'assessment' interviews with children (see e.g. Metropolitan Police and Social Services Bexley, 1987; Home Office, 1989). The Cleveland Inquiry report had been critical of the way in which many interviews were conducted during the Cleveland crisis, referring to a frequent presumption that abuse had occurred, insufficient expertise, over-enthusiasm, and a lack of awareness from the interviewers of the extent of the pressure placed on the children during the interviews (Secretary of State for Social Services, 1988, p. 209). The root of such problems was seen to lie in confusion about the purposes of the interview – whether it was to ascertain the facts, or for therapeutic purposes, or for a mixture of both (Secretary of State for Social Services, 1988, p. 208). The 1992 *Memorandum* is emphatic on this point: 'The interviews described in this Memorandum are not and should never be referred to as 'therapeutic interviews'. Nor should the term 'disclosure interview' ever be used to describe them' (Home Office, 1992, p. 3; the term 'disclosure interview' is now seen as undesirable because it implies that there is actually something to 'disclose', thus precluding the possibility that abuse may not have taken place).

At first sight the introduction of video-recorded evidence appears to offer substantial advantages in terms of the welfare of the child, by reducing the stresses of lengthy or repeated court appearances. A closer study of the *Memorandum* from a discourse perspective, however, uncovers significant tensions between the requirements of welfare and law (and also – from the managerial perspective – exposes the *Memorandum* as yet another attempt to prescribe and control the activities of social workers, in keeping with the nine volumes of 'Guidance and Regulations' on the Children Act). The *Memorandum* offers detailed advice on the structure of the interview and on complying with the rules of evidence (e.g. avoiding the use of 'leading questions', hearsay, and references to the bad character of the accused: Home Office, 1992, pp. 26–32). Its aim is to ensure that the interview produces acceptable evidence for use in court, and its whole orientation is to satisfy the legal criteria to achieve this. There is, however, a danger that the welfare of the child will be lost in the search for sound evidence on which to base legal proceedings, which becomes apparent in three respects.

First, the *Memorandum* gives social workers a major role alongside the police in the gathering of evidence for criminal proceedings; counselling and therapy take second place to this investigative responsibility (Home Office, 1992, pp. 2, 23). Second, the expectation in the *Memorandum* is that it should be possible to gather this evidence in a single one-hour interview (Home Office, 1992, pp. 12, 13); it does not regard the child's telling about abuse as part of a long-term process in which the worker and the child gradually and carefully build up their relationship. Thirdly, the *Memorandum*'s strong arguments against the use of leading questions do not recognise that the child may need help to recount what has happened to him/her. The Cleveland report acknowledged that techniques to help the child to tell might be appropriate in certain circumstances, even though these might undermine the evidential value of the interview; nevertheless, they could be the only way to get to the truth of the matter and thereby protect the child from further harm (Secretary of State for Social Services, 1988, pp. 206, 208). The *Memorandum*, with its sights firmly set on securing legally sound evidence, makes no such concession.

The preliminary findings of research into the implementation of the *Memorandum* reveal some significant problems (see Davies *et al.*, 1993). One example is that there have been very great differences across the country in the number of video-recorded interviews carried out by different local authorities/police forces. During the first year of the Criminal Justice Act 1991 approximately 14,000 interviews were conducted under the *Memorandum*, but some forces made over 1,000 whilst others made none at all (Davies *et al.*, 1993, p. 4). This discrepancy has largely been attributed to difficulties in funding the necessary interview facilities, technical equipment and specialist training for staff. It is not all attributable to resource shortages, however, and other factors include the history of joint police/social work investigations in the area concerned, and the present state of relations between the two organisations.

Another important issue concerns the number of video-recordings which have actually been shown in court. Although video-recorded interviews are now becoming a regular part of social work investigations into suspected abuse, very few of them end up being used as evidence in criminal proceedings. During 1993 there were only 299 applications to show video recordings in the Crown court, and eventually only 109 were played (source: Lord Chancellor's Department). Judges may refuse to allow a video to be shown if they are of the opinion 'having regard to all the circumstances of the case, that in the interests of justice the recording ought not to be admitted' (Criminal Justice Act, 1991, s. 32A). Reasons could include failure to observe the rules of evidence, or poor technical quality (although it should be noted that some videos may not be shown, even after an application has been made, because of a late guilty plea from the defendant). Further research is needed into the reasons why such a small proportion of recordings is ultimately used in criminal trials, but the early figures cast doubt on whether the *Memorandum*'s single-minded focus on producing evidentially valid recordings for legal proceedings is even a realistic goal, as well as whether it best serves the welfare of children.

CHILDREN'S RIGHTS

We have seen that a central feature of the Children Act is the attempt to strike a 'balance' between the duties and powers of social workers, the responsibilities of parents and the needs and welfare of the child. The underlying tensions behind these balances are apparent in much of the day-to-day work of social workers. In identifying the discourses of law, welfare, the market economy and managerialism we have presented a framework for understanding how the role of social work, in child welfare in general and child protection in particular, is being redefined by political, professional and social forces. In this section we

91

use the framework to discuss a further important aspect of current social work practice – the discourse of children's rights and its relevance to the principles of the Children Act.

Social work has traditionally been concerned with ensuring that children in need receive the basic care and welfare necessary for their development. For this reason, children's rights from a social work perspective have been interpreted within the terms of the welfare discourse; that is to say, in terms of their needs and the right to have these needs met. For example, the United Nation's Convention on the Rights of the Child, which the UK ratified in 1991, includes the right of children to protection from abuse, neglect and exploitation. The NSPCC has also adopted a child protection agenda where the rights of children are defined in broad terms of their needs, and in general most organisations which are concerned with children's welfare tend to think about children's rights in terms of vulnerability in relation to adults.

There is, however, another dimension to children's rights. Children's rights are increasingly being defined in legal terms, where the child is seen not just as being in need of protection, but as an individual with the right to legal representation and to having a say in decisions which affect their welfare. From this perspective, children are seen as being able to make choices, take decisions, and exercise responsibilities, and if their right to do so leads to conflict with their parents or other adults, then the courts are the arbiters who decide the issue. However, there are problems with the trend to define children's rights in legal terms – for example, it is argued that the complexities of social relations, particularly in institutions such as the family where conflicts exist alongside strong emotional attachments and moral obligations, are not reducible to legal decisions of right and wrong or transgressor and transgressed (King and Piper, 1990; King and Trowell, 1991). Additionally the enforcement of rights inevitably involves empowerment, and the question of how much power it is possible for children to have in order to control their lives has profound moral and political implications – for instance the possible effects of enhanced children's rights on the future of the family and parent–child relationships.

The contrast between an adult-defined needs-based approach to children's rights, and a child-defined choice-based approach are aspects of the tensions between the welfare and legal discourses. The legal children's rights perspective places an emphasis on the child as an independent and competent individual, capable of exercising judgement. Taken to its extreme, this position rejects the notion of childhood as a developmental process in favour of a theory which sees children as oppressed by adult control and therefore in need of rights to overcome that oppression. A welfare perspective sees children as essentially dependent and vulnerable beings who benefit from the protection and guidance of adults. An extension of this position could see the period of protection as continuing well beyond the commonly accepted legal age of adulthood. Whilst there are advocates for the extremes of both these positions, most would agree that the ideal lies somewhere in between – although where this middle-ground is to be found is far from clear.

Early social work education and training did place an emphasis on obtaining children's wishes when planning for their future, but with the increasing focus on child protection and the bureaucratisation of social work agencies in the 1980s, the basis for intervention became more explicitly needs-led. Where account was taken of children's wishes and feelings concerning their future, corresponding action was all too often lacking, despite some persistent efforts by social workers to advocate on behalf of the children, particularly where adolescents were concerned. The Children Act seeks to rectify this omission and explicitly states that children's wishes and feelings should be taken into account in decisions which affect their lives. This has had the effect of reintroducing the issue of children's rights, even though the term 'rights' in relation to children, or for that matter families and state agencies, is deliberately omitted in the Act itself (e.g. the replacement of 'parental rights and duties' by 'parental responsibilities'). The Act stresses that the welfare of the child is to be the court's 'paramount consideration', but this is with regard to 'the ascertainable wishes and feelings of the child' (Sec. 1(3)). In spite of the Act not referring to the wishes and feelings of the child as rights, the emphasis is clear – for the first time there is an acknowledgement of the wishes of children as a central feature of child-care legislation and this has prompted new debates about children's rights in social work practice and the courts. We use four examples to illustrate some of the issues which underlie these debates.

First, a child's right to make choices is limited by the range of choice available, which may be seen as a reflection of how social work practice is shaped by the market economy discourse. Social workers who are seeking to accommodate a child may well find that the wishes of the child do not accord with the resources available – for example, the wish of a child to be placed in a foster home in a particular locality may not be practicable. In the past, resource-led decisions which have ignored the wishes of the child may have gone no further than records in case notes, but there is now some evidence to suggest that the child-centred principles of the Act are beginning to produce results that go beyond the tokenism which was so often a feature of the past. An example is a decision by councillors in Leeds to close a children's home in 1992 which was postponed by the action of the young people who lived in the home. The children successfully argued that they had not been adequately consulted and that their views had not been taken into account. The decision to close the home therefore contravened the Children Act's requirement to seek the views of children before taking decisions about their future. The children's right to be consulted on a matter which concerned resources exemplifies the tension between the welfare principles of the Children Act to provide better services (which therefore require adequate resources) and the government's continuing attempts to curb local authority spending (the market economy discourse) (*Community Care*, 21 November 1992, p. 3).

Second, the wishes of a child may not always coincide with legal powers and entitlements. A child who wishes to stay with an abusing parent, as some children do, may find that this is not possible if an Order is obtained to remove him/her from the home. A 14-year-old who wishes to work full time instead of going to school cannot exercise this 'right'. The way in which the law limits children's rights to make choices illustrates the distinctions society makes between children and adults, although many of these distinctions appear arbitrary and contradictory the nearer adolescents are to adulthood. Evidence of the confusion which abounds on issues concerning children's rights and the law was highlighted in early 1993 by a public outcry over how to treat persistent juvenile offenders, particularly so-called 'joy-riders'. This outcry led to proposals for the reintroduction of custodial sentences for under-14-year-olds, although strongly criticised by many of the organisations involved in working with young offenders. Underlying this debate are the wider moral and social questions of what age and under what circumstances children should be treated as adults.

Third, a child's choice in a matter may have directly harmful consequences. Where this is the case, parents, social workers and the courts are reluctant to allow them to carry out their choices. This was highlighted in the summer of 1992 by the case of a 16-year-old girl who was in the care of a local authority. She was suffering severely from anorexia nervosa, and the authority wanted to move her to a hospital for specialised treatement. The young woman refused to go, and the authority applied to the court for authorisation to place her in the hospital, and for her to be given medical treatment without her consent if necessary. In the first instance, an Order was made in those terms, but the young woman appealed. The matter was settled in the Court of Appeal by the drawing of two important distinctions – first, between the giving of consent to treatment and the refusal of consent, and second, between the powers of people with parental responsibility and the powers of the court. It was held that consent to treatment from any 16 or 17-year-old, or from a younger child who is deemed to be of sufficient intelligence and understanding to make an informed decision, could not be overridden by anyone with parental responsibility, but could be by the court. A refusal to give consent, on the other hand, can be overridden by consent from someone who has parental responsibility, as well as by the court (Re W (a minor) (refusal of medical treatment) (1992) All ER 627; 10 July 1992). This decision appears to undermine the Children Act's emphasis on the wishes of children, particularly their right to refuse medical examinations or assessments under Emergency Protection Orders or interim Care Orders (s.44(1) and s.38(6)). The court got round this problem by distinguishing between 'assessment' and 'treatment', arguing that the provisions of the Children Act applied only to the former.

The dilemma of upholding children's rights which may have harmful consequences is not only one which is dealt with by the courts. A child whose 'right' to choose is overridden by adults often ends up in conflict with parents and adult authority, whilst many parents are faced with the difficulty of relaxing their controls in the knowledge that their child may be exposed to potential dangers. These dilemmas are acutely felt by social workers who work with adolescents in local authority homes. The local authority is responsible for children in their care, but allowing them to carry out their own choices – to exercise their rights – could result in danger to the child, whilst refusing them their choices is itself likely to provoke a potentially harmful reaction.

Finally, children do not necessarily have the capacity to exercise the responsibilities that follow from their choices. Acquiring the knowledge and social skills which are needed for responsible actions is a gradual process which is closely linked with chronological age, and not all children have the capabilities to foresee the consequences of their choices. From a welfare perspective, it is therefore necessary for adults to make some judgement concerning the child's ability to make decisions and to cope with all the consequences, intended or otherwise, that will follow.

Evidence about the extent to which children are now able to make their voices heard in social work decision-making is far from clear. The Children Act required local authorities to set up complaints and representation procedures for parents and children, but the DH report on the first year of the Act shows that there had been only 542 complaints from children in England by the end of June 1992. In some local authorities there had been none at all (DH, 1993, p. 44). The questions raised here are whether children in care have not made formal complaints because they fear doing so would only make matters worse; or because they fear the complaint would have no effect; or because they are not aware of their rights to do so; or because their grievances are resolved informally, before the formal complaint stage.

Since the introduction of the Children Act, media attention has been captivated by the possible social changes in adult–child relationships which may result from the developing legal children's rights perspective. At the heart of the matter is whether society is ready to accept the empowerment of children and its consequences. As with many social issues, it is the media which plays a large part in defining and influencing social problems. For example, there has recently been an element of moral panic concerning the choices of several children to live apart from their parents. The term 'child divorce' has been adopted with its connotations of the erosion of family values and the disempowerment of parents, in spite of the fact that 'parental responsibility' towards children is a central feature of the Act. Social workers are finding that these elements of children's rights are introducing new roles to their work, such as advising children how to seek legal representation on their own behalf where there are no grounds for the local authority to institute proceedings. The confusions about children's rights are exemplified in two comments from the Minister of Health Virginia Bottomley, both reported in the social work journal *Community Care*. In the first, talking about children's rights to initiate court action on their own behalf, she expressed the view that 'the status of children has changed from being passive victims or recipients of service, to people with rights as individuals, the right to be heard, believed and trusted' (*Community Care*, 12 November 1992). The context of the second comment was the media and political debate about the treatment of persistent young offenders; on this occasion, Virginia Bottomley said 'there is concern among the wider public that we may have gone too far in stressing the rights of children at the expense of upholding the responsibilities of parents and professionals in supervising them' (*Community Care*, 11 March 1993).

CONCLUSION

In this chapter we have highlighted some of the major changes in social work practice in the fields of child protection and children's rights. These changes are the outcomes and reflections of wider debates about the proper basis and manner of state activity in relation to family life – about the balance between state and parental responsibilities, social workers' powers and family autonomy.

If it was ever intended that the Children Act should produce any solutions to these dilemmas, this has clearly not been achieved. The fields of child care, child protection and children's rights are and will always remain contentious, because the issues involved are political and moral as well as legal.

The longer-term outcome of the changes to social work remains to be seen, but the indications are that the welfare dimension is in danger of being lost to the demands of other discourses – notably law, the market economy and managerialism. We doubt whether social work will be adequately able to protect children, let alone actively promote their best interests, if welfare ceases to be the defining element.

PART II

Adult Abuse

CHAPTER FOUR

Domestic Violence: An Overview

Norman Johnson

INTRODUCTION

When the title of this chapter was being considered, there were several terms that might have been used to describe violence against women by their partners or ex-partners. The truth is that there are no entirely satisfactory terms: each has its own dangers and shortcomings. 'Marital violence' and 'spouse abuse', for example, presume that the partners are married, and fail to recognise that violence between partners is overwhelmingly male violence against women. The term 'battered women' identifies the victim accurately, but appears to restrict the violence to physical assault, and is ambiguous in that it gives no indication that the violence occurs within the context of private relationships. 'Battered wives' avoids this confusion, but has the added disadvantage of excluding unmarried couples. Pahl (1985) points to the significance of the use of the term 'battered wives' rather than 'violent husbands': the effect is to shift the focus from the perpetrators to their victims. The term 'domestic dispute' is far too weak since disputes do not necessarily involve violence.

The term chosen for this chapter is 'domestic violence' which, as Smith (1989, p. 1) indicates, 'helps to emphasise – in a way that the terms "abuse" and "disputes" do not – that what is being examined is violence, not arguments or minor altercations, but violence'. It does not clearly identify, however, who is the victim and who the perpetrator.

The main reasons for settling on 'domestic violence' are largely pragmatic. This is the term used by government departments, notably the Home Office, and by the House of Commons Home Affairs Committee. Some of the relevant legislation also uses the term. Lastly, the major voluntary organisations working in this field – for example,

Women's Aid Federation (England), the corresponding organisations in Northern Ireland, Scotland and Wales, and Victim Support – find the term acceptable.

THE POLITICS OF DOMESTIC VIOLENCE

Politics is about power, but power itself takes many forms ranging from force and coercion at one end of the spectrum to persuasion and authority at the other. Between the two extremes are inducement and manipulation.

Force and coercion imply the imposition of sanctions or the threat of their imposition. At the macro level, states frequently use violence to achieve their ends and, for a while at least, whole populations may be intimidated. However, the power of the state is not necessarily expressed through the use or threat of naked force. It also has the capacity to control information and to determine the political agenda.

This has direct relevance for domestic violence. As Dobash and Dobash (1980, p. 2) observe:

'In 1971, almost no one had heard of battered women, except, of course, the legions of women who were being battered and the relatives, friends, ministers, social workers, doctors and lawyers in whom some of them confided. Many people did not believe that such behaviour actually existed, and even most of those who were aware of it did not think that it affected sufficient numbers of women or was of sufficient severity to warrant wide-scale concern.'

The comparative 'invisibility' of domestic violence can be explained in part, perhaps in large part, by a patriarchal state controlled by men. For a variety of reasons, domestic violence was kept off the political agenda until the 1970s.

Patriarchy has been a prominent feature of feminist writing since the late 1960s. One of the earliest, and still one of the most compelling, discourses on patriarchy is that by Millett (1969) who claims that relationships between the sexes are characterised by 'dominance and subordinance' in which 'males rule females' (p. 25). Millett argues that

'This system ... tends to be sturdier than any form of segregation, and more rigorous than class stratification, more uniform, certainly more enduring. However muted its present appearance may be, sexual dominion obtains nevertheless as perhaps the most pervasive ideology of our culture and provides its most fundamental concept of power.'

(p. 25)

Millett maintains that patriarchy is sustained by both ideological and structural factors. The ideological support stems from a system of socialisation which conditions both men and women to accept male domination as 'natural'. Women are socialised into adopting compliant, submissive and passive roles and accepting their essentially subordinate position. Structural constraints reinforce this order. Millett identifies the family, the class system and the economic and educational systems as the main structural bulwarks of patriarchy.

Dobash and Dobash (1980) also emphasise the central importance of the ideology and structures of patriarchy in creating and maintaining women's subordinate position:

> 'One of the means by which this order is supported and reinforced has been to insure that women have no legitimate means of changing or managing the institutions that define and maintain their subordination. Confining women in the home, banning them from meaningful positions outside the family, and excluding them from the bench and the pulpit is to deny them the means of bringing about change in their status.'

(p. 43)

But if, as Millett (1969, p. 25) claims, government is patriarchal and serves the interests of men, how do feminist issues such as domestic violence get on to the political agenda? How are governments convinced that a social problem exists and that it is significant enough to warrant some official response? The answer lies in the process by which social problems come to be identified and defined.

The process by which an undesirable condition is converted into a social problem or, to use the terminology of Mills (1970), the process by which an individual trouble becomes a public issue, is a complex one. Spector and Kitsuse (1977) argue persuasively that the identification of social problems should concentrate on the process of definition rather than on the adverse conditions themselves:

> 'Our definition of social problems focuses on the process by which members of a society define a putative condition as a social problem. Thus we define social problems as the activities of individuals or groups making assertions of grievances and claims with respect to some putative conditions.'

(p.75)

One of the advantages of this definition is that it directs our attention to the essentially political nature of social problems. As Tallman (1976,

p. 18) says: 'a social problem is a social condition that has been politicised'.

In the 1970s domestic violence became a political issue. The beginning of the battered-women's movement in Britain is well known. In the words of Dobash and Dobash (1992, p. 25): 'It emerged in a rather unexpected manner, beginning with a campaign to protest against the elimination of free school milk and ending with a refuge for battered women.' The moving spirit behind the campaign was the charismatic Erin Pizzey. In the course of the campaign Erin Pizzey and her associates came into contact with many young mothers whose main complaint was isolation and loneliness. To combat this problem a plan was formed to set up a community centre for women and their children, and eventually a small condemned house was obtained for this purpose from Hounslow Borough Council. In 1972 the house was opened under the title of Chiswick Women's Aid.

Very soon the group found itself dealing with the problems of women who had suffered violence at the hands of their male partners, so that the house in Chiswick came to be used as a refuge. The work they were doing for battered women received a great deal of publicity in the press, on radio and on television. A book written by Erin Pizzey (1974) was given extensive media coverage.

This publicity served both to make the Chiswick group well known and to bring the problem of domestic violence to the attention of a much wider public. A legal battle with Hounslow Borough Council about over-occupation of the refuge, which went as far as the House of Lords, further increased public interest. In the midst of this legal wrangle, the Chiswick women occupied the Palm Court Hotel in Richmond.

Some of the members of Chiswick Women's Aid travelled round the country giving talks and encouraging the establishment of local Women's Aid groups. The first national conference was held in 1974 and in 1975 a national organisation, the National Women's Aid Federation, was set up. The second conference in 1975 was the occasion for a split in the Women's Aid movement. Such splits, not uncommon in relatively new social movements, are an amalgam of personality clashes, a struggle for power and disagreements over matters of principle. Spector and Kitsuse (1977, p. 8) say that disputes arise out of the competition between groups 'for control of the definition of a problem'. The split in Women's Aid shared the main characteristics of other disputes of this kind. Dobash and Dobash (1980, p. 224) say that 'the contentious issues leading to the split involved differences in philosophy, organizing principles, leadership styles, and the definition of the problem of battered women'. The dispute was between Erin Pizzey and her supporters, and the remainder of Women's Aid. Part of the explanation was undoubtedly Erin Pizzey's fears that her hitherto undisputed leadership of the Women's Aid movement was being threatened. She was also uncomfortable with the egalitarian and democratic principles which her opponents so passionately espoused, and she rejected the link with Women's Liberation and with other elements of the Women's Movement. The Chiswick group and one or two other groups withdrew from the National Federation.

The consequence of this split was that the national influence of Chiswick Women's Aid sharply declined and the National Women's Aid Federation emerged as the leading organisation in this field. Initially, the National Federation covered the whole of the United Kingdom, but in the 1970s each of the individual countries established their own organisations so that we now have: Northern Ireland Women's Aid, Scottish Women's Aid, Welsh Women's Aid and Women's Aid Federation England (Home Affairs Committee, 1992, p. 76).

One of the objectives of any social movement or pressure group must be to force their concerns on to the political agenda and keep them there. To achieve this, groups have to try to convince those who take decisions that a problem exists and that solutions must be sought and they must try to influence public opinion generally. As Tallman (1976, p. 33) explains in a general discussion of social problems, groups 'must make the problem visible and seek to create an aura of moral concern'.

The Women's Aid Movement has been undoubtedly successful in bringing the problem of domestic violence to government and public attention. The official attention may be gauged by the number of reports and statements issued by parliamentary, government and quasi-government agencies. Among the earliest publications was the influential Select Committee Report on Violence in Marriage (Select Committee, 1975). During the late 1970s and early 1980s the Department of Health and Social Security funded a number of research projects and made attempts to bring researchers together. More recently, there has been an inter-departmental ministerial group on Women's issues (1989–92), a Home Office study (Smith, 1989), and reports from the Law Commission (1992) and the House of Commons Home Affairs Committee (Home Affairs Committee 1992). The Law Commission, the Lord Chancellor's Department and the Home Office all presented evidence to the Home Affairs Committee.

It would not be true to say that all of this activity is attributable to Women's Aid pressure, but a good measure of it is. Women's Aid has campaigned tirelessly, making skilful use of the media, organising marches and rallies, lobbying and negotiating and conducting research. What is remarkable about this is that Women's Aid has combined vigorous campaigning with direct service provision. It is all too easy, as Schechter (1982) observes, to be diverted from social change to service provision. That political authorities and human-service professionals sometimes encourage and welcome such a change of focus is demonstrated by Morgan (1985, p. 66) who writes:

> 'Refuges, formerly run by small collectives of feminist activists, often with a strong community base, were replaced by larger 'service' centers administered by boards of directors and staffed by professionals ... Where once the impact of gender domination was raised as a way of understanding violent abuse of women, now the focus is on individual pathology ... and the psychological profile of the victim.'

Morgan is writing about the United States, where the threatened domination of professionals has proceeded further than it has in Britain. Even in Britain, however, the power of those employed in the helping professions is considerable (Hugman, 1991; Witz, 1992), and professional redefinition of the problem of domestic violence has to be resisted. In this context, Dobash and Dobash (1992, p. 47) make a useful distinction between 'visionary' or 'activist' professionals and 'occupational' professionals. The difference between these two types of professionals is that whereas 'the former seek meaningful change in society using their field of work, the latter simply seek work.'

One of the reasons for the success of Women's Aid in keeping domestic violence on the political agenda, and at the same time avoiding domination by professionals, is their close association with the wider women's movement. Maynard (1993, pp. 99–100) emphasises this link:

> 'The higher profile afforded to the issue of male violence against women in recent years is almost entirely due to the political practice of activists in the women's liberation movement and feminist research deriving from this. ... As feminism developed momentum in the late 1960s and early 1970s, the significance of violence in women's lives started to emerge.'

Finkelhor (1988) argues that much less research would have been done into violence against women and child abuse, and much less attention would have been paid to it, had there not been expanding child welfare and women's movements. Feminist writers in the nineteenth century

106

(Cobbe, 1878) addressed the issue of domestic violence as did the early suffragettes (McLaren, 1909). As feminists began to direct their energies more and more towards suffrage, the problem of violence was given less attention. It did not again surface as a public issue until the resurgence of the women's movement in the late 1960s.

There are, of course, different forms of feminism and not all of them have demonstrated a concern with domestic violence and a willingness to take political action to oppose it. For example, libertarian feminists of the new right emphasise liberty through the market and have nothing to contribute to the debate about male violence, and liberal feminists are largely concerned with equal opportunities. It has been radical and socialist feminists and, more recently, black feminists who have taken the lead in highlighting violence as an issue of central importance to the women's movement. Radical, socialist and black feminists accept the feminist dictum that 'the personal is political', and they are agreed on the importance of power and oppression to an understanding of violence against women. There are inequalities of power between men and women generally, but these inequalities are compounded when women are members of other groups who experience discrimination – especially poor people and ethnic minorities.

The empowerment of women has always been an explicit aim of the women's movement; and Women's Aid attaches particular importance to it because battered women are very often powerless. From the beginning, therefore, Women's Aid espoused the principle of self-help on the grounds that 'for women to involve themselves in providing a solution to their plight and to take control of their own lives is a fundamental reversal of their previous situation – powerlessness in the face of male violence' (Clifton, 1985, p. 43). In their evidence to the House of Commons Home Affairs Committee, Women's Aid Federation (England) stated that all agency responses to domestic violence 'should be enabling and empowering to women, and should be based on the principle of listening to and respecting women's choices' (p. 93).

RECIPIENTS AND PERPETRATORS OF VIOLENCE

In the previous section prominence was given to the role of Women's Aid and to the women's movement generally. The only reference to men was as aggressors. This bias is defensible on two grounds: (i) the politics of domestic violence has been dominated by Women's Aid who have managed to influence, if not set, the political agenda; (ii) the balance of evidence strongly suggests, as we shall see, that most domestic violence consists of the abuse of women by their male partners or ex-partners.

A heated debate about the gender division among the perpetrators of domestic violence was sparked off by two publications by Steinmetz in 1977 and 1978 (Pagelow, 1985). She wrote of a 'battered husband syndrome' and claimed that 250,000 American husbands were battered by their wives each year. Straus, Gelles and Steinmetz (1980), in a study of 2,143 married couples, concluded that wives were only slightly less likely to use violence against their husbands than the other way around. Shortly after the completion of the initial study, Straus (1980b) reworked the data looking at *severe* attacks only. This new analysis showed that severe assaults by husbands on non-violent wives outnumbered by three to one severe assaults by wives on non-violent husbands. This suggests that violence by wives is often defensive rather than offensive, and Staus believed that wives resorted to violence when they themselves had suffered repeated attacks over a considerable period. When Straus and Gelles (1986) replicated the earlier study, they obtained similar results: wives and husbands were almost equal in their use of violence, but this needed to be qualified by distinguishing between defensive or retaliatory violence and offensive violence.

Two memoranda of evidence submitted to the House of Commons Home Affairs Committee (Home Affairs Committee, 1992) suggest that violence by women on their male partners is greater than is commonly appreciated. The argument in both pieces (one from the organisation, Families Need Fathers, and the other from George, a physiologist at Queen Mary and Westfield College) is that male victims have difficulty in talking about their situation and that the problem is ignored by the media and most helping agencies.

There can be no doubt that some men are treated violently by female partners and that the problem is under-reported, but the evidence is insufficient to substantiate claims that female-instigated violence is as extensive as violence by men upon women. Most of the research into female violence has concentrated on physical violence, but sexual violence would present a very different picture in which men would emerge as almost the sole perpetrators. In relation to physical violence, it may be pointed out that men are more muscular than women, and that their greater economic independence makes it easier for them to avoid violence by simply leaving.

I am in agreement with Smith (1989, p. 15) when she states that 'with the exception of the work of Straus *et al.* (1980) most research testifies to the fact that in the overwhelming majority of cases, domestic violence is perpetrated by men against women'. This holds true across the United Kingdom in different cultural and ethnic groups. Mama (1989, p. xiii), in the first major study – and at the time of writing the *only* major study – of violence against black women in the home, writes:

'While black women as well as black men are subjected to the physical violence and abuse of race attacks and coercive inner-city policing, black women are also expected to show sympathy and understanding when the men that live with them also turn violent. The prevalence of violence against women in black communities illustrates the full meaning of triple oppression along the dimensions of race, class and gender.'

Mama, in this quotation, raises the issue of social class, but points out that the men who were violent to the women in her study 'came from all socio-economic classes'. There has been some discussion about the relationship between domestic violence and social class. Some studies, for example Gelles and Cornell (1985), have reported a greater prevalence of domestic violence among working-class couples. However, there is much stronger evidence suggesting that domestic violence is not the preserve of any one social class (Martin, 1976; Walker, 1978; Dobash and Dobash, 1980; Pagelow, 1981; Andrews, 1987).

In some of the research, working-class couples would be in the majority simply because of the sample used. If, for example, studies draw their sample from the women in refuges or from police or welfare records, then working-class families are bound to be over-represented. The lower socio-economic groups are more visible and the areas in which they live have a greater police presence. Furthermore, as Smith (1989, p. 15) points out: 'It may be ... that middle class families are less willing to admit its (domestic violence) occurrence, are less willing to draw outsiders' attention to problems they experience and make more use of private medical care and other resources.'

Research into domestic violence and effective responses to it have been hampered by the lack of reliable statistical data. In its memorandum to the Home Affairs Committee the Domestic Violence Intervention Project notes that 'hard data on the extent and incidence of domestic assaults are in short supply. None of the available figures are reliable, and they cannot be regarded as anything other than very rough estimates.' We are little nearer to having an accurate picture than we were in 1975 when the Select Committee on Violence in Marriage concluded: 'Despite our efforts, we are unable to give any estimates of what the likely numbers are; several witnesses talked in terms of the tip of the iceberg, and this seems to us to be correct.' All researchers are agreed that even if a composite figure, using a variety of sources, is produced, it is likely to seriously underestimate the size of the problem. The main reason for this is that domestic violence, by its very nature, takes place in the privacy of the home and most of it is not reported to anyone at all. Even when incidents are reported, they frequently go unrecorded or they are recorded in such a way that they cannot be separately identified. In *Criminal Statistics,* for example, domestic assaults are categorised together with assaults in general. Prospects for changing this practice are slight: an attempt in 1979 to introduce new categories for domestic violence was abandoned in the following year, and in its evidence to the Home Affairs Committee (1992, p. 3) the Home Office says: 'The introduction of a new system would have to be considered carefully with the police and its potential usefulness weighed against the additional costs of collection.'

Police statistics are flawed by the practice, now gradually being abandoned, of 'no-criming' what they have traditionally described as 'domestic disputes' (Edwards, 1989; Bourlet, 1990).

Judicial Statistics, published by the Lord Chancellor's Department, include injunctions granted under the Domestic Violence and Matrimonial Proceedings Act, 1976, but injunctions obtained in matrimonial proceedings are not included, unless they have powers of arrest attached, and injunctions made within a tort action for damages for assault or trespass are similarly excluded. The number of orders made under the Domestic Proceedings and Magistrates' Courts Act are published in *Statistics of Domestic Proceedings in Magistrates' Courts.*

Figures derived from divorce proceedings have some, but limited, value. The most common ground for divorce is 'unreasonable behaviour' which obviously includes violence. Parker (1985) states that in 1980 one-third of all petitions for divorce were on grounds of unreasonable behaviour and women were the petitioners in 89 per cent of these cases. Parker contends that the majority of cases included allegations of violence.

I have deliberately avoided giving figures derived from each of these sources. They are so beset with problems; there are huge gaps, and so many qualifications have to be made that any calculation based on them is bound to be misleading. A good treatment of the problems in measuring the extent of domestic violence is to be found in Smith (1989) who concludes: 'The individual and collective problems posed by the various sources of information mean that there is simply no reliable estimate of the extent of domestic violence.' The problem of non-reporting may mean that it will never be possible to have a wholly accurate picture of the prevalence of domestic violence, but the situation could be improved by more helpful and more accessible official statistics.

THE NATURE AND EFFECTS OF DOMESTIC VIOLENCE

Domestic violence may take many forms. The main categories are usually identified as physical, sexual, and emotional or psychological; but this classification is fairly crude and there are endless variations within each category. Women's Aid Federation (England) (Home Affairs Committee, 1992, p. 97) says:

> 'Violence can mean, among other things: threats, intimidation, ma-nipulation, isolation, keeping a woman without money, locked in, deprived of food, or using (and abusing) her children in various ways to frighten her or enforce compliance. It can also include systematic criticism and belittling comments.'

The different forms of violence are closely interlinked in two senses:

1. repeated physical or sexual assaults are certain to have emotional and psychological consequences, and psychological violence results in physiological deterioration;
2. it is unusual for any one form of violence to occur singly.

Most of the publications on domestic violence include horrifying descriptions of particular episodes, very often based on the victims' own accounts (Dobash and Dobash, 1980, 1984; Pagelow, 1981; Kelly, 1988; Mama, 1989; Hoff, 1990; Victim Support, 1992). There would be little point in repeating these descriptions here, but some idea of the seriousness of the offences must be given. The first characteristic is that the violence we are talking about is never restricted to a single incident and it becomes more frequent and more severe over time (Gelles, 1974; Carlson, 1977; Dobash and Dobash, 1984; Pahl, 1985). The violence may continue over many years. In a study of 656 women living in refuges, Binney, Harkell and Nixon (1981) found that some of the women had been abused for thirty and even forty years, the average being seven years.

The physical violence may include slapping, punching, kicking, choking, butting, biting, burning, pulling hair, pushing down stairs and the frequent use of weapons of one sort or another. According to Gayford (1978), Pagelow (1981) and Andrews (1987), physical violence, especially punches in the abdomen, are more common during pregnancy. Many studies have identified sexual violence as a recurrent

111

aspect of violent relationships: rape, involving both vaginal and anal penetration, is reported frequently (Russell, 1982; Bowker, 1983; Frieze, 1983; Wilson, 1983; Walker, 1985). Often rape is accompanied by a beating, and verbal abuse is constantly present.

Dobash and Dobash (1980, 1984) have analysed what they call the violent event, starting with the antecedents and finishing with the aftermath. Two-thirds of all incidents were preceded by an argument, half of them lasting five minutes or less. The men concerned sometimes deliberately provoked arguments as an excuse for violence. The specific causes of arguments, some of which might appear trivial to an outsider, formed part of a long-standing pattern of underlying resentment. Dobash and Dobash (1980 pp. 101–2) argue that the immediate antecedents of a violent episode

'can be understood only in the context of the authority hierarchy and wider expectations of men and women living in violent relationships. One can sustain the contention that these altercations are trivial only if one examines and considers just their superficial appearance. The specific factor or factors preceding the violence may seem insignificant and the violent response totally unrelated to the context in which it occurs when the confrontations are analyzed without due consideration of the ongoing relationship.'

Sexual jealousy was the most common cause of a violent episode, followed by confrontations about money and complaints about the woman's housekeeping, meal preparation and child care.

The effects of repeated and prolonged violence on the women can be divided into the physical and the psychological. The physical effects are serious injury, sometimes permanent, and a great deal of pain. A more general deterioration in physical health is almost certain.

The psychological effects include high rates of anxiety and depression. Women live in constant fear. They know that when their partner returns from his night out at the pub they will be beaten or raped and possibly both. Almost as bad as the certainty of a beating is uncertainty and unpredictability: not knowing when the next attack will take place or which of their actions will be used as an excuse for it. Women have to be constantly on their guard about what they say and what they do, in the knowledge that whatever they do appears to be wrong.

Isolation, lack of personal contacts with friends and family, creates further stress. Very often the isolation is imposed by the partner who may even confiscate or destroy the woman's clothes. Her trips to the shops are strictly timed and she is forcibly restrained, by threats or worse, from seeking help or even medical treatment. Sometimes the isolation is self-imposed because of shame and an unwillingness to reveal what is happening.

Violence and constant criticism lead to a loss of self-esteem and confidence. If a woman is constantly told that she is worthless, she may come to believe it and begin to blame herself for the situation she is in. Paradoxically, the abused woman may feel guilty. This is partly a consequence of the unfair responsibility often placed upon women in a marriage or partnership for its emotional health and stability.

Suicide or attempted suicide or at least thoughts of suicide are referred to in a number of studies (Gayford, 1978; Stanko, 1985; Hoff, 1990). Hoff (1990, p. 49) in her detailed study of nine abused women says: 'The most extreme manifestation of the women's self-blame, recrimination and internalizing the conflict is their tendency to self-destructiveness ... all nine women had self-destructive tendencies at varying levels of dangerousness.' When asked what kept them from killing themselves, three of the women referred to their children.

The presence of children in a violent relationship creates additional stress for a woman, who may fear for their safety, but what of the effects on the children themselves? The Women's Aid Federation (England) (Home Affairs Committee, 1992, p. 99) have this to say about the effects upon children:

'From our work in refuges we have identified a number of difficulties which children who have survived domestic violence may experience. This has been backed up by research undertaken in Canada by Peter Jaffe and his colleagues (Jaffe et al., 1991). Effects may include: stress related illnesses, confused and torn loyalties ..., lack of trust, unnaturally good behaviour, taking on the mother role, an acceptance of abuse as 'normal', guilt, isolation, shame, anger, lack of confidence, fear of a repeat or a return to violence, and so on.'

The work by Jaffe et al. confirms earlier findings by the same team of researchers (Wolfe et al., 1985; Jaffe et al., 1986). There is a relationship, too, between domestic violence and child abuse. Gayford (1975) found that over one-half of the men who used violence against their wives also abused their children. This is confirmed by Stark and Flitcraft (1985) who argue that violence against women is the major precipitating context of child abuse. Children whose mothers are 'battered' are more than twice as likely to be physically abused as are children whose mothers are not 'battered'.

EXPLANATIONS

A common approach to a variety of social problems is to focus on the individual. This appears to be simply common sense. Domestic violence, for example, is perpetrated by individuals and it seems to follow that explanations and solutions should focus on individual aggressors. There are two main kinds of explanation focusing on individuals: physiological theories, and psychoanalytic or psycho-social approaches.

There are several variants of physiological theory. One focuses on evolution and the genetic characteristics that predispose men to violence. Others emphasise brain structures, chemical imbalances, dietary deficiencies and hormonal factors such as testosterone. Genetic and hormonal explanations offer reasons for the greater predisposition towards violence in men than in women, but this does not apply to chemical imbalances or dietary deficiencies. Physiological theories are not context specific: they purport to explain all forms of violence and they contribute little to the understanding of specifically domestic violence. Their main deficiency, however, is that they play down both individual responsibility for violent acts and the influence of structural and political factors. Such theories, always more commonly encountered in the United States than in Britain, are now deservedly out of fashion.

Another individualised explanation of domestic violence is to attribute it to the psychopathology of the perpetrator and/or the victim. Perpetrators are said to be weak, pathologically jealous men (Gayford, 1975) with low self-esteem and experiencing insecurity, especially about their masculinity (Roy, 1982; Harris and Bologh, 1985). Other researchers emphasise the perpetrators' rigid notions of male and female roles (Moore, 1979; Sinclair, 1985).

Some interesting work with male perpetrators has been started in recent years. An example is the Men's Centre in London which has links with social services departments and the medical profession. Another example is an organisation based in Stirling called Change: Men Learning to End Their Violence Against Women. Change provides a criminal-justice-based re-education programme for men who are violent to their female partners. It has also developed training programmes and educational materials for use by other agencies.

Several researchers attribute male violence to aspects of the woman's personality or behaviour; a classic case of blaming the victim. In his evidence to the Select Committee, Gayford, a psychiatrist connected with Chiswick Women's Aid, said that many battered women 'have a degree of inadequacy' and that

'A few women present as extremely damaged personalities who will need long term support with their children. Often they need protection against their own stimulus-seeking activities. Though they flinch from violence like other people they have the ability to seek violent men or by their behaviour to provoke attack from the opposite sex.'

(Report from the Select Committee on Violence in Marriage, Vol. 2, 1975, HMSO, p. 37)

A year after giving this evidence, Gayford (1976) described ten types of battered wives using such debasing stereotypes as 'Fanny the Flirt', 'Tortured Tina', and 'Violent Violet'.

Pagelow (1981) refers to the contradictory nature of the evidence which claims to identify the characteristics of women that give rise to violence from their partners. She refers to earlier work conducted by Snell *et al.* (1964) which diagnosed a small number of battered women 'in contradictory terms as passive, aggressive, indecisive, masculine, domineering, masochistic, frigid, overprotective of their sons, and emotionally deprived people who needed periodic punishment "for her castrating activity" ' (p. 20).

Walker (1979, 1985) talks of immobilising terror leading to learned helplessness. Dobash and Dobash (1992, pp. 229–30) reject the notion of 'learned helplessness' which has 'negative implications for public perceptions and actions associated with the problem of violence against women' and is 'based on false premises and unsubstantiated evidence regarding the predicament and actions of women experiencing persistent violence.'

Pizzey and Shapiro (1982) go further than simply asserting that women provoke violence by their behaviour or personal characteristics. They claim that battered women are addicted to violence; they need and enjoy it, deriving sexual excitement from being abused. It is difficult to explain Pizzey's change from being almost a lone champion of battered women to the position she took in 1982. Three years earlier she took part in an interview jointly with Gayford and McKeith in which battered women were said to be suffering from serious mental and emotional disturbance (Bowder, 1979).

Social learning theory, while still concentrating on individual perpetrators, introduces a social element by attempting to explain men's violence towards women as learned behaviour. This phenomenon is variously referred to as a 'cycle of violence' or as 'inter-generational transmission of violence'. What it purports to demonstrate is that those who witness violence between their parents, or who themselves experience abuse as children, are likely to resort to violence in adulthood (Steinmetz and Straus, 1974; Straus, Gelles and Steinmetz, 1980). Stark and Flitcraft (1985) reject the notion that violence is transmitted from one generation to the next; they argue that the studies which claim to show this are methodologically flawed and base their conclusions on inadequate evidence and unsound interpretation. Widom (1989) also points to methodological weaknesses in the research, including its retrospective nature and the lack of an adequate control group. Women's Aid Federation (England) are characteristically unequivocal:

'The experience and analysis of Women's Aid workers leads to a rejection of the cycle of violence theory as providing neither a useful nor an adequate understanding of domestic violence and its effects on children. This theory ignores the gender divisions and inequality that exist in our society, and offers men who abuse an excuse for their behaviour.'

(Home Affairs Committee, 1992, p. 101)

Other explanations give more prominence to socio-structural factors as causes of domestic violence. Among those favouring such an explanation are Steinmetz and Straus (1974), Straus and Hotaling (1980), Straus (1980a), and Gelles (1983). Smith (1989, p. 25) says that such authors see domestic violence as 'a response to frustration, stress and blocked goals'. Among the possible sources of stress are 'economic conditions, bad housing, relative poverty, lack of job opportunities and unfavourable and frustrating work conditions'. Men and women are socialised into particular roles to which are attached a set of socially determined expectations. If structural factors prevent these expectations from being realised, frustration results and violence may ensue. Furthermore, in a variety of ways violence is socially legitimated.

It should be observed, however, that while stress resulting from poverty, inequality and various forms of deprivation may be contributory factors in domestic violence, only a small proportion of those who experience such conditions behave violently towards their partners, and many of those who do behave violently are neither poor nor deprived.

The identification of structural factors gives a more political flavour to explanations of domestic violence. Consider, for example, the immense political implications of a study by Straus (1987) in concluding: (i) that there was a lower incidence of domestic violence where

116

the inequalities between men and women were less marked, and (ii) that weaker social bonds gave rise to increased domestic violence.

We have already noted the political significance of the women's movement, and feminist explanations of domestic violence are essentially political in nature. As Smith (1989, p. 27) says:

'At the core of feminist explanations is the view that all violence is a reflection of unequal power relationships: domestic violence reflects the unequal power of men and women in society and also, therefore, within their personal relationships.'

This is a view strongly expressed in the report of the National Inter-Agency Working Party convened by Victim Support (1992) which uncompromisingly states that 'it is woman's unequal position in society, too often still dependent on men, socially and economically, which makes them vulnerable to domestic violence' (p. 2). Similar sentiments are expressed by all four national Women's Aid groups. Male violence, or the threat of it, is seen as a means of controlling women and of maintaining the domination of men and the subordination of women (Dobash and Dobash, 1980, 1992; Pahl, 1985; Kelly, 1988; Mama, 1989; Hoff, 1990).

Pahl (1980, 1989) has identified more precisely than most the close relationship between the control and management of money in marriage and the exercise of power. Wives were likely to have greater decision-making power if they were in paid employment. Research by Kalmuss and Straus (1981) shows that women's economic dependence is a mediating factor in violence against wives; the greater the dependence, the greater the risk of serious assault. Homer, Leonard and Taylor (1985, p. 91) have also studied the control and management of money in violent relationships, and concluded that 'the exercise of the power of the purse and the force of the fist coincided in the lives of the vast majority of the women interviewed'.

There can be no doubt that feminist analyses have added greatly to our understanding of domestic violence by viewing it in the context of power relationships and the more general position of women in society. Mama (1989, p. 4), however, says that 'Western feminists ... have focused too narrowly on patriarchy and sexual oppression, and therefore failed to consider class, racial and cultural oppressions.' Black women are developing new approaches that challenge 'the ethnocentrism and essentialism' of much of the feminist work of the recent past.

Feminist approaches to domestic violence reject explanations based on individual pathological behaviour. In doing so, they bring domestic violence firmly into the political arena. Individual therapy may have a place, but the violence will continue so long as women are denied equal access to power and resources.

RESPONSES

Other chapters in this volume cover the medical and social work responses to domestic violence. This section will therefore be restricted to a consideration of the role of the police and to the important question of the provision of secure accommodation.

The police

The police response to domestic violence has come in for a great deal of criticism (Dobash and Dobash, 1980; Pahl, 1982; Faragher, 1985; Johnson, 1985; Edwards, 1989; Bourlet, 1990). This is of some significance because women frequently turn to the police for help (Pahl, 1978; Binney, Harkell and Nixon, 1981) and police action is crucial in providing adequate protection for women threatened with violence.

Distilling the work of the writers cited above, the following criticisms of the police response to domestic violence can be briefly identified:

1. A general reluctance to intervene in 'domestic disputes'.
2. The categorisation of violence under the general heading of 'domestic disputes' conceals the fact that violence has occurred and trivialises the offence.
3. A belief that dealing with 'domestics' is 'not real police work'.
4. The treatment of domestic violence as an aspect of the duty of the police to keep the peace, rather than emphasising their duty to enforce the law.
5. A general preference for reconciliation rather than prosecution.
6. Records of domestic incidents are often sketchy and there is too great a readiness to assign violence to the 'no-crime' category. If the decision is to take no legal action then a 'no-crime' report is filed.

Limited space precludes a full discussion of these criticisms, but it is important to record that recent changes in police policy and practice may have begun, but only begun, to blunt their force. Some of the changes stem directly from Home Office Circular 60/1990 which contained new guidelines and was sent to every police force. The general principle informing the guidelines was that domestic violence was to be regarded as a serious crime and that assaults within the home should be treated in the same manner as assaults in the streets; the 'no-criming' of domestic violence was condemned. The guidelines emphasised the overriding need to protect victims and recommended that all forces should formulate clear and unequivocal policies in respect to domestic violence. A more positive interventionist approach was recommended and a strong reminder was given that arrest and prosecution should always be given serious consideration as one of the options. One of the priorities identified by the Home Office was 'the need to ensure that the perpetrators of domestic violence are brought to justice' (Home Affairs Committee, 1992, p. 1). The Home Office Research and Planning Unit is monitoring rates of arrest, charging, prosecutions and convictions. Two changes in the law, though not originally intended to deal with domestic violence, may make it easier to achieve prosecutions of perpetrators. Until 1986 a wife could not be compelled to give evidence against her husband. The Police and Criminal Evidence Act of 1984, which came into effect in 1986, removed this immunity. The second change was the creation of the Crown Prosecution Service under the Prosecution of Offences Act, 1985. Decisions to prosecute now lie with the Crown Prosecution Service; this clearly somewhat limits police discretion in these matters.

The evidence so far indicates that 'no-criming' is declining fairly substantially and that rates of arrest and prosecution are increasing. The Home Office claims that by 1991 'all police forces in England and Wales had formulated clear policies on domestic violence, and that most had also introduced specific improvements in their response to incidents of violence in the home' (Home Affairs Committee, 1992, p. 2). This compares with Bourlet's (1990) finding that in 1985 only 20 per cent of forces had a specific advisory policy or force order.

Not all recent developments stem from the Home Office Circular. A number of police forces had already taken action to improve their practice, and in many respects the Home Office was drawing on examples of existing good practice. The Metropolitan Police were at the forefront of many developments, introducing a force order on domestic violence in 1987 and in the same year establishing the country's first Domestic Violence Unit.

Bourlet (1990) warns against measuring change simply on the basis of published policy statements and force orders. There may be a gulf between chief officers and police constables on the beat:

'The chief officer constructs or devises a policy, ... but it is the police constables who translate that policy into practice. Without the commitment of the officer to follow his or her chief constable's policy line, the policy might just as well have not been created.'

(p. 71)

Improvements there have undoubtedly been, however. The Inter-Agency Working Party on Domestic Violence (Victim Support, 1992) welcomed 'the growing concern of the police over matters of domestic violence in recent years and the many recent innovations and improvements in their guidelines and practice' (p. 11). The Working Party recognised, however, that change was proceeding slowly and that it was patchy.

Accommodation

The provision of safe, secure accommodation is one of the prime requirements for women experiencing violence at the hands of their partners. The lack of such accommodation may result in women reluctantly staying in a violent relationship. There are three areas to be considered: protection in the family home, the provision of alternative accommodation, and refuges.

There are three pieces of legislation which afford some degree of protection and security when abused women remain in the family home: the Domestic Violence and Matrimonial Proceedings Act, 1976 (DVMPA); the Domestic Proceedings and Magistrates' Courts Act, 1978 (DPMCA); the Matrimonial Homes Act, 1983 (MHA).

The DVMPA, which relates only to proceedings in the County Courts, made three changes to the existing law. The three changes were that injunctions were no longer available only as ancillary to other matrimonial proceedings; the availability of injunctions was extended to cohabitees on the same basis as married women; the police were now to be involved in the enforcement of injunctions when powers of arrest were attached. The remedies available under the Act are non-molestation injunctions and ouster injunctions. The latter has the effect of excluding the partner from the 'matrimonial' home or an area which includes the home. The DVMPA also allows judges to grant emergency orders for immediate protection and injunctions which require the man to allow his partner to return to the home if she had been forcibly ejected. Powers of arrest may be added to an injunction.

There are several weaknesses in the operation of this system. The first is that an ouster injunction will only be granted for three months at a time and the same time limits are also often applied to non-molestation injunctions. The second problem is the difficulty of enforcing injunctions in what may be a difficult area to police. Enforcement might be easier where powers of arrest are attached, but such powers are sparingly used and frequently refused. There is considerable variation between courts in their readiness to grant powers of arrest. Even when an injunction with power of arrest is breached, the police do not always make an arrest. The National Inter-Agency Working Party (Victim Support, 1992, p. 27) recommends that 'a power of arrest should be added as a general rule whenever there has been actual bodily harm' and that arrests should be made when a man is in breach of an injunction

The DPMCA, which relates to magistrates' courts, is intended to provide a speedier and more informal way of gaining protection. Although the magistrates can grant both personal or family protection orders and exclusion orders, the DPMCA is more limited than the 1976 Act in that it applies, illogically, only to married women, and it deals only with physical violence whereas the earlier Act also includes cases involving mental cruelty and harassment.

The MHA gives to the courts the power to regulate the respective rights of spouses to occupy the matrimonial home. Under this Act, a married woman can protect her right of occupation by obtaining an exclusion or ouster order against her husband. Non-molestation orders are not available.

By now the non-legal reader will be inclined to ask why three pieces of legislation with overlapping provisions are necessary and how does one decide which statute to invoke? In 1983 Lord Scarman in the *Richards* v. *Richards* judgement described the present arrangements as:

'A hotchpot of enactments of limited scope passed into law to meet specific situations or to strengthen the powers of specified courts. The sooner the range, scope and effect of these powers are rationalised into a coherent and comprehensive body of statute law, the better.'

This quotation is employed in the memorandum of evidence submitted to the House of Commons Home Affairs Committee by the Lord Chancellor's Department (Home Affairs Committee, 1992, p. 11). The same document describes the present system as 'unnecessarily complex and inefficient' and says that 'for each case there is likely to be a confusing choice of jurisdiction, influenced by a variety of factors which may have little to do with the essential nature of the case' (p. 11). The Law Commission (1992) has recommended the repeal of the present legislation and its replacement by a single code giving all family courts the same jurisdiction to make non-molestation and occupation orders, to protect the same group of victims, and on the same grounds. This would certainly simplify the system and remove some of the present anomalies. The Commission also recommends that non-molestation orders and occupation orders between entitled parties should be capable of being made for any specified period or until further order. Another important recommendation is that courts should be *required* to attach powers of arrest to all orders in cases where there has been violence or threatened violence, unless there are good grounds for believing that adequate protection can be afforded without a power of arrest. The Lord Chancellor's Department has welcomed the report, but says that 'detailed consideration is required before any firm decision can be made as to whether the Report as a whole or any parts of it should be implemented' (Home Affairs Committee, 1992, p. 12).

If the protection afforded by the current three statutes is inadequate the woman will need to seek safe alternative accommodation. Women may apply for rehousing under the provisions of Part III of the Housing Act of 1985. If a woman is forced to leave her home because of violence or the threat of it she is defined as homeless under the Act. The next step is to try to establish 'priority need'; this applies to women with children or who are pregnant or who are vulnerable on account of age or disability. If the woman is in priority need, then the local authority has a duty to provide temporary accommodation while enquiries are made. If the local authority is satisfied that the woman meets all the criteria, it has a duty to provide permanent accommodation. Until recently, it was possible for local authorities to evade their responsibilities by claiming that women who left a home because of violence were intentionally homeless. In 1991, however, relevant sections of the Code of Guidance which accompanies the Act were tightened in order to close this loophole. Another provision of the Act is that applicants may be asked to demonstrate that they have a local connection. This would be a foolish requirement for women trying to escape domestic violence by moving away from their home area, and the Act specifically forbids the application of the local connection criterion in the case of women who are homeless because of violence.

Local authority housing departments find themselves in a very difficult position. There has been a very severe cut in government expenditure on housing – 79 per cent between 1978/79 and 1989/90. Between 1971 and 1980 the annual average addition to local authority housing stock was 111 thousand; between 1986 and 1991 the average had fallen to 19 thousand. In addition 1.5 million local authority houses have been sold under the right-to-buy arrangements and the stock has been reduced still further by various provisions of the 1988 Housing Act. Between 1979 and 1991 the number of homeless households increased from 57,000 to 160,000. In 1991, 64,000 households were in temporary accommodation – 13,000 in bed-and-breakfast establishments.

This is the background against which local authorities are expected to meet their obligations to homeless people. This hits women experiencing violence particularly hard, because their need for secure accommodation is so desperate. Many of the best houses have been sold, and the choice available to abused women is restricted. Normally only one offer is made and the women may not be consulted about their requirements. Some local authorities are encouraging women to seek injunctions and return home. An improvement might be achieved by giving statutory force to the Code of Guidance, but this would not solve the problems arising from the reduced stock of public sector housing.

The shortage may mean a longer period spent in temporary accommodation, such as a refuge – another resource in short supply. In 1975 the Select Committee on Violence in Marriage estimated that at least one refuge place for every 10,000 of the population was needed, and in spite of the rapid spread of refuges since the opening of the first in 1972, only about a third of the number of places recommended eighteen years ago are currently available. Each year approximately 30,000 women and children make use of refuges in the United Kingdom. There are twenty-four refuges specifically for black women of which seventeen are for Asian women. Most, though not all refuges are attached to the 200 local Women's Aid groups affiliated to the National organisations.

Refuges provide emergency and safe accommodation, but this is by no means their only function. They also offer specialist help and support and are an invaluable source of information, advice and advocacy; they provide help with financial arrangements, with legal proceedings and with the problems associated with securing permanent accommodation. The range of services will vary from one refuge to another, partly dependent upon resources. Above all, however, refuges offer an environment which facilitates mutual support and in which problems can be shared. Women's Aid refuges are run on self-help principles; their aim is to empower women and help them to regain control of their own lives. Successfully doing things for themselves bolsters residents' self-esteem and gives the necessary confidence to build new and independent lives.

Shortage of funds is a constant problem; as the Women's Aid Federation England says:

'The existing funding of refuges is arbitrary and piecemeal. Refuges have totally different funding patterns, depending largely on geographical location rather than need. No one body has a clear responsibility for refuges, and consequently each potential funder sees it as some other department's responsibility, with the result that many refuges receive a totally inadequate level of grant aid.'

(Home Affairs Committee, 1992, p. 112)

Differences in the level of funding lead to differences in the standards and facilities of refuges in different parts of the country. Many refuges suffer from inadequate space for families, insufficient play-space for children, and low staff–resident ratios. It is difficult to overestimate the value of refuges as part of an effective response to domestic violence, but it could be even more effective if adequate statutory funding was more readily and uniformly available.

CONCLUSION: STAYING, LEAVING, SURVIVING

Women often stay with their violent partners for many years. Some would undoubtedly see this as evidence that either the violence was not so serious as claimed or, like Pizzey and Shapiro (1982), that the women needed and enjoyed the violence. I have no intention of discussing the preposterous claim of Pizzey and Shapiro: it is based on very little evidence and it flies in the face of the experience of all those who work in this field. The claim that if women do not leave then the violence must be bearable, demonstrates a marked lack of sensitivity and a refusal to try to understand the position the women are in. We must look elsewhere for the real reasons, accepting that a complex interplay of sometimes contradictory factors is at work.

Hoff (1990, p. 56) says that 'the women's reasons for staying are embedded in social norms and beliefs about women, marriage, the family and violence'. Hoff asked the women in her study why they remained after the first incident of violence, and she comments: 'it is apparent that they loved their partners, tended to excuse the negative behaviour, and acted on their commitment to make the marriage work' (p. 40). The women may cling to the hope that the man will change. They give him the benefit of the doubt when he promises it will not happen again.

A complicating factor is the feelings of guilt and shame which abused women sometimes experience. If the marriage or relationship is not working, they may look for the fault in themselves, accepting the view that women are responsible for maintaining and nurturing relationships. The feelings of shame may prevent the woman from seeking help, even from friends, neighbours and relatives.

There may also be an element of fear, or at least apprehension, involved. The fear may be that the man will find them and become even more violent, the apprehension is connected with the uncertain future and perhaps doubts about their ability to manage on their own. Being constantly subjected to violence and abuse damages self-esteem and diminishes confidence. Furthermore, the woman may be unsure about the availability of help.

To feel safe it may be necessary for the woman to move to an unfamiliar neighbourhood, leaving friends and relatives and virtually all her possessions behind. The possible effect on the children may be an additional worry; they too must come to terms with living in a new neighbourhood, finding new friends and changing schools. Finding suitable housing is not going to be easy and unsatisfactory temporary accommodation may be the best that can be hoped for: a lone woman with children and possibly meagre resources is in a weak position in the housing market. If the woman is black, her position may be even more precarious. We know very little about how different ethnic groups in the population perceive and experience the breaking away from a violent relationship, and about the different levels and sources of help available to them before and after leaving.

After reviewing some of these difficulties, the report of the National Inter-Agency Working Party on Domestic Violence (Victim Support, 1992, p. 8) says that 'the wonder is not that women find it hard to leave the scene of the violence but that so many find the courage to do so'. Hoff (1990, p. 62) notes the complexity of the process involved in deciding finally to leave:

'For each woman the circumstances and events leading to that decision were unique to her situation: the fear that he would kill her; that she would kill herself; fear for her children or her family; recognition that there is no hope for change; the shock of a particular beating; the horror of being beaten while pregnant.'

It is interesting that Hoff does not mention the woman's fear that she might kill him. Some justification for Hoff's omission might be found in the figures relating to the murder of partners: each year in Britain, 12 to 15 women kill their partners, as compared with 70 men. There has been considerable controversy surrounding the way in which the legal system treats women who kill their violent partners. About 40 per cent of the women are convicted of murder compared with 25 per cent of the men. Heavy prison sentences are imposed on some of the women, and there has been much pressure from various sections of the women's movement for the law to be changed to allow women to plead mitigating circumstances when they have been subjected to prolonged domestic violence (Pilkington, 1993).

It may be that more women than in the recent past will now leave violent relationships, simply because of the publicity given to the problem and the greater knowledge of the help available.

Finally, I would not wish to finish without questioning the commonly held perception of abused women as helpless victims. This is far too negative a view and is a denial of the enormous courage and resourcefulness shown by many of the women. The term 'victim' is an appropriate one, but it does not need to imply helpless fatalism. These women are not only victims; they are also survivors, and a number of writers (Gondolf, 1988; Hoff, 1990; Dobash and Dobash, 1992) are now emphasising this more positive aspect of the women's lives. The books by Gondolf and Hoff are both entitled *Battered Women as Survivors*. Hoff describes the women in her study as 'crisis managers rather than helpless victims' (p. 56). Dobash and Dobash (1992) categorically reject the notions of learned helplessness and a battered woman syndrome. If we wish to empower women who have experienced, or are still experiencing, domestic violence, we must begin by recognising the undoubted strengths they already have.

CHAPTER FIVE

Health Professionals and Violence Against Women

Jan Pahl

Abused women are more likely to be in touch with the health service than with any other agency. Yet research has suggested that health service professionals, such as general practitioners, health visitors and nurses, very often fail to help them. This may because the professionals never learned of the abuse, because they learned of the abuse but did not know how to help, or because what they offered was not perceived as helpful by the woman herself.

The aim of this chapter is to throw light on the problems which health service professionals face in giving assistance to abused women. How many victims of violence is the average health service professional likely to meet in the course of his or her work? What symptoms may indicate abuse, even if a women herself is evasive about how her injuries occurred? What can health service professionals do to help abused women? And what can be done to prevent the problem, as opposed to patching up its effects? These are the sorts of question with which we shall be concerned.

THE EXTENT OF THE PROBLEM

The problems involved in estimating the prevalence of wife abuse have already been discussed by Norman Johnson in Chapter 4. It is even more difficult to give precise figures for the numbers of abused women who contact health service professionals. The result is that information from health service records produces very different estimates from data drawn from other sources. For example, a study of the community response to marital violence collected information from health visitors, general practitioners and accident and emergency departments (Borkowski et al., 1983). The conclusion was that all these professionals see cases of marital violence relatively infrequently. When 45 health visitors were asked to complete a form recording the size of their caseload and the numbers of known or suspected cases of marital violence, the results suggested that one in every 56 women, or 1.8 per cent of the health visitor caseload, fell into this category. About a tenth of general practitioners reported that they saw an abused woman at least once a fortnight, while half reported that they were likely to see an abused woman at least once a month.

Evidence from accident and emergency departments suggested that examples of wife abuse constituted only one in every 3,000 cases. However, the researchers commented that they knew of at least one victim of marital violence, who went to one of the accident and emergency departments where the research was carried out and who told them how she had sustained her injuries, but whose case was not recorded (Borkowski et al., 1983). Other emergency department studies have suggested that between 2 and 4 per cent of women presenting with traumatic injuries are diagnosed as victims of domestic violence (Victim Support, 1992, p. 20).

However, epidemiological approaches produce very different figures from case records held by practitioners. One study estimated that serious violence occurs in up to 5 per cent of marriages in any one year (Marsden, 1978). Another concluded that between one in five and one in three of all couples experience physical violence at some point in the course of the marriage (Borkowski et al., 1983). In a random survey of working-class women in London, one in four women reported having been the victim of domestic violence at some time or other in their lives (Jones et al. 1986). Self report questionnaires completed anonymously by women waiting in accident and emergency departments showed that 24–35 per cent had experienced violence (Victim Support, 1992, p. 20). Crime statistics give some idea of the size of the problem. Almost half of all homicides of women are killings by a partner or ex-partner. One in five of all murder victims is a woman killed by a partner or ex-partner (Smith, 1989).

The evidence suggests that health professionals routinely fail to identify physical abuse in women. This reflects both the women's reluctance to admit how their injuries were caused and health professionals' unwillingness to probe. Research in the United States has shown the benefits of a more positive approach. The research involved training staff in emergency departments to use a protocol containing direct questions about the women's experience of abuse (McLeer and Anwar, 1989). The questions elicited a trauma history and asked if the women has been injured by someone. The majority of women responded readily to the questions in the protocol and seemed to be relieved that someone had directly asked them how they had been hurt. Those who had been battered were given information regarding community resources available to them. The majority of women who had not been battered did not appear to mind being asked if they had been hit or injured by someone. Following a full year of using the protocol, the records for every fourth case of female trauma were reviewed. Cases were classified as positive for battering whenever a woman stated that her injuries were caused by her having been beaten by someone with whom she was or had been intimately involved.

The results showed that the percentage of women identified positively as having been battered increased from 5.6 per cent to 30 per cent, following staff training and use of the protocol. An unexpected but significant finding concerned the relationship between age and battering: the records showed that 42 per cent of female trauma cases in the 18-to-20-year age span had been battered, 35 per cent of the women aged 21 to 30 years, and 18 per cent of women aged 61 years and older. The researchers suggested that directing staff attention to the identification of battered women through the use of a protocol can increase the positive identification of injuries caused by battering. The finding that 42 per cent of female trauma victims between the ages of 18 and 20 were positively battered raises questions regarding the prevalence of battering among teenage girls. Finally, the geriatric population is one characterised by frequent injuries subsequent to accidents. With 18 per cent of injured women over 61 years of age admitting that they were injured in the course of being beaten, it becomes essential to increase professional awareness of the risk in this age group. The researchers concluded that unless emergency department staff maintain a high index of suspicion for battering among female trauma patients, large numbers will go undetected and untreated. They suggested that doctors and nurses working in emergency departments should introduce the use of standardised protocols in order to provide adequate care to this group of women (McLeer and Anwar, 1989).

These figures suggest that though many health professionals see abused women in the course of their work, relatively few identify the real cause of the woman's injuries or distress. There are striking similarities between Britain and the USA in terms of the gap between the numbers of abused women recognised as such by health professionals and those discovered by more direct questioning. Increasingly, violence against women is also being seen as a public health issue (Shephard and Farrington, 1993). Thus, for example, the Australian government policy statement on women's health identifies violence against women as a priority, together with reproductive health and sexuality, health of ageing women, emotional and mental health, occupational health and the needs of carers (Commonwealth Department of Community Services and Health, 1989).

THE EFFECTS OF ABUSE

Studies of women who have been abused have documented the damaging effects on both physical and mental health. The violence experienced by many wives is both prolonged and severe. In my own study, 62 per cent of the women had been subjected to violence for three or more years, and the injuries they had suffered ranged from cuts and bruises, through broken bones and damaged eyesight, to a ruptured spleen, stab wounds and a fractured skull (Pahl, 1985). The findings of this small study were confirmed by the results of a much larger survey, undertaken at the same time in all the refuges of England and Wales (Binney, Harkell and Nixon, 1981). This larger survey found that 73 per cent of women in refuges had put up with violence for three or more years; a third of the women had suffered life-threatening attacks or had been hospitalised for serious injuries. The rest of the sample had experienced assaults which included being kicked, pushed into fires or through glass, being thrown against walls or downstairs, being punched and having hair pulled out; two-thirds said that mental cruelty was one of the reasons why they left home.

In the Islington crime survey almost all the women who were the victims of domestic violence had experienced punching or slapping; three-fifths had been kicked. In just under a quarter of the incidents reported weapons had been used, ranging from bottles and glasses to knives, scissors, sticks, clubs and other blunt instruments. Nearly all the victims had suffered bruising to the skin or eyes; just under a half experienced cuts and a tenth had their bones broken. Nearly half the women had sought medical advice and a quarter of these had been hospitalised at least overnight (Jones *et al.*, 1986). These figures remind us that domestic violence is a crime, as well as a cause of morbidity and mortality. If these assaults occurred between strangers in the street they would immediately be reported to the police. In providing medical and nursing care it is important not to lose sight of the criminal nature of the violence.

In addition to the physical injuries sustained, it is common for women to suffer psychological damage. Many report symptoms of stress, such as lack of sleep, weight loss or gain, ulcers, nervousness, and irritability, and some women report thoughts of suicide (Stanko, 1985; Mullen *et al.*, 1988), Walker (1985) documented high levels of anxiety, fears and panic attacks, depression and other clinical symptoms, including an increased sensitivity to further impending violence. Jaffe *et al.* (1986) showed that women who had experienced domestic violence had significantly higher levels of anxiety and depression than a comparable sample of women (matched for family income, length of marriage and number of children) who were not victims of domestic violence. Andrews (1987) demonstrated that women who are the victims of domestic violence are more likely to be depressed than non-victims. Again, she characterised the classic symptoms as weight and sleep disturbances, a sense of hopelessness and lack of concentration. Thus abused women have many reasons for contacting health services professionals.

There is growing evidence about the harmful effects on children of growing up in a violent home. This was summarised by Jaffe, Wolfe and Wilson (1990). The effects include increased levels of anxiety and sadness, psychosomatic illnesses such as headaches, abdominal complaints and asthma, and lower ratings in social competence, especially for boys. There is some evidence that a boy who grows up in a violent home is more likely to use violence when he is an adult, while a girl who sees her father abuse her mother is less likely to leave a violent relationship herself (Straus, Gelles and Steinmetz, 1980; Gelles, 1976). However, this conclusion must be set in context by remembering that most of those who grow up in violent homes go on to have loving and non-violent relationships as adults, while many violent husbands grew up in non-violent homes. Women's refuges play a crucial part in enabling women to leave violent relationships and in undoing some of the harmful effects on children. As one child who had spent fourteen months in a refuge commented, 'If it weren't for refuges there'd be a lot of funerals.' The evidence on this topic was drawn together by Saunders (1993). His review underlined the fact that children make up two-thirds of the refuge population, and that more than 15,000 children pass through Women's Aid refuges in England every year (Women's Aid Federation England, 1991).

HEALTH SERVICES HELP FOR ABUSED WOMEN

It is important to emphasise that many different professionals, in many different agencies, are potentially in a position to help an abused woman and her children. If she has injuries she is likely to need medical and nursing care. She has been the victim of a crime, so the police may be involved, and she may have to go to court to get an injunction to prevent her husband from assaulting her again. Many husbands are not deterred by legal action, so the woman may decide to leave home to protect herself and her children. Leaving home because of violence, or threat of violence, gives a woman with children priority right to local authority accommodation, so the housing department may become involved. Many women in this position find themselves without a source of income, so are forced to contact the social security office. In a search for solutions to her many problems the woman may get in touch with the social services department, who in turn may refer her to the local women's refuge. One reason why abused women fail to get the help they need is that, because there are so many agencies in a position to offer partial help, each one refers her onto the next: there is a danger than no one professional considers the woman's situation as a whole.

Qualitative interviews with 109 abused women explored help-seeking in considerable detail (Dobash, Dobash and Cavanagh, 1985). The interviews showed that the women made at least four different types of requests for assistance. These included requesting assistance in stopping a particular attack, seeking a sympathetic person to listen and give moral, medical or material support after an attack, trying to involve others in the ongoing negotiations with the man in order to stop the continuing violence, and, finally, attempting to gain the material assistance, such as accommodation and financial support, necessary to escape from the violent relationship. Although the particular requests varied in nature they were all oriented in some way to the woman's attempts to stop the violence. An examination of these requests revealed that they all contained elements that were supportive of the woman, but only some embodied more direct and explicit challenges to the violence.

In order to understand the complex dynamics of the process of seeking help, the women's requests were classified on the basis of whether they were looking for support or for a challenge to the violence. Supportive responses meant those where, for example, the woman seeks a sympathetic listener and is heard, given credence and treated sympathetically, but no attempts are made to confront the violence itself. Challenging responses included such things as advising the woman about her rights and assisting her in acquiring them, attempting to stop an attack in progress, speaking to the man about the unacceptability of the violence, referring to agencies and assisting the woman to escape. Where the response was both supportive and challenging, it was defined as challenging. Although these two general characterisations were sufficient to define the requests, they were not sufficient for the responses. These included a third type, negative actions such as denial, negation, victim-blaming and refusal to assist.

The results of the analyses showed that the nature of the requests made by the 109 women changed over time, from those that were mostly supportive to those that were mostly challenging. For example, after the first assault a total of 113 contacts were made with third parties: of these 73 per cent were requests for supportive forms of assistance, and only 27 per cent challenged the violence. By comparison, a total of 371 contacts were made after the most recent assault and 66 per cent of these were for challenging forms of assistance (Dobash, Dobash and Cavanagh, 1985, p. 156). These results mean that a professional who is concerned with helping women must listen carefully to the nature of the requests each one is making.

Black women who have been abused by their male partners experience similar problems to white women, but in addition have to cope with the racism of some white professionals. The struggles of black women have been vividly documented by Mama in her study of statutory and voluntary sector responses to violence in the home (1989). Like other researchers she found that abuse took place among all social classes; however, black women experience many additional difficulties. It is important that health professionals who are consulted by black and Asian women take some responsibility for helping these women to overcome the barriers which racism can erect.

Within the health service the main sources of help are general practitioners, health visitors, practice nurses, and doctors and nurses working in accident and emergency departments. In examining the contribution of these professionals I shall draw on two main sources of information: quantitative data from a number of studies and qualitative data from my own interviews with abused women. Tape-recorded interviews mean that we can listen to the voices of the women themselves talking about their encounters with various professionals.

HELP FROM GENERAL PRACTITIONERS

If we consider the prevalence of wife abuse in the general population, and the fact that in the United Kingdom almost every adult is registered with the family doctor, it becomes clear that every doctor's list will contain a proportion of battered women. It is impossible to say how many of these will consult their doctor about the violence or its consequences, since we have no population-based data, but we do have evidence from women living in refuges about their previous attempts to seek help from professionals.

In one study of 636 women, living in refuges throughout England and Wales, 52 per cent of the women had contacted their general practitioner for help with the problem. However, 44 per cent had not found the contact helpful (Binney *et al.*, 1981). A study of 109 women, interviewed in refuges in Scotland, revealed that while 80 per cent of them had been in touch with their general practitioner, only 25 per cent had mentioned the violence to which they were being subjected (Dobash and Dobash, 1980). Many of these women found that the response was unsatisfactory. General practitioners rarely seemed to challenge the violence; instead their responses were confined to treating wounds, prescribing psychotropic medications and sometimes referring women to psychiatrists. The researchers concluded that the medical profession's failure to understand the problems of abused women must be understood against a background of patriarchal assumptions about women and marriage, and a professional training which seeks to fit complex social, psychological and physical problems into neat, clear-cut, physical symptoms that can be defined as treatable (Dobash, Dobash and Cavanagh, 1985).

My own study involved tape-recorded interviews with women who spent time at a refuge in south-east England. Of the 50 women who were interviewed, 32 had talked to their general practitioner about their marital problems and about the violent behaviour of the man with whom they were living. By comparison, 35 of the women had called in the police at one time or another and 40 had discussed their problems with a social worker (Pahl, 1979). In many incidences the general practitioner was the first person, apart from family and friends, to hear about the violence. The general practitioner was also likely to have a continuing part to play, since if the woman was to prosecute for assault, get an injunction to protect herself, apply for local authority housing or initiate a divorce or separation using the violence as evidence, she would need a medical certificate to support her case. Thus it seemed as though doctors would inevitably find themselves involved in the problems of abused women.

Some of the women visited their general practitioners but did not mention the violence, often because they felt ashamed or because they did not expect to meet with a sympathetic response. The study suggested that doctors should become more sensitive to the concealment of wife abuse, as they have become sensitive to the concealment of child abuse. Here is one woman, whose doctor was aware of this possibility, but who still did not learn the truth:

> 'On Valentine's Day he beat me up so much – I crawled up the stairs to Eve – I was near enough done in. He threw me across

the room – he kept kneeing me in the gut. And I had great big bruises like that all over my body. When the doctor saw my bruises he said "How did you get those?" And I said to him "I fell over". And he said "Are you sure?" And I said "Yes".'

Q. 'Why couldn't you talk to him?'

'I don't know. I was embarrassed. It made me feel I was in the wrong. You never expect a battered wife to be living in Broadstairs with all the old people.'

Another woman said of her doctor:

'I didn't feel I could talk to him. They always seem to rush you. So I used to say I'd fallen downstairs or that the wardrobe had fallen on me.'

Of the women who had talked to a general practitioner, 18 (56 per cent) said that he or she had been either 'very helpful' or 'quite helpful'; 14 (44 per cent) said that he or she had not been helpful. The most frequent response of these 'unhelpful' general practitioners was the prescribing of anti-depressants and tranquillisers. One woman said of her doctor's use of tranquillisers that 'He dishes them out like Smarties'. Many of the women saw such treatment as an inappropriate, stop-gap measure which could well postpone their achievement of a satisfactory long-term solution.

Another source of dissatisfaction was the recognition that the wrong patient was in the consulting room. It was not possible to interview the men who had committed the assaults and so nothing can be said here about their need for medical or psychological treatment; a few of the women mentioned that their husbands had received treatment at psychiatric hospitals, but many more commented that their husbands perceived the violent behaviour as normal. Some general practitioners clearly considered the possibility that it might be more appropriate to treat the man than the woman, but recognising the impossibility of this, seemed to be unable to help the woman either. The following woman was echoed by many others when she said:

'The doctor recommended psychiatric treatment for my husband – but I was much too frightened to tell him what the doctor had said.'

Another described how:

'I used to go to the health centre all black and blue, and my legs all black and blue and my knees all puffed up where he had kicked me. But they never bothered. They talked about it, but they didn't do anything to help.'

Q. 'What sorts of things did they say?'

'They just said "Is he ill in any way? Does he need help?" I think he does, with these tempers and that, because it's not normal, bad tempers as violent as that. And I told them about his violent temper and they said they couldn't do nothing about it. Because they don't like to interfere.'

Sometimes the husband would go to the doctor with his injured wife, so that she was unable to talk about how the injuries had occurred. As one said:

'I couldn't talk to him about it. Well, when I used to go and see him usually John was with me anyway. He's very jealous like that, even though the doctor is an old man.'

Other women were dissatisfied because the general practitioner's advice seemed to them to be inappropriate, irrelevant or unsympathetic. One woman, whose husband was eventually judged by the court to be so violent that he was not allowed any access at all to their children, said of her general practitioner:

'My doctor said that he didn't want to appear for me. He'd seen a lot of the beatings and the bruisings, but he didn't want to appear for me. My solicitor was going to force him, you know, sub poena him, but my doctor's attitude was that I wanted to change my husband and that I never would do, that I should learn to live more tolerantly with him.'

Another woman said:

'The doctor wasn't sympathetic at all. Actually I wasn't looking for sympathy. I was wondering if he could advise me of anywhere to go. But he just sort of said "Take these tranquillisers and you'll be alright." I said to him "I've come for help. I don't know who to go to but I read in many magazines that people go to their doctors." I said this to him. And he asked me what was wrong, and I said "I'm feeling very depressed and I'm having a lot of problems with my husband, and I would like some advice." But he just wrote out a pre-scription and said "Well take these and you'll be alright." He said something like he hasn't got the time, or he's not paid to do what the social services should do. So I said "Who are the social services?" And all he said was "Go to the town hall." I sat down for two weeks and I thought "Going to the town hall seems silly." '

One woman had talked to two different general practitioners:

> 'The first one I went to – I could have swung for him. He said "What do you think this is – a bloody marriage guidance council?" He just wrote out the prescription and that was it.'

Q. 'A prescription for what?'

> 'Valium.'

Q. 'And what did you talk to the other doctor about?'

> 'I told him everything. He was so good, you know. He sat down and really listened. He said "I think you'd be better off without your husband." He said "Keep pushing the council for a place of your own!"'

General practitioners who were seen by the women as 'helpful' had many characteristics in common. The women described how these doctors listened carefully, approached the problem sympathetically, offered appropriate advice, both medical and non-medical, kept careful records of their injuries and so on. Helpfulness in general practitioners was not so very different from helpfulness in other health service professionals, so we shall return to this topic in more detail later in the chapter.

HELP FROM HEALTH VISITORS

Health visitors are responsible for visiting all new babies and for giving advice and support to families with children under five. In my own study 90 per cent of the families had a child under five years old in the family at some time or other during the years when the violence was taking place (Pahl, 1982). Looking back to the time when the violence first began, in a third of the households there was a child under two years, while in another third of the households the woman was pregnant when the violence began. Clearly, then, health visitors are potentially one of the most immediately available sources of help for abused women.

The children were one important reason why women endured the violence for so many years. Often the relationship between father and children was satisfactory. Men who batter their wives do not normally batter their children; however, men who batter their children are quite often also wife batterers (Bowker *et al.* 1988). Women who had been ill-treated by their husbands were unwilling to leave their children behind when they fled, yet they also hesitated before removing them to the poverty and loneliness of life as a single parent family, even though this would mean greater safety for themselves. As the years passed, however, it often became clear that the violence was affecting the children. Many women said that it was when the eldest child started to notice what was happening between the parents that they decided that it was time to leave home. About half of the women said that the children had been distressed by the marital problems of their parents, and that this was one of the chief reasons for making a determined effort to leave by going to the refuge.

There seemed to be three main reasons why the women in the study did not find health visitors as helpful as one would have expected. The first of these was that many of the women saw the health visitor as concerned primarily with the children. When the health visitors were said to be helpful this often referred to their helpfulness over the children's problems, such as bed-wetting or slow development, rather than over problems in the woman's own life.

Secondly, some husbands prevented their wives from receiving help. Many were suspicious of all visitors to the house, particularly if they appeared to come from any of the welfare agencies. One wife said:

'I was offered home help because I was a bit ill after the baby was born and the health visitor said that I needed help for a little while. My husband was away then in London. She got me the home help; he came home and he said "No you're not. You do your own housework." And he wouldn't let me have any home help. The doctor wanted to put me on tranquillisers but I still had to get up and look after the kids and do the housework. The health visitor tried to be helpful, but everything she said he said "No".'

Another woman, who was savagely beaten by her husband over many years, had to make clandestine arrangements for meeting her health visitor. This woman's difficulties were exacerbated by the fact that her husband owned a cafe where she was expected to work for her keep and where she was rarely out of his sight. She said:

'Three days after we were married, he said "If you want to leave, don't ever think about it. Because I'll kill you before you leave me." I wanted to leave my husband a long time ago, but I've got nowhere to go. I couldn't tell the health visitor my problems because he would just sit there and listen. I'd got to say "Yeah, I'm alright, children's fine, yeah yeah." So I went to my doctor and said "I can't speak with the health visitor." So I arranged to meet her somewhere else. And

138

she said "You've got to get out of that house. Sooner the better. You've got to leave him." Then I had a new health visitor and she started coming to the cafe as a customer, because my husband didn't know her. Then we started talking. Of course, any time he comes along we've got to stop. But she made a report.'

Some wives were beaten for talking to outsiders about their marital problems. Indeed, the combination of fear, shame and guilt made wives remain with violent husbands long after one might have expected them to leave. As one wife said:

'I don't know who can help me and who can advise me. I said to the health visitor about it and she said about the social services coming in. But I'm always frightened about anyone coming in to see him, in case he starts on me. And I'm afraid of going to see anyone because of that – I'm afraid that he's going to start on me.'

Thirdly, some women who managed to talk to the health visitor about their marital problems still did not feel that they had been helped. Often this was because the health visitor responded inappropriately, for example by urging the wife to 'try harder', by implying that the violence was her fault, or by working for reconciliation when the wife was asking for support in challenging the violence.

For years before going to the refuge, many of the women had desperately needed detailed advice about the possible courses of action they might take, and support in making decisions on behalf of themselves and their children. One said:

'I went to the police because he gave me a black eye, but when he found I'd been round there I got another hiding. Anyway they just said "Go back and make it up." I said "I've tried for two years to make it up." I talked to the health visitor about it too but she didn't do nothing about it. She just said "Why don't you go home and try to make it up?" But I said "You don't know how hard it is to do that really." She said that he does need some help, and I'm sure he does because no normal bloke would do that. She said "I'll be round tomorrow." But I never saw her since.'

Some health visitors seemed to behave as though the wife had no claim to be helped in her own right, as though her welfare was subsumed under the heading of the welfare of the family or of the children. It is important to recognise that married women may have needs of their own which are quite separate from, and different from, those of the husband, of the children, or of the family as a whole. This point may seem trite: nevertheless it lies behind much of the pressure exerted upon abused women to remain in their homes.

ACCIDENT AND EMERGENCY DEPARTMENTS

There is very little information about the treatment of abused women in accident and emergency departments in Britain. However, a study carried out in the United States produced some every interesting results (Stark, Flitcraft and Frazier, 1979). The data for the research were drawn from the medical records of 481 women who were treated for injuries in the emergency department of a major hospital. The records noted all the women's previous visits to the emergency department and were used to classify them into four categories.

Positives: at least one injury was recorded as inflicted by a husband, boyfriend or other male intimate.

Probable: at least one injury resulted from a punch, hit, kick, shot or similar and deliberate assault by another person, but the relationship of assailant to victim was not recorded.

Suggestive: at least one injury was inadequately explained by the recorded medical history.

Reasonable negative: each injury in the medical record was adequately explained by the recorded etiology, including those recorded as sustained in muggings or anonymous assaults.

Physicians working in the emergency department were asked to estimate the numbers of abused women they encountered in their work and their answers were compared with the data from the records. During the sample month, physicians identified 14 battered women (2.8 per cent). However, from the full medical histories, almost 10 per cent of the 481 women could be positively identified as battered at least once, and an additional 15 per cent had trauma histories pointing towards abuse. This means that where physicians saw one out of 35 of their patients as battered, a more accurate approximation was one in four. What the physicians described as a rare occurrence was in reality an event of epidemic proportions.

The study documented the ways in which medical and nursing staff responded to abused women. It showed that when a battered woman first came to the emergency service her discrete, individual injury was defined as the only appropriate object for care. The fact that the injury was caused by a 'punch' seemed to be no more significant than if it resulted from a 'fall', and if the cause was recorded there was no comment. One important difference between abused and non-abused women was in the extent to which medical staff treated them for psychi-atric symptoms. Thus 24 per cent of the abused women were prescribed minor tranquillisers or pain medication, compared with only 9 per cent of non-abused women. Psychiatric referrals were noted in 15 per cent of the records of abused women but only in 4 per cent of other records.

These findings led the researchers to investigate the links between abuse and psychiatric disorder. They posed the question like this: Does battering primarily arise among women who suffer significant psychi-atric disorders or, to the contrary, do these disorders evolve during the course of an abusive relationship and, indirectly, as a consequence of inadequate service intervention? The data from the medical records showed that prior to the onset of abuse there were no statistically significant differences between battered and non-battered women in their rates of psychiatric disorder, mental health service utilisation, or in the appearance of psychosocial labels in their medical records. However, the records showed that as women returned again and again to the emergency department with new injuries, each one treated without regard to the context in which it occurred, they began to develop psychiatric symptoms. Thus, during the time covered by the records, one of every four abused women attempted suicide at least once, more than one in three were referred to community psychiatric services, while one in seven was eventually institutionalised at the state mental hospital. In the vast majority of cases such problems emerged only after the first incident suggestive of abuse.

The conclusion was that, far from helping to solve the problems of abused women, the staff of the emergency department were part of the process by which their problems were created. By treating the injuries, but ignoring the context in which the injuries occurred, health service professionals were actually exacerbating the difficulties the women faced (Stark, Flitcraft and Frazier, 1979; see also Hadley, 1992).

The researchers suggested that the patterns they had identified could be understood as part of a more general failure to respond to male viol-ence against women. Male professionals, in particular, may be reluctant to challenge a situation which they define as a private matter between husband and wife. Their failure to challenge male control of women individualises what is essentially a social issue. We shall return to this topic in the conclusion of this chapter.

PSYCHOTHERAPEUTIC APPROACHES

There has been considerable controversy over the value of the psy-chotherapeutic approach to domestic violence. Psychotherapy can be focused on the women, as in individual counselling or women's support groups, or on the men, as in programmes for batterers. In the United States there is now a vast array of such initiatives, with at least 200 programmes for batterers in existence in 1992; in many cases attendance at these programmes is ordered by the court (Dobash and Dobash, 1992). In general the psychotherapeutic approach to domestic violence is more widespread in North America than in Europe, reflecting different attitudes to individualism and to the development of therapeutic ideals and interventions. The spread of this approach to violence, and the forms it takes, were discussed by Dobash and Dobash (1992). They pointed out some of the dangers of the therapeutic focus, which can reduce the social problem of violence against women to a narrower concern with the troubles of individual men, women and families.

Some of the difficulties involved in using psychotherapeutic techniques have been summarised by Goldner (1992). She draws on her own experience as a therapist to consider the family systems approach in the context of feminist critiques. Family systems theory focuses on exploring the dynamics of family life and the relationships between individuals within families; it emphasises the strengths of families and their right to self-determination, in the context of increasing interference by the state into family life. Feminists challenge this approach on the grounds that it ignores power differentials and conflicts of interests within families. They argue that the idea of protecting the family from external control masks the control which men can have over women and children by dint of their greater physical, social and economic power.

TRAINING FOR HEALTH PROFESSIONALS

Wife abuse should be specifically included in the training of all the relevant health service professionals. This includes medical and nursing staff and the relevant reception and administrative staff. A study in North America of the curriculum content in accredited medical schools found that no instruction about domestic violence was provided in just over half of the 117 schools that responded. The others provided an average of 1.5 sessions lasting 1.9 hours (McIlwaine, 1989). At present there is no equivalent information about the content of medical training in Britain.

Training courses for nurses, midwives and health visitors in Britain all deal with gender issues and with violence in the family. However, the specific content of this part of the course is decided by each individual college or course organiser. Recent research at the University of Detroit has shown that effective training can lead to changes in attitudes as well as in knowledge (Mandt, 1993). Students following the degree level course in nursing at Detroit work primarily in large urban hospitals and clinics. These settings see large numbers of victims of violence. The course, Nursing and Crisis Intervention for Victims of Family Violence, was developed as a senior level clinical course. The focus of the course is on the integration of biopsychosocial and nursing concepts and principles to enable the nurse to deliver care to the individuals, families and groups experiencing crises arising out of family violence. The didactic portion of the course emphasises theories of violence, grief and crisis intervention, integrated with nursing theory. Students apply these theories in a variety of settings, including shelters for battered women and children. Recognising the high emotional impact of the content of the course, a significant amount of time is devoted to group discussion.

The first few weeks of the course often prove quite unsettling, because students have the same stereotypical attitudes about battered women that prevail in the general population. With no theoretical understanding of the problem, many still believe that such women somehow bring the violence on themselves, want it, probably deserve it, or could simply leave any time they wanted to. Within a few weeks the conflict between old attitudes and newly acquired knowledge becomes apparent, as students struggle to incorporate what they have learnt into their own clinical practice. By the end of the course all students invariably report that their professional practice has been reshaped, with assessment skills sharpened, empathy increased and previously unknown interventions now integrated into their daily practice.

Many students reported that they frequently saw women whom they believed to be abused, but all they did prior to this course was to treat the results of the physical violence, patch up the wounds, and send the victims on their way. Frequently, women whose injuries were suggestive of abuse said that the injury was sustained in a fall or in some other benign way. These students reported that they were satisfied with whatever explanation the woman gave, since they did not really feel that it was their business to 'pry'.

The course opened their eyes and enabled them to view violence itself as a health problem. As one student reported:

'I never felt it was any of my business to ask a woman directly if a spouse or partner had beaten her up. I just thought if she wanted to tell me she would and I shouldn't pry. This course has taught me otherwise. Just the other day a young lady came into the department with a large laceration on the head. She had the tell-tale bruises on her arms that indicated a defensive posture. I came right out and asked her "Did your husband hit you?" She broke down and started to cry. We talked and I gave her some information I had learnt. I told her about the extent of domestic violence, hoping she would know she wasn't the only victim. I told her about the shelters and gave her some phone numbers to call if she wanted. I don't know if I did any good, but I do know I never would have even asked her the first question if I hadn't taken this course.'

(Mandt, 1993, p. 45)

The students who followed this course became much more understanding of the woman's inability to leave the situation and found that they were able to interact in a much more non-judgmental fashion. They reported that, prior to the course, they viewed the woman in such a situation as foolish, and felt that if she kept going back for more abuse, it was impossible to have much sympathy. After the course they had a much greater understanding of the difficulties which women face in leaving abusive relationships and a better knowledge of possible sources of help.

RECOMMENDATIONS FOR GOOD PRACTICE

There is much that health service professionals can do to help abused women. Good practice can be summed up under four different headings:

1. *Respecting the woman's account.* This may simply mean taking seriously what she says about how her injuries occurred and acting appropriately. A woman who admits to being abused is likely to feel both distressed and ashamed: in these circumstances reassurance and support are appropriate responses. In other instances a woman may be reluctant to admit to what happened. Professionals should be aware that the majority of abused women do not disclose the cause of their injuries unless they feel confident that they will meet with sympathy, privacy and a non-judgmental approach.

2. *Knowing the relevant information.* The most helpful health professionals are often those whose vision extends beyond the health service. For example, every health professional should know how to contact the local women's refuge and should be aware that the 1985 Housing Act gave local authority housing departments the duty to offer accommodation to all women with children who have to leave

144

home because of violence or threat of violence. It is also important to be able to give women information about income maintenance: many remain with violent men simply because they do not think they have any financial alternative. Professionals should be able to advise women about claiming Income Support from the local social security office. Knowing something about the relevant law may also be helpful, and in particular about the process of getting an injunction to protect the woman from further violence.

3. *Keeping careful records* Careful documentation of injuries and easy access to such documentation are often essential for successful legal proceedings or to prove a right to rehousing. Lacking such evidence a women may find herself being advised, in effect, to go home, get beaten again, and then present herself with the evidence of the beating. Careful records made on her first visit about the nature and the extent of the injuries, even if not immediately useful, may in the long run save her additional suffering.

4. *Giving enough time.* Finding a solution to family and marital problems can take a long time, both in terms of each individual session, and in terms of the months and years needed to make decisions about divorce. In my own study one of the women who was most enthusiastic about the helpfulness of her general practitioner described how he frequently arranged for her to have the last appointment of the surgery so that time should not be limited. One of the most helpful health visitors learnt not to call at the house when the husband's van was parked outside: her many visits were all made when the husband was out.

More detailed guidelines have been developed by Jezierski (1992). These are intended to provide directions for health professionals; specific items in the guidelines may apply more to some professionals than others. The guidelines deal with the principles which should underpin work with abused women, with identification and assessment, and with appropriate intervention.

Jezierski sets out five general principles for health services professionals when intervening in situations involving possible or actual physical, sexual or psychological abuse of a client:

1. Be aware of the possibility of abuse whenever someone has been injured.
2. Respect the woman's account of what happened and her decisions about what actions she will take.
3. Be aware that giving help will involve offering relevant information, as well as providing nursing or medical care.

4. Keep careful records of the woman's injuries.
5. Give enough time for the woman to tell you what has happened and to discuss what she should do.

Assessment involves not only recognising signs of abuse but also giving the woman an opportunity to talk about the context in which the abuse took place. Assessment is likely to begin with a head-to-toe, front and back, physical assessment. The clinician should note any signs of both old and new trauma, including bruising, scarring, deformities and so on. Assessment should include palpation and auscultation of the chest, phalanx and abdomen, as well as examination of ribs, extremities, skull and pelvis to identify areas of possible fracture. Signs suggestive of domestic abuse include the following:

1. The injuries do not match the history.
2. The patient's behaviour may include distant or vague responses to questions, poor eye contact or flinching in the presence of husband or significant others.
3. The physical injuries may include multiple injuries and injuries in different stages of healing, while the patient may complain of seemingly insignificant trauma even though she has come to the emergency department.
4. The woman's history may include a substantial time delay between the time of injury and the point at which she sought health care, abuse as a child, vague references to 'having had a bad time lately', or pregnancy (battering often increases with pregnancy). She may have records showing past visits to the casualty department for various physical problems or chronic somatic complaints.
5. Her husband or partner seems very attentive, but is reluctant to allow the patient to answer questions for herself.

The appropriate intervention is likely to vary depending on whether or not the woman denies the abuse and whether she plans to return home or to leave the abuser. Table 5.1 gives the protocol that was developed in North America for use by medical and nursing staff who suspect that a patient is being abused (Jezierski, 1992); it has been adapted to make it suitable for use in the United Kingdom.

A comprehensive review of nursing care for survivors of family violence has been produced by Campbell and Humphreys (1993). This covers violence against children and elderly people, as well as violence against women, and it sets practice firmly in a theoretical framework. Male violence is seen as having its roots in machismo and patriarchy, which set the stage for men to learn and use abusive behaviour.

Table 5.1 *Intervention by nursing and medical staff*

A. *Patient denies abuse*	B. *Patient admits abuse: will return to abusive environment*	C. *Patient admits abuse: plans to leave abusive environment*

– Make an affirmative statement to patient that includes nonjudgemental interest and concern
– *If* patient is an abuse victim she has every right *not* to be abused
– *If* patient is an abuse victim she is *not* to blame
– Ask the patient in a gentle but firm manner if she has been hurt by someone[*]
– Write phone number of battered women's refuge or solicitor on plain paper
– Discuss refuge and other resources available
	– Discuss protection and safety plan[a]
	– Provide emergency kit information[b]
	– Instruct patient on plan for emergency escape[c]
	– Provide for follow-up medical care
	– Offer resources such as social services, refuge, support groups
	– Make affirmative statement as in Column A
		– Assist with contacts:
		    police
		    solicitor
		    social security
		    housing department
		    refuge
		    relatives
		    friends
		– Assess for any physical needs (food, clothing, transportation)
		– Provide for follow-up medical care
		– Social services
		– Make affirmative statement as in Column A

[*]Suggestion for phrasing of questions by assessing nurse: "The injuries you have are like bruises and lacerations people get when someone hits them. Did someone hit you? Are you afraid?"

[a] 1 When abuse is occurring, protect abdomen and head, curl up into a ball and put hands over head.
2 Remove potential weapons or instruments that are harmful from the home setting.
3 Yell loudly and continually when being hit.
4 Arrange with a nearby neighbour that if cries are heard, the neighbour will call 999.
5 The victim or her children can call 999.

[b] Emergency escape kit
1 Any necessary documents that could prove useful in court, in going to welfare agencies, in setting out on her own.
2 Money, to be used for phoning, travel, accommodation or other maintenance expenses.
3 Change of clothes.
4 Clothes for children.
5 List of necessary phone numbers including:
   a women's refuge
   b social services
   c emergency 24-hour phone lines/police
   d support system – friends, family members, clergy and so on.
   e solicitor (if she has one)

[c] Advise the victim to plan ahead for what she will do next time an abuse incident occurs. This should include how she will escape – by what mode of transportation, where she will go, whom she will take, and where the emergency escape kit will be for easy access. Advise her to prearrange sanctuary with friends.

Source: Adapted from Jezierski, 1992, p. 299.

CONCLUSION

When health services professionals fail to help abused women the explanation often lies in their attitudes to women, to marriage and to family life. These attitudes include assuming that women could leave if they wanted to, while taking for granted male dominance within the home, male control of finances, and women's responsibility for any marital problems. The effect is to lay the blame for the violence on the woman and to ignore the perpetrator of the violence and the context in which the violence took place. There were many examples of this process in the interview material presented earlier in this chapter: 'I'm not a bloody marriage guidance council' said one doctor; 'Why don't you go home and try to make it up' said a health visitor; 'Take these tranquillisers and you'll be alright' said one doctor; 'Learn to live more tolerantly with him' said another. The cumulative effect of these sorts of remarks is to disempower women, while allowing the violence to continue.

As we have seen in this chapter, there are many short-term actions which health professionals can take to help the abused women whom they meet in the course of their work. However, finding long-term solutions to the problem of wife abuse means giving more power to women, both individually and collectively. This was the point which emerged at the end of the United Nations expert group meeting on the topic. The report on the meeting concluded:

> 'Violence against women is the product of the subordination of women. Short term measures may have a short term effect ... but it is certain that no long term measure will be successful unless there is a fundamental change in the social and economic structures that maintain the subordination of women within marriage and in the wider society.'
>
> (United Nations, 1989, p. 105)

Health professionals may not feel in a position to alter the social and economic structures which support male dominance, but they should recognise that this is the context in which abused women approach them for help.

CHAPTER SIX

Social Work and Domestic Violence

Siobhan Lloyd*

INTRODUCTION

In August 1993 two reports relating to the social work response to violence within the family were discussed at a Scottish social work committee (Grampian Regional Council, 1993). The first recommended approval for the appointment of a senior manager with responsibility for identifying the 'nature and quantification of the extent of such violence ... for a considered strategy to be developed'. A background paper in support of the proposal noted the forms of violence which would be studied if approval was given for the appointment – marital violence between spouses or partners, abuse of elders and 'some forms of physical abuse of children'. The paper went on to suggest that, as part of the job remit, the post holder would consult with a range of agencies including health and legal professionals, the housing department and voluntary agencies. It did not, interestingly, refer to Women's Aid at any point in its text, either as a specific point of contact or as an agency with particular expertise and knowledge in the field of domestic violence.

The second report concerned the staffing of child care teams within one division of the department. It noted current difficulties with the recruitment of child protection social workers and the need for financial incentives and support to develop and maintain stability in this staff group. It referred to low morale, the pressure generated by the work and the paradox whereby child care teams need experienced workers but are limited by their ability to attract less experienced, newly qualified staff.

Taken together, the reports illustrate some of the current issues for social work in relation to violence in the family. Firstly, there is the

149

question of how the issue is defined, and by whom. The reports also raise questions about assuming that all forms of violence in the family can be adequately understood and researched in the same way. This has obvious implications for the nature of the social work response both at the level of the individual worker and departments as a whole. Secondly, they highlight the question of awareness among politicians and social workers at all levels about the specific and interrelated needs of specific groups – older people, partners and children. Thirdly, the way in which social work practitioners and managers are trained and supported for working with family violence is raised but not addressed. Finally, there are the issues relating to the way in which policy relating to domestic violence is developed, implemented and evaluated.

This chapter will address these issues in respect to one specific aspect of violence in the family – the violence perpetrated on women by their male partners, its effects on the women and their children and the social work response to it. The chapter will make a brief examination of the contexts in which social work as a profession responds to domestic violence. It will outline the experience of women who have contacted social workers for help and support and look at specific issues for women with children and for men who are violent towards their partners. It will consider the implications of this evidence for policy-making, social work practice, the training of staff and inter-agency working . Throughout the chapter, the main focus for discussion will be the experience of women with children. These women's experiences have been more thoroughly researched, partly because of the potential for statutory intervention when children are involved and because their voice has been most clearly heard through their contact with non-statutory agencies, especially Women's Aid. This is especially important because giving a voice to women who have experienced violence as children or adults has been a significant gain of the women's movement. As one report succinctly put it.

'The starting point for any approach to violence against women must be the actual experience of women.'

(NALGO, 1991, p. 3)

The need to ensure that the voice of women is heard is supported by research which consistently finds that the majority of violent crimes against women go unreported, especially when the crimes are of a sexual nature and/or have been committed by a man known to the woman (Dobash and Dobash, 1981; Chambers and Millar, 1983;

150

Borkowski et al., 1983; Hanmer and Saunders, 1984; Edwards, 1985; 1986). This body of research also confirms that societal and professional attitudes to violence against women are based on myths and stereotypes which deny the true extent, nature and effects of that violence. Continuing to dispel these myths and challenge their ensuing stereotypes are important prerequisites to devising effective strategies for countering violence against women and children and working with the men who perpetrate it.

Although there are features common to all violent behaviour by men towards women, black and ethnic-minority women, women with disabilities, lesbian women and older women have particular experiences and needs. The specific forms of discrimination faced by them are also reflected in the lack of understanding of and provision for their needs within statutory and voluntary sector agencies. Mama (1989) argues that the treatment of black women, for example, 'epitomises grudging reluctance and even refusal of British society to meet their basic needs' (p. 6). There is some irony in this stance, since the development of many health and welfare services in Britain has relied on the labour of black women. Black women also face the pressure of racism from within their own communities. This is manifest in coerced loyalty towards partners who are violent. There is also the fear that by reporting domestic violence they may add to racist stereotypes of black men being more prone to violence. A black woman who has come to live in Britain and is subsequently abused by a white man has the additional burden of fear that he, rather than she, will be believed. The threat of deportation, fear of her family's response if she returns to her country of birth and the stigma of a 'failed marriage' are also strong (Maguire, 1988). For women with little English, leaving a violent partner poses additional difficulties of communicating her distress so there may be cultural pressures to stay in the relationship (Scottish Women's Aid, n.d.). Mama (1989) also documents incidents where the collective pressure of an extended family decreases the likelihood of a woman leaving. A colour-blind response to domestic violence fails to take these cultural aspects into account, minimising or ignoring the different pressures they place on women who live with violent partners or on women living in violent homes.

Older women too have specific needs and they can also face prejudice and discrimination from agencies including social work departments. If they have spent many years in a violent relationship they may not know who to contact if they decide to leave. Fear of change if they do leave can also be a major deterrent. An older woman who has become the carer of an abusive partner can also face pressure from health and social services agencies to continue caring; children can exert a similar pressure, especially if they are unlikely to fulfil this role (NALGO, 1991; Hughes and Mtezuka, 1992). The issues for lesbian women are no less complicated. Lesbians acknowledge their sexuality at different stages in their lives; some may have been in a heterosexual relationship which was violent and their sexuality may have been used by a male partner to justify his violent behaviour. Lesbians with children have added difficulties relating to custody and maintenance if they do leave. Lesbian partners are not immune from the violence of a former male partner either, although this is an area in which there is little or no research (Lobel, 1986; Cosis Brown, 1992).

Women with learning difficulties or disabilities face difficulties too if they get to the point of leaving a violent relationship. Purpose-built resources for them are almost non-existent, with few accessible refuges or emergency accommodation. They may have additional problems relating to communicating with professionals, access to relevant information is often poor and stereotyping of their needs and abilities can lead to professional abuses of their self-respect. The outcome can be discriminatory practice on the part of social workers (Williams, 1992).

SOCIAL WORK PRACTICE AND DOMESTIC VIOLENCE

The way in which social work agencies and their staff understand and respond to domestic violence is the result of a number of interrelated factors:

- social workers' understanding of the issue;
- their training for working in this area;
- departmental organisation which encourages or inhibits a sensitive response to the issue;
- the development of a clear social work policy on domestic violence;
- support for non-statutory organisations working with domestic violence.

There are two core issues which underpin all of these themes. Firstly there is the question of the prevalence of domestic violence in social workers' caseloads, where it is identified, how it is understood by the worker, how it is recorded and the response made to it. It is difficult to estimate the extent of domestic violence encountered and identified by social workers, since contact with a department may be for other reasons, most notably when there are issues relating to the welfare or safety of children. A study of social work case records in Boston in the early part of the twentieth century found that 34 per cent of the cases involved wife-beating (Gordon, 1989). An estimate of one-third of the 103 cases analysed in a more recent study involved domestic violence (Maynard, 1985). Interestingly, these figures are contrary to the expectations of social workers themselves that researchers would find very few cases (Borkowski *et al.* 1983; Maynard, 1985). One feature of all the studies on this theme suggests that the figures which are estimated and recorded by social workers greatly underestimate the full extent of the problem.

Maynard also found that despite the high level of violence against partners identified in case records, other factors were held responsible by social workers for 'the source of the problem'. Violence was regularly ignored as a causative factor in family problems and as the primary cause of distress in the women concerned in almost all of the cases analysed in her study (Maynard, 1985). In only 12 per cent of cases were physical abuse by a partner seen by social workers to be central to the problems of the woman and her children. Social workers in only three cases in the study felt obliged to visit specifically because of a man's violence to his partner. This research raises questions about the training of social workers for domestic violence work and the way in which they place the needs of women secondary to the needs of children, rather than responding to the needs of both.

The prevalence and identification of domestic violence as a cause of problems within families lead to a second important theme. The way in which domestic violence is understood by social workers is critical in the response made to it both by agencies and individual social workers. One of the achievements of the women's movement has been the defining of domestic violence as a social problem rather than a phenomenon of violent individuals or relationships. This has ensured that women who are abused in this way have been supported by organisations such as Women's Aid in having their voices heard. Women have always found ways to resist battering by male partners, but throughout the latter part of the twentieth century they have begun to resist it ideologically and politically in a more public arena (Gordon, 1989). The establishment of Women's Aid in the early 1970s was a key factor in this process. It was followed in the 1990s by Shakti, Gryffe and Southall Black Sisters all of which have responded to the specific needs of black women and their children. These organisations have provided much of the political impetus for changes in the response of police, social work and health agencies to domestic violence and they have provided vital research material on which to base their arguments for change.

UNDERSTANDING DOMESTIC VIOLENCE: THE SOCIAL WORK PERSPECTIVE

It remains curious that despite the advent of anti-discriminatory practice and the development of feminist practice, the social work response to domestic violence still adheres to pathologising or family systems models (Central Council for Education and Training in Social Work, 1989; Dominelli and MacLeod, 1989; Hanmer and Statham, 1988; Langan and Day, 1992; Phillipson, 1992; Wise, 1984). The main reason for this is because women in violent relationships are still seen by many social workers as 'clients in need of therapy, rather than people in need of alternatives and choices' (Dobash and Dobash, 1992, p. 234). Jones (1989) in a review of literature relating to agency responses to domestic violence reiterates this point and goes further, suggesting that,

> 'agencies including social services departments, different branches of the medical profession, local authority housing departments ... all point in the same direction – domestic violence is condoned to a certain point ... only when violence exceeds the limits [sic] does the condemnation become overt.'

> (p. 102)

Gordon (1989) provides a useful historical perspective on the issue. She argues that the social work response to wife-beating in the early twentieth century was negligible or, at best, framed in terms of child protection. She suggests that there is an historically consistent thread in the social work response to domestic violence, recorded from the earliest casenotes. These show a marked reluctance to afford women time in their own right to talk about violent partners. Women turned to child protection agencies because of the inadequacy of police protection for themselves and their children. The records show how women wanted separation and maintenance agreements which the police could not provide. The social workers to whom the women were referred were faced with a contradictory set of constraints – attempting to shore up two-parent families, and failing, because of the lack of options open to them, to reform violent men. As a consequence of their inability to respond in a positive way, many social workers found themselves ignoring wife-beating. They were then able to redefine the problem with which they were confronted in this way:

154

'when it could not be ignored, caseworkers, especially those with a therapeutic emphasis, began to define it as a problem for the woman to work on.'

(Gordon, 1989, p. 280)

Social workers need to be able to identify when domestic violence is happening in a family. Some indicators of potential abuse are outlined in Table 6.1 and these may be a helpful when a worker suspects that a woman is being abused in this way.

Table 6.1   *Possible indicators of domestic violence*

In a woman:
- self directed abuse
- depression
- anxiety
- describes jealous, possessive partner
- hit, slapped, punched or kicked by partner
- minimises injuries received from partner

- violent nightmares
- insomnia
- alcohol or drug abuse
- defends partner's behaviour
- frightened of partner's behaviour

In a man:
- explosive temper
- constantly criticising or denigrating
- controlling of partner
- breaks or throws objects when angry
- makes all decisions about family matters

- over-protective
- jealous
- suspicious
- has hit, slapped or punched partner
- defensive about partner's injuries

In children:
- school difficulties
- poor attention span
- withdrawn
- increased fears
- violent behaviour, especially in boys

- unexplained injuries
- somatic or emotional problems
- behavioural problems
- sleep problems

Gordon documents how, during the 1930s, there were further attempts to make women responsible for the violence perpetrated against them. She shows how social workers started by trying to reform violent men but, since professional casework concentrated on office visits, fewer men were seen. Women, by comparison were seen as 'more introspective and critical and therefore more productive in casework' (Gordon, 1989, p. 282). In the search for ways to help 'troubled families' it soon became acceptable to focus on the members of the family – women and children – most open to the influence of social workers. This had the effect of pathologising women rather than locating responsibility with violent men. The legacy of this perspective is still widely prevalent in social work today.

After the Second World War there was a further shift in emphasis with attention focused on 'wife and gender maladjustment' (Gordon, 1989, p. 296). One standard text of the time on marital conflict categorised problems which resulted in domestic violence into several categories, four of which referred to women's 'faults' (excessive pressure, the need to suffer, rejection of femininity, and sex response) and three to external pressures (interfering relatives, cultural differences and economic factors). There was no reference to any responsibility on the part of the man for the violence. Gordon emphatically rejects such explanations and concludes,

'One assault does not make a battered woman: she becomes that because of her socially determined inability to resist her escape, her lack of economic independence, law enforcement services and lack of self-confidence.'

(Gordon, 1989, p. 284).

We may wish to believe that attitudes and assumptions among social workers have changed; that they no longer blame the women whose partners are violent; that they will support women in challenging male violence and finding an alternative to destructive relationships for themselves and their children. It does not appear, however, that we have yet reached this point. The explanations which are given for men's violent behaviour are discussed elsewhere in this volume: their significance for social workers lies in the way they reinforce familial values and role expectations for both women and men. Intergenerational theories, for example, have an important part to play in the social work canon, especially since they sanction intervention 'for the sake of the children'. The argument here is that children who experience and witness violence are socialised to accept violence as a way of life and as a legitimate solution to their problems. Gelles supports this view when he asserts.

'not only do families expose individuals to violence and the techniques of violence but the family teaches approval for the use of such violence.'

(Gelles, 1974, p. 98)

It is worth noting that 'family' in this context is curiously non genderspecific. This is a feature of much social work literature on the family, especially in relation to the care of children. It ignores the fact that the responsibility for child care still lies predominantly with women. An alternative perspective is offered by Moore (1975) who reports that social workers attached to one sample of families where the man was violent, considered that more than 80 per cent of the children were adversely affected by it, making them jumpy, nervous and anxious. Children are also burdened by feeling that they are in some way responsible for the abuse or for not trying to stop it. The long-term effects of witnessing the abuse of one parent by a partner are discussed later in this chapter. For the moment it can be noted that many children witness or hear the violence perpetrated on women within their families. Dobash and Dobash (1979), for example, found that almost half the violent incidents in their study happened in front of observers, more than 60 per cent of whom were children in the care of the couple.

A further theoretical perspective which has had an important and potentially damaging implication for the social work response to women in violent relationships is the theory of 'learned helplessness' (Walker, 1978; 1979; 1984). The theory purports to explain why women become victims of violence in the first place and it offers one explanation of the reasons why women find it difficult to leave. In common with other approaches which concentrate on the 'victims' it traces the roots of victimisation in a woman's background rather than in that of the violent man. It suggests that, once planted in childhood, the seeds of the condition take root in all women's relationships with men. The theory proposes that women in violent relationships do not identify what is happening as the perpetrator's problem. They reinterpret violent events as a consequence of their failure as partners, they become more shamed and humiliated with each incident and silence is their final response. Walker argues that once women perceive themselves to be helpless they start behaving in ways in which reinforce their helplessness, passivity and submissiveness. In an effort to explain why women do not leave violent partners, the theory offers a view of women as helpless and hopeless, held captive by a combination of their psychology and gender socialisation (Dobash and Dobash, 1992).

Ferraro and Johnson (1982) present an alternative view. They argue that women are only ready to leave a violent relationship when they are psychologically ready to stop denying or minimising the abuse. Once this happens they are ready to choose an alternative to remaining in the relationship. Catalysts which prompt this to occur include an increase in the severity and visibility of the violence, the external definition of the problem by an 'outside' party such as a social worker and a change in the woman's available resources which encourages her if she is in the process of leaving a violent man. This last point is reiterated by Dobash and Dobash (1992) who present a summary of the evidence that the most important factors in women's efforts to leave a violent relationship are her economic and employment status. They argue that the theory of learned helplessness renders it impossible to tell

'whether a woman suffering [from learned helplessness] finds it impossible to seek help or whether she begins to pursue help and then stops because she suffers from this psychological ailment.'

(Dobash and Dobash, 1992, p. 227).

They point to dangers in adhering to this static model, suggesting instead a dynamic process of change in women's perceptions of the nature of the violence, their predicament and in their patterns of help-seeking. They argue that theories which rely on a partial understanding of women's psychology are rigid in their categorisation, seeing people as either healthy (acting consistently and deliberately) or unhealthy (suffering from a condition which makes it impossible for them to do so). If the latter is the case then it follows that women

'cannot be hesitant, confused or ambivalent. Women either leave or stay. They, like everyone else, cannot engage in diverse, even contradictory action.'

(Dobash and Dobash, 1992, p. 233)

The issue is even more complicated in cases where learned helplessness has been used as part of the defence of provocation when a woman has murdered a violent partner (Kennedy, 1992). In these cases the defence presents evidence to support the view that the woman has been so psychologically battered that her violent response is excused on the grounds of diminished responsibility rather than justification for a reasonable act. This again places the woman firmly in the role of victim.

The implications for social work practitioners are clear. If social workers understand women's condition and behaviour in any of these ways, the help they offer is likely to perceive women as victims and clients in need of therapy. It will concentrate primarily on the needs of children and on women's reconciliation to or accommodation of violent partners. Women's own needs are ignored, their strengths minimised and once again attention is diverted from the root of the problem – violent men and the social and political structures which support male violence.

Social workers respond in a variety of ways to a disclosure of domestic violence and they still appear to have no clear idea about the sort of assistance they might give. Maynard (1985) reported that little was immediately done to help the woman. The presenting problem of a partner's violent behaviour was usually defined as a matter of concern for child welfare. A common response is to 'talk about the problem' rather than to give practical assistance and outline the available options for a woman and her children irrespective of whether she chooses to leave or to remain in the relationship (Bowker, 1983).

Maynard (1985) found cases where a woman was blamed for a man's violent behaviour. Her perceived 'failings' were expressed by social workers in terms of poor housekeeping and not meeting her partner's sexual demands. These were regarded by social workers as 'understandable' reasons for the domestic violence. Indeed, one casenote quoted in the study noted 'it seems her nagging is a trigger for domestic violence'.

In general terms it appears that social workers' responses to domestic violence are determined by workers' own value systems and their perception of women's roles within the family rather than as individuals in their own right. Their responses are also the result of adhering to stereotyped images of women who experience domestic violence and the beliefs of individual social workers about why it occurs. There are also contradictory messages relating to the privacy of home and family life for adults and the challenging of that privacy when there are questions raised about the protection of children. The consequence for women in violent relationships is that there is a greater readiness by social workers to give help and assistance once a woman has made the break from her own home. Only then does there appear to be a greater willingness to define the woman's needs in her own right and to re-categorise her as 'deserving'. The situation is neatly summed up by Borkowski *et al.*, (1983, p. 72):

159

'The irony is that privacy contributes to and reinforces the intimacy and sense of solidarity in family life that society values, whilst it also nurtures and protects 'the conditions' in which conflicts and violence develop.'

Jones (1989) summarises the social work response to domestic violence into two main categories. First there is a concern with keeping families together and, second, putting the needs of children first. This was confirmed by Dobash and Dobash (1979) who noted that social workers gave practical assistance on housing and legal issues only when children were perceived to be in physical danger. Even in these cases women can be caught in a double bind, feeling threatened with the potential loss of their children into care because they do not have adequate or secure accommodation. This threat can, in turn, be enough to make them return to the family home with the possibility of further violence perpetrated on themselves and their children. Jones (1989) attributes the primary concern for reconciliation to a context of social work training courses which stresses working within the family context to solve problems occurring in families. This perspective pays little account to the different experiences of individual family members and it fails to locate responsibility for the problem of domestic violence with the violent man.

FREQUENCY OF CONTACT BETWEEN BATTERED WOMEN AND SOCIAL WORKERS

It is now well established that women in violent relationships, far from remaining passive, engage in an active process of seeking help, referred to as 'staying, leaving and returning' (Dobash and Dobash, 1979). Relatives, especially mothers, are often the first to be contacted for support; social workers are not immediately thought of as a source of help and many women, in common with the general population, do not have a clear idea of what they might offer (Jones, 1989). In Mama's (1989) study of black women's experiences in two London Boroughs, when women were asked if they had contacted social services departments, some said yes, they had found it necessary to seek assistance from the Department of Social Security. This showed a general and very common confusion about the respective roles of social workers and Department of Social Security staff.

Despite this lack of understanding, many women do contact social services departments when they are in a violent relationship, if they are on the point of leaving it or if they have left and are seeking alternative accommodation. One study found that 95 per cent of women in its sample had contacted social workers during a violent relationship, 5 per cent making contact after the first attack and 20 per cent after the most recent attack (Dobash and Dobash, 1979). A later study noted an increase in the level of contact with social services from the first attack (7 per cent) to the most recent attack (43 per cent) (Pahl, 1985). This research confirms earlier studies with the finding that 75 per cent of the sample had contacted a social worker for practical assistance and emotional support before seeking refuge outside the family home. It is also known that for many women, family friends and relatives are the main support as they struggle with trying to make sense of their experiences. They often widen their help-seeking network to include social workers once they have made the transition from seeking help in trying to make the relationship work to seeking help in ending or leaving it (Bowker 1983).

Mama's study of two London authorities (1989) provides a graphic illustration of the reluctance of social welfare agencies to meet the basic needs of black women leaving violent relationships. Thirty-three per cent of her sample had made contact with social services departments and there were marked differences between ethnic groups. Half of all the Asian women had made contact, 2 per cent of the Caribbean women and only two of the six African women in the sample. There were also marked differences in women's descriptions of their experiences of social work contact, with none of the Caribbean women seeing it as positive and only a small number of Asian women doing so.

It is important for social workers to understand the difficult and tentative way in which women begin to come to terms with the fact that they are in an abusive relationship. They often feel an enormous sense of personal failure, they can have fears about 'going public' on a matter of such private personal concern and they can have justifiable fears about their own safety and that of their children. They may also be concerned about the reaction of social workers to a disclosure of domestic violence. The way in which a woman is interviewed plays an important part here (Chaplain, 1988). If she feels that she is believed and responded to in a supportive and sympathetic way this can facilitate her recovery from the traumatic events which have led her to seek help. Table 6.2 outlines some suggestions which can be employed by social workers in this respect.

Social workers themselves exhibit variety in their response to domestic violence but research shows that they appear to have no clear idea of what sort of assistance they might give to women in this situation. Maynard (1985) reported that little is immediately done by social

161

Table 6.2   *Helping a woman to disclose domestic violence: some guidelines for social workers*

- Try to conduct the interview in a quiet, private place away from the violent partner and the family home.

- If the woman's children are present, try to have them looked after while the interview is taking place.

- Be aware that the woman is checking out how safe you are to tell. She has every right to do this.

- Be aware that you may be the first person, particularly the first professional, to acknowledge problems she has experienced.

- If she discloses domestic violence, validate her experiences and the difficulties she now faces.

- Find out if she has any other sources of support e.g. family, friends, colleagues and how she plans to use them.

- Ask what *she wants* to do rather than give a view on what *you think* she ought to do. Remember how difficult it is for a woman to leave her home and that she may have taken many years to get to this point.

- Ensure that up-to-date information on local sources of help, especially Women's Aid and legal help, is available.

- Be prepared for her to return to a partner who is violent; many women make attempts over a number of years to leave before finally doing so.

workers to provide practical help and the presenting problem is immediately redefined as a matter of concern for child welfare rather than support for the woman. An additional factor here is the perception of social work contact by other professionals (Johnson, 1985). Borkowski *et al.*, (1983) found that social work intervention is not seen as helpful by other practitioners including health visitors, doctors and solicitors.

Again and again we are presented with three facts: that social workers are seen as a source of help but women are unclear about what they can offer and their role is often confused with that of the DSS; the social workers themselves are unclear about their role, that their response is often to reframe the problem in terms of child protection and that they can unintentionally precipitate a woman's return to a violent partner. If a social worker conveys to a woman whose self-esteem and energy are already low that she should put up with the violence for the sake of her children, her sense of failure is compounded.

WHAT WOMEN SAY ABOUT SOCIAL WORK'S RESPONSE TO DOMESTIC VIOLENCE

Despite these limitations in the response of social workers to women seeking help, there appears to be a relatively high level of satisfaction from women themselves with the response they receive. Binney *et al.*, (1981) noted that of the 50 per cent of a sample who had sought help from social workers, more than half were satisfied. Pahl (1985) and Bowker (1983) confirm these levels of satisfaction, with Pahl noting that satisfaction was higher if the woman felt that a social worker helped in securing practical successes such as a place at a refuge. Indeed, both of these researchers have found that social workers are the most common source of referrals to Women's Aid refuges.

At initial contact with a social worker, women stress the importance of having up-to-date, accurate information, help with finding accommodation and learning about a refuge. Later they use social workers for support in making a new home and coping with life as a single parent. The most consistently valued support from social workers is their perceived ability to 'work the system' on a woman's behalf, advising on available services, sharing knowledge of relevant legislation and negotiating on the woman's behalf with other agencies. On the other hand, women who have made a number of attempts to leave violent partners may be prevented from seeking help from social workers because of previous unhelpful contact or because an individual social worker is negatively influenced if a woman has returned to the violent relationship in the past (Homer *et al.*, 1984).

SOCIAL WORK, HOUSING AND WOMEN'S AID – A CRUCIAL LINK FOR WOMEN

Women who are experiencing violence within their own homes are likely to have two immediate and basic housing requirements – access to safe emergency accommodation should they make the decision to leave, with or without children, and safe permanent housing in a suitable area in the longer term. In Scotland, under the provisions of the Matrimonial Homes (Family Protection) (Scotland) Act 1981, a woman can secure an exclusion order which puts the violent man out of the home, even if they are joint owners or tenants. The Act aimed to give women the choice whether to leave the family home or not and it does not affect women's rights under Part 2 of the Housing (Scotland) Act 1987. This legislation entitles women with children who have experienced violence to be classified as unintentionally homeless and, as such, to be eligible for accommodation from the local authority. The Act is important in listing both the potential for violence and a woman's fears of violence as sufficient evidence of her situation. Of course the Act is open to local interpretation and it can be difficult when a woman has no obvious local connection or if she is seeking accommodation during the night.

The true extent of women's homelessness because of violence or fear of violence remains unknown since national figures are not recorded by gender (Victim Support, 1992), so the true extent of this particular aspect of the problem is itself problematic. Binney *et al.* (1981) noted in their study of 114 refuges that women reported the lack of accommodation as the single most significant obstacle to leaving a violent partner. Relationship breakdown and domestic violence were noted as the biggest cause of homelessness among single women noted by Watson and Austerberry (1986), yet these women may find it more difficult to secure temporary accommodation from a local authority and a refuge may not be the most appropriate location for their needs to be met.

Mama (1989) notes some of the specific issues for black women in relation to housing needs: she points out that throughout the history of public housing provision there has always been the exclusion of particular groups, one of which is black people, especially women. Racial stereotyping and racist attitudes among housing officials and politicians have contributed to black women's access to public housing being severely restricted and circumscribed, with significant consequences for the longer-term well-being of women and their children.

There are three important issues in the provision of immediate or emergency accommodation for women in violent relationships. The first is the consistent implementation of homelessness legislation nationally, so that all women are treated equally. Secondly, there is the issue of funding for Women's Aid refuge space, both in real terms and in the quality of the accommodation offered. Binney *et al.* (1981) found that almost half the Women's Aid groups surveyed by them reported poor maintenance by a local authority landlord, despite being charged full rent. The poor condition of property was also exacerbated by severe overcrowding. Thirdly, there is the provision of safe permanent accommodation and the support available to women and children from social services, Women's Aid and other agencies, if and when it is secured. Some of the recommendations outlined in the Convention of

Scottish Local Authorities (COSLA) Report (1991) would greatly help here. These include:

- adopting the principle of refuge leases being held by Women's Aid;
- consultation with Women's Aid on the development and implementation of housing policies as they relate to women and children;
- a contact officer within housing departments;
- a commitment to reducing the time-lag between allocation of refuge space and secure accommodation;
- a commitment to increasing refuge space for women and children;
- increasing the options for women without children who have experienced domestic violence.

The potential for the combined role of social work, housing and Women's Aid is obvious; their individual practical, emotional and legislative resources have yet to be brought together in a way which helps to ensure that women, with or without children, are given a speedy response at a time when their need may be greatest.

CHILDREN, DOMESTIC VIOLENCE AND SOCIAL WORK

It is crucial for the subsequent well-being of women and their children that social workers, especially those with responsibility for child protection, are aware of the ways in which children experience the violence perpetrated on their mothers. There are a number of aspects to this issue. Firstly, it is important for social workers to understand and be aware of the ways in which children can be involved in the violence. Secondly, they need to have an understanding of the effects of domestic violence on children. Thirdly, they need to be more aware of ways in which women can be supported to care for children who may exhibit a range of disturbed behaviour and they need to challenge the view that all children who witness violence will themselves become violent in their adult relationships. There is also a clear need for child protection guidelines to take account of protecting children from abuse in the context of domestic violence. Finally, there are issues relating to social workers' own experiences of violence in relationships and their personal values in relation to the issue.

What children know and remember about domestic violence varies, and in contrast to adults who have been sexually abused as children, the long-term effects of their experiences are less well documented (Hall and Lloyd, 1993). Sometimes children are directly involved in the violence and they can be hurt in trying to protect their mother. Children may be forced to watch or participate in the abuse, they often hear the violence and they can see its effects on their mother. There is no doubt that living in an atmosphere of fear and tension can be damaging for children and this is heightened if they see their mother being beaten or abused in other ways (Women's Support Project, 1991).

One review of the literature summarised the effects of domestic violence on children (Jaffe *et al.*, 1991). Sleep disturbance, bullying, temper tantrums and an inability to concentrate were common. Some children's behaviour fluctuates from extreme passivity to sudden and unprovoked aggression. Others express feelings of acute anxiety, powerlessness and guilt about their inability to prevent assaults on their mother. Others exhibit the watchful behaviour of an abused child or they become exhausted from being kept awake at night. It has also been suggested that girls show a higher tendency to internalise the distress they feel with symptoms indicating depression and anxiety. The response of boys may be compounded by their greater likelihood to act out their distress by becoming aggressive or defiant at school or with peers (Jaffe *et al.*, 1986). Children can also be used by violent men to control or manipulate women after they have left a violent partner. O'Hara (1993) cites a number of examples of this, including verbal abuse, threats towards women and children at access visits and the abduction of children in an effort to force women to return to the relationship. Many children who live in families where women are being assaulted by their partners experience physical abuse themselves. Bowker *et al.* (1988) found that 70 per cent of men who beat their wives were also physically violent towards children living in the same house, and O'Hara (1993) cites a number of studies which give figures of between 28 and 70 per cent.

There may be additional problems if a pregnant woman is being battered by her partner. It is now known that battering may start or intensify during pregnancy, that it may lead to miscarriage and that 45 per cent of all women who experience domestic violence do so during pregnancy (Helton, 1986). In these situations it is vital that social workers do nothing which reinforces a woman's fear or her low self-esteem. Finding out about alternative housing, counselling and welfare resources on her behalf will help her to feel less isolated and more in control of her life.

All of these issues are important from a child protection perspective. Child protection guidelines which relate to the protection of children from abuse have little to say about their protection in the context of domestic violence. Two recent cases provide a sobering illustration of this issue. The first was the death in early 1992 of three-year-old Toni Dales. Toni was killed by the man in whose home she lived, after her skull was broken when he threw her across a room. The report which investigated her death noted how social services had not made contact with the child who was in the care of a man with a long record of violence towards women, including her mother (Cleveland County Council/National Children's Bureau, 1993). This information had been passed from the police to the probation service who were involved because of the man's separate conviction for violence. Nursery staff had noted the child's disturbed behaviour; the police were informed but concluded that there was not enough evidence to prosecute. At no time did professionals meet to pool information which could have protected her. The report on Toni's death noted with chilling dispassion,

> 'The likelihood is of the existence of domestic violence. It appeared to be perceived as "acceptable" without clarification of details of the assault.'

(Cleveland County Council/National Children's Bureau, 1993, p. 33)

Social workers' awareness of the nature and extent of domestic violence and the ways it can be linked with violence against children was also highlighted in the report on the death of Sukina Hammond in 1988 (Avon County Council and Department of Health, 1989). She died at the age of six, the result of a physical attack by her father. Her mother was also attacked trying to protect Sukina. Nine months previously Sukina's father tied her mother to a chair and beat her for many hours. The report on her death notes that this was described at a case conference as 'a domestic incident'.

Four themes emerge from these cases. First, they both demonstrate a lack of understanding of what the behaviour of both children was indicating; second, they show little understanding by social care professionals of the nature of domestic violence; third, there was poor co-ordination of the statutory response to repeated incidents of domestic violence; and fourth, there was a marked reluctance of statutory authorities to intervene. This appears to have been partly based on a weak understanding of domestic violence.

The implications for social work policy-makers and practitioners are clear. In the first instance it is vital to improve training for social workers on the cause, nature and consequences of domestic violence for women and their children. There is also a need for training to see women not as victims but as survivors with courage, strengths and personal resources which they can use for themselves and their children. Secondly, there is a strong argument for incorporating issues relating to child protection and domestic violence in child protection guidelines and for establishing local co-ordinating groups for professionals and activists working in this area. The report on Toni Dales's death made this point when it argued for a concentrated local effort to tackle the issue of violence against women. There is also a vital role for carers who work with children who have lived in violent households so that their isolation and fear are reduced. Letting them know that other children feel the same and they too feel frightened when the abuse is going on can be enough to stop children blaming themselves. All of this has implications for the training of staff of family centres, nurseries and child-care social workers.

SOCIAL WORK AND WOMEN'S AID

A report produced by the Convention of Scottish Local Authorities (COSLA, 1991) noted tensions in the relationship between social work departments in Scotland and local Women's Aid groups. Social workers are the main source of referrals to Women's Aid, yet social work departments provide few resources for women living in or leaving violent relationships. There may always be tensions between these two agencies: one based firmly in the voluntary sector, operating from a clear, unambiguous feminist perspective with a value base which is collectivist, empowering and autonomous; the other perceived by it as a patriarchal institution which has, by its inactivity in the past, been seen to condone male violence towards children or, at best, put the needs of children before those of women – at the expense of both.

Women's Aid recognises that it can only meet a fraction of the needs of battered women and their children. It is, however, the 'expert voice' in the field of domestic violence, yet it is frequently marginalised and ignored by social work departments. This is well illustrated by its consistently low, intermittent or irregular level of funding from this source. In 1990–91, 17,257 women approached the Scottish Women's Aid network of groups for help (Scottish Women's Aid, 1992). Table 6.3 shows an increase in referrals of 1,781 over the previous year and also shows the large number of women turned away because of the lack of an available space in a refuge.

Many of these women returned, in the absence of a viable alternative for themselves and their children, to the violence of their home. Others may have approached the homelessness section of their local housing department where the reaction to their situation depends on the availability of resources and the definition of 'unintentionally homeless' adopted by the housing authority.

Sustained, regular and realistic levels of funding for Women's Aid is clearly a priority. In addition, however, there is a need for a clearer un-

Table 6.3   *Referrals to Women's Aid in Scotland 1989–91*

	1989–90	1990–91
Refuge places	237	254
Women in refuge	1,888	1,810
Children in refuge	3,002	2,886
Women turned away	3,396	3,896
Women seeking info/help	10,192	11,549
Total	15,476	17,257

Source: Scottish Women's Aid (1992) Annual Report for 1991.

derstanding of the role of Women's Aid and of the service which it provides to women and children. The training of social workers by
Women's Aid staff, many of whom are themselves women who have
left violent relationships, is another way of improving communication
between the two agencies. This can also help to ensure that women who
make contact with social work departments are not faced with disbelief
or shame (Gondolf, 1988). There is also the potential for social workers
to develop groups for women who are in or have left violent relationships. Again, these have the potential for making a women feel less
isolated, reducing her feelings of guilt and for increasing her self-
esteem (Horley, 1988; Ni Carthy, 1984).

MULTI-AGENCY APPROACHES TO DOMESTIC VIOLENCE

Some local authorities are beginning to co-ordinate initiatives to
respond to domestic violence through education, joint investigative
practice, working parties on specific topics and research initiatives with
local academic institutions. Most of these initiatives bring together a
range of departments and non-statutory agencies in the same geographical area, with the aim of ensuring that policy and practice are conducted in a consistent and well-informed way. In theory, this sounds
straightforward; in practice, there are issues of competing interests, professional rivalry and resource allocation within and between agencies.
These initiatives can, as in so many other areas of joint work, make the
process of inter-agency collaboration infinitely more complicated.
There is an additional underlying difficulty which relates to the understanding of the nature of domestic violence and the most appropriate
response to it.

In 1991, NALGO published a report reviewing local authority initiatives to combat violence against women (NALGO, 1991). The report's title *Responding with Authority: Local Authority Initiatives to Counter Violence Against Women* suggests a more proactive approach to the issue and its contents give a useful blueprint, with examples, of how some local authorities have developed and implemented initiatives. The document notes that successful multi-agency initiatives are characterised by two features: a willingness to share expertise and build up links, and a well-defined and realistic set of tasks. It is suggested, for example, that one approach might be to restrict the activities of multi-agency groups to information exchanges and co-ordinating the existing response to domestic violence. Another is to break down the areas of responsibility within working parties or groups and examine the response of each participating agency within that context.

The London Borough of Hammersmith and Fulham provides an example of one approach. In 1987 the Community and Police Committee investigated the incidence of domestic violence in its geographical area and the responses of all local agencies to it. The report of the investigation (Hammersmith and Fulham Borough, 1988) then formed the basis of widespread changes in council policy in housing and social service provision for women and children who experience domestic violence. This was followed in 1989 by a multi-agency group which looked specifically at the police response to the issue. Representatives from the police, Women's Aid, Victim Support, a local law centre, women and equal opportunities officers and a specialist police unit were all involved. Information was gathered and analysed and a number of recommendations for change were made. This example shows how one initiative can lead to other developments, all with the aim of making improvements in agencies' response to women in violent relationships.

The impetus for a joint agency initiative can come from any source. Individual workers who are concerned about domestic violence, a women's health project, the police, a local incident or increased media attention all have a role to play. A day conference can be a useful means of starting multi-agency discussions and raising awareness of issues relating to violence against women. Such events can also play an important part in public education. A good example comes from Edinburgh where, during 1992–3 a series of conferences, public debates and a highly visible poster campaign were instigated by the regional council in conjunction with local organisations, community groups and academics. The combined campaign is called 'Zero Tolerance' and, drawing on experience from Canada, took as its main theme the simple idea that violence against women and children should not be tolerated in a civilised society. A number of conferences were planned and opened to the public; they debated a wide range of issues relating to domestic violence and other forms of violence against women; agency responses were challenged and possible ways ahead were debated. At the same time the poster campaign, which used simple and direct images on key sites throughout the city, demonstrated the extent of violence against women and children in Scotland. The campaign was the first major advertising campaign in Britain with the aim of attempting to challenge societal attitudes towards the physical and sexual assault by men of women and children. It also carried a strong message about the need for men to change their behaviour.

The campaign has now been taken up in other Scottish local authorities, led by women's or equal opportunities' units. In London it has been reworked to focus on domestic violence alone and the images it uses are of male perpetrators rather than the women they abuse. This has aroused considerable debate in relation to the contrast in images between Edinburgh's empowering presentation of women and children in everyday situations and the London campaign's images of perpetrators who are variously angry and pathetic. There is also a substantive difference in the slogans used by the two cities; Edinburgh posters have the line 'Male abuse of power is a crime' on every display, whilst the London posters have adopted the softer slogan 'It's not just a fact of life, it's a crime'. A final point of note is that the Edinburgh campaign deliberately opened with an issue which was impossible for the public or institutions to oppose – that of child abuse – and it gradually worked towards the final slogan in a way which was desensitising and challenging. As Riddoch (1994) notes, 'Domestic violence has been accepted for centuries. It takes a persuasive approach, not a prescriptive one, to get real change happening.' An evaluation of the Edinburgh campaign has concluded that it has been successful in attracting attention and generating debate about the issues it highlights. It has also caused people to reflect on the power which they have as adults and as men and it has also challenged some misconceptions about domestic violence and child abuse (Kitzinger and Hunt, 1994).

Local authorities in Scotland produced a joint report which made a number of recommendations in relation to the response of all local authority departments to domestic violence (COSLA, 1991). The report noted that little had been done to assess the extent of domestic violence in Scotland; indeed only one district authority has made any systematic attempt to gather information of this kind (Aberdeen District Council 1990). Most authorities rely on referrals to Women's Aid as a guide, whilst acknowledging that these figures represent only a fraction of the problem.

Calling for a corporate response, the report outlined a number of recommendations for a positive multi-agency response. These include:

- producing an information leaflet on the range of services available to women affected by domestic violence;
- undertaking research to assess the extent of the problem in any geographical area before assessing the most appropriate multi-agency response;
- setting targets for action within and between agencies and instigating a monitoring and review system in conjunction with Women's Aid;
- encouraging the development of a multi-agency approach with the inclusion of health professionals, the Department of Social Security and the voluntary sector;
- more preventive work through education in schools and in the community;
- training in all aspects of domestic violence which is undertaken in conjunction with Women's Aid;
- the nomination of a senior member of staff in each agency as an initial contact person for domestic violence issues;
- an examination of ways of improving liaison between individual departments and between local authorities and Women's Aid.

Change in the way organisations respond to the issue of violence against women has been, and will continue to be slow, but change is occurring. Another potential area for innovation is in joint training and joint work. Social workers and police are already undertaking joint investigations in the area of child abuse. There is, as yet, little evidence that this will happen for domestic violence but the establishment of specialist units within police forces may point the way ahead. At present these units adhere to one of two models – either for the investigation of adult sexual offences or as specialist child abuse investigation units (Burman and Lloyd, 1993). In Scotland none of these units has a remit for domestic violence, although there are separate units for this purpose in some English police forces.

SOCIAL WORK PROGRAMMES FOR VIOLENT MEN

The small increase in programmes for violent men has two potential effects on social work policy and practice. On the one hand they offer the possibility of men being forced to focus on their violent behaviour and, in the process, to change their behaviour so that choices other than violence are made (Sonkin and Durphy, 1989). On the other, they raise important questions about resources. If more money is allocated to the setting-up of programmes for battering men, it is argued, this could detract from the existing, if limited, support for women who experience their violence.

There are also questions relating to the most appropriate form of intervention in men's programmes. Eisikovitz and Edleson (1989) provide a clear account of the alternatives at present in operation, with a critique of the methods they employ. Within the criminal justice system, the use of arrest in reported cases of domestic violence has produced evidence that it produces a reduction or cessation in violence (Dobash and Dobash, 1992). A counter-argument here is that arrest and prosecution of violent men increases women's vulnerability (Sherman and Berk, 1984). An evaluation of conciliation and mediation schemes also show that they are inappropriate for dealing with wife assault (Lerman, 1984).

During the 1980s, diversion schemes were introduced in Scotland as a means of directing offenders from the criminal justice system prior to prosecution. Violent men were diverted to social work programmes and, more recently, to conciliation and reparation schemes. Strong objections to both approaches were voiced by Scottish Women's Aid, who pointed out that diverting at the pre-prosecution stage demonstrated to an offender, their partner and society at large that domestic violence is an offence not worthy of legal sanction. As a result, some agencies have now reconsidered their policy on the issue and have opted for diversion from the criminal justice system after a case has gone to court (Moody, 1983).

Similar reservations have been expressed about the usefulness of family therapy and couple therapy, two models of work often employed by social workers. Here, the intervention focuses on the interactions within the family system rather than on challenging male behaviour (Maynard, 1985). Men often fail to attend family therapy sessions so the woman can again be left feeling responsible for the violence. Further isolation and self-blame often ensue. There is an additional danger here, with the implication that violence is a 'family problem' rather than something which is the responsibility of the perpetrator. This can also convey a message to the woman that couples should stay together. There is also the potential for an increase in violence by the man when the woman talks openly about her experiences and feelings when the couple are still living together (Adams, 1988).

A more radical model which is currently being implemented in Scotland focuses on two main areas – the man's violent behaviour and an unequivocal rejection of it. Its central tenet is that domestic violence is never justified and that it is a serious crime (Adams, 1988; Pence and Paynar, 1990). The work with offenders does not entail any couple therapy, which might inadvertently transfer responsibility for the violence to the woman. Instead, the offender is the joint responsibility of the courts and local social services departments. Using the Duluth model, which was first conceptualised and implemented in Duluth, Minnesota (Dobash and Dobash 1992), men are processed through the courts and are required to attend re-education sessions which are aimed at ending their violence. Failure to comply with these conditions results in the offender being returned to court.

A programme based at the Centre for the Study of Violence at the University of Stirling builds on the Duluth model by aiming to improve men's understanding of their violent behaviour; it also aims to help them change it. The programme uses a method of confrontational group work which means that men must face and accept responsibility for their violent behaviour and their need to change it. The focal point for the work is the man's violence. Violent events are described and re-enacted in a group setting, showing that these events are not the result of uncontrolled urges. Re-enactment provides a useful insight into feelings and emotions to the point at which the man made the choice of violence. Analysis of this 'critical moment' allows the man to consider the way in which the violent incident progressed and developed, to re-enact the event and to consider choices he could have made at the moment when he chose violence (Dobash and Dobash, 1992).

These and similar programmes have increased our knowledge about men who abuse women and children. Social workers involved in them have confirmed that violent men have little empathy for others, that they use violence to coerce, control and dominate women and children and that they reject responsibility for their actions by trying to deflect this responsibility onto others. The programmes also offer men the possibility of finding more positive ways of dealing with anger, gaining insight into their emotions and improving empathy and self-control (Dickie, 1989). There is the risk, however, that they attract resources away from support for women because of their statutory nature. They will need to be carefully monitored and evaluated.

GENDER ISSUES IN WORKING WITH DOMESTIC VIOLENCE

The question of who works with violent men and women who have been subject to their violence remains a topic for debate (Beagley,

1987). On the one hand, it is argued, only male workers can truly understand men who are violent. The counter-argument demands proof that men can be entrusted with this responsibility. There are also issues relating to the collusion of men with each other, however inadvertently, in domestic violence work. It has, therefore, been suggested that, especially for programmes involving violent men, good practice entails women and men working together to provide a positive role model. This is an obvious area where training can be of great use. A related concern is the funding of programmes for violent men and for the support of women abused by them. There may be a risk that the former will drain resources from the already limited amount of financial assistance for women who have been abused by their partners.

SOCIAL WORK AND DOMESTIC VIOLENCE: A WAY AHEAD?

We have seen that, whilst local authority social work departments do not have a statutory responsibility for women who have experienced or are experiencing domestic violence, many women who are trying to leave a violent relationship approach social workers for advice and assistance. Neither the women themselves nor the social workers whom they contact have a clear idea of what can be provided. Support, information on legal, housing, welfare and access issues all fall within the remit of social workers. Women and children have very different needs in relation to domestic violence and it is impossible to respond to both their sets of needs in an innovative way if resources are limited or absent. In addition, social work managers are understandably reluctant to take on new responsibilities at a time of scarce resources.

There are, however, a number of measures which can be easily and effectively implemented at an organisational level and by individual social workers. These measures might include:

By the social work agency:
- Showing concern for the woman. Although there are major concerns relating to the needs of children who are living in families where a man is violent, women can be supported and responded to in ways which acknowledge their considerable personal strengths and resources. The presence of a social worker who is prepared to listen, believe and validate a woman's experience cannot be underestimated.
- Providing accurate and up-to-date information on local sources of practical and emotional support for women. This may be needed in a variety of languages and should be widely distributed and displayed.

- The identification of a specific, trained person within a social work department who has responsibility for liaison with other local authority departments, health professionals and Women's Aid.
- A twenty-four-hour point of social work contact for women living with or in the process of leaving a violent man. This could be publicised as part of the service offered by an out-of-hours social work team.
- Adequate material resources for support, advice and counselling services in the voluntary sector dealing with domestic violence and other forms of violence against women.
- Consulting with and including Women's Aid in matters of training and the development of policy for the social work response to domestic violence. In particular, issues relating to pre-court diversion of violent men and the resourcing of programmes for them merit discussion with Women's Aid.
- Undertaking regular training in conjunction with Women's Aid to ensure that social workers are aware of the reality of domestic violence and its effects.
- Monitoring the extent and nature of domestic violence in social work caseloads. This could be done simply by revising the categories on intake or referral records.

By individual social workers:
- Recognising signs which indicate that a woman is experiencing violence from her partner. Social workers need to be able to recognise the possible source of injuries when they have been inflicted by a partner.
- Recognising the effects of domestic violence on a women over time, the consequences for her self-esteem and her emotional and physical well-being.
- Validating a woman's experience by recording violent incidents in casenotes.
- Valuing a woman's strengths in surviving in the relationship and for protecting her children as best she can.
- Being clear about confidentiality, especially when the work includes child protection issues.
- Being realistic about the support which can be offered by a social worker to a woman immediately and in the longer term.

It is clear from the preceding discussion that social workers can offer a great deal to women and children who have been subjected to domestic violence. There are issues relating to policy-making, training and the attitudes and values of staff; the question of the different needs of women and children needs to be addressed and the whole area of multi-agency collaboration merits further discussion. Finally, it is interesting to note that the police, who have been heavily criticised in the past for their response to domestic violence, have begun to respond in a more positive way. The time is surely right for social work to follow their example.

* Thanks to Margaret Taylor, National Worker for Scottish Women's Aid, for helpful comments and suggestions on this chapter.

PART III

Elder Abuse

CHAPTER SEVEN

Elder Abuse: A Critical Overview

Chris Phillipson and Simon Biggs

INTRODUCTION

In the mid-1970s, a new phrase entered the lexicon of the caring professions – that of 'granny-battering' (Baker, 1975; Burston, 1977). In Britain, doctors and social workers began, from this period, to document cases of people subject to often severe instances of cruelty and neglect. Mervyn Eastman (1983; 1984; forthcoming), who was to become a leading figure in the debate, produced a monograph detailing numerous cases from his own records and from other contacts with older people and informal carers. Few could doubt, from the nature of his descriptions, that an important area of concern had been identified. Yet, shocking as the cases he identified certainly were, it might be argued that they made little immediate impact, either on the community of professionals concerned with caring for older people, or on the wider society. The reasons for this were threefold. First, for the professions involved with older people, adjustments were still being made to the various other forms of family violence identified in the 1960s and 1970s (notably child abuse and violence to women). Set in this context, the problems of 'battered grannies' (a term which hardly promoted the cause) struggled to gain a public hearing. Added to this was the low status of professionals concerned with caring for older people, who were often the least well qualified and worst paid in their respective groups (Phillipson, 1982; Biggs, 1993). Both the above factors limited the extent to which the issue of abuse would be taken seriously or treated with any degree of urgency. A second reason, however, was the status of older people in post-war British society. Fennell *et al.* (1988, p. 6) have described the 'welfarisation' of older people in this period, this involving they suggest a subtle mixture of diminution and patronage. The authors write:

'There may be nothing wrong with welfare, as such, but there is a risk that the people we welfarize, we do not allow fully human stature: they are not quite whole people, not people like us. They are only one step removed from the "poor dears" in nursing homes whom other elderly people are said to patronize in the subtle stratification system of the disadvantaged.'

The idea of the 'abused elder' seemed to fit, therefore, an existing stereotype which emphasised the marginality of the old. Indeed, it was difficult to separate cause and effect: were the old marginalised because of experiences such as abuse? Alternatively, was abuse all of a piece with the pathology of ageing, the 'inevitable' spiral of physical and mental decline faced by older people?

A final factor which hindered the debate on abuse was the term itself. Very few commentaries in this field can resist expressing concern at the range of definitions of abuse and/or their lack of precision (Johnson, 1991; Pitt, 1992; Ogg and Munn-Giddings, 1993). However, it would be more surprising if there was clarity and agreement in this area given the nature of the subject-matter. We are dealing, after all, with covert and overt conflict in social relationships, both private (in domestic settings), semi-public (in the special settings of residential homes and related forums), and public (in the wider society). Placing the nature of this conflict into precise concepts will always be difficult: there will always be a degree of selectivity in who we decide is being abused, and on what we see as representative of abuse. Moreover, as Glendenning (1993) remarks, definitions of the problem will always vary according to who is expressing concern: the victim, the carer, the physician, the nurse, the social worker, and so on. None of this is to say that the concept is worthless or to trivialise the experiences of those older people affected. It is, however, to suggest a degree of caution in terms of how we interpret issues in the debate about abuse and to recognise the difficulties of both analysis and intervention.

The purpose of this chapter is to explore a range of issues concerned with the concept of abuse: its definition, its prevalence, theories for its existence, and policy responses. The chapter will provide an assessment of current debates in this area. Because of the extensive literature now becoming available on this topic, the chapter provides a critical analysis of the concept of abuse as well as a review of the various dimensions associated with this phenomenon.

THE RE-DISCOVERY OF ABUSE

If elder abuse struggled to find a secure footing in professional concerns in the 1970s, it had certainly arrived by the mid-1990s. In Britain, in this period, the first detailed texts were published (Decalmer and Glendenning, 1993; Bennett and Kingston, 1993); practice guidelines emerged from the Department of Health (DoH/SSl, 1993); specific training materials began to be developed (Pritchard, 1992; Phillipson and Biggs, 1993), and pressure groups were formed (notably Action on Elder Abuse). This mounting concern for an issue which had been identified at least twenty years earlier needs a brief explanation. The reasons are complex but may be summarised as follows. First, in contrast to the situation in the 1970s, it almost certainly reflects the increased confidence and power of what Carroll Estes (1979, p. 2) describes as 'the aging enterprise – the programs, organizations, bureaucracies, interest groups, trade associations, providers, industries, and professionals that serve the aged in one capacity or another'. This group became more assertive in the 1980s and was able to push a range of issues concerning older people further up the agendas both of a number of professions and of society more generally. This was also supported by the expansion in the academic study of ageing, with findings from US research in the field of abuse influencing a number of British practitioners and academics (Bennett and Kingston, 1993; Decalmer and Glendenning, 1993).

Second, attention to abuse was also assisted by the growth of community care policies (Ogg and Munn-Giddings, 1993). Here, the emphasis on de-institutionalisation produced concern with, on the one side, the pressure faced by informal carers (Dalley, 1988); to, on the other, the potential for neglect and inadequate care of vulnerable groups such as very elderly people: the question of the 'informalisation of care' as a factor in the social creation of abuse is an issue we shall return to at the end of this chapter.

Third, acceptance of the idea of abuse was assisted by a critical debate concerning prevailing ideologies about, and services for, older people. In the 1970s, the idea of abuse was almost too shocking. Society – in the form of the welfare state – had focused on the old as one of the groups it was most concerned to shield from harm and misfortune. It was one thing that research had already revealed vast amounts of poverty and material deprivation (Townsend and Wedderburn, 1965): that at least could be explained and responded to with reforms (albeit inadequate). The idea of the old being subject to physical violence or financial exploitation in their own homes seemed to go too far: destroying in one go the mythology surrounding the post-war family (Seccombe, 1993). By the 1980s, however, the idea of violence as endemic in society was widely accepted (Dobash and Dobash, 1992), as was the view that older people were still losing out in the provision of services and support (Phillipson, 1982). Added to this was the view from critical perspectives within gerontology that dependency in old age (which abuse was clearly bound up with) was not a given, but was socially structured though a range of policies and professional ideologies (Estes, 1993). In this sense, the phenomena of abuse was no longer surprising in the 1990s: it could now be explained by prevailing theories and recognised as a social fact. Developing appropriate responses was, of course, another matter.

DEFINITIONS OF ABUSE

Enough has been said to indicate that the issue of defining abuse is one of considerable complexity. In the literature, the term 'granny bashing' has long been replaced by that of 'elder abuse' and 'elder neglect'. Other terms include 'elder mistreatment', 'inadequate care', and 'miscare' (Bennett and Kingston, 1993). Johnson (1986; 1991) has attempted to identify the different elements within the umbrella term of 'elder mistreatment'. She identifies four elements: first, an 'intrinsic definition' which conceptualises the phenomenon; second, a 'real definition' which indentifies the main elements of mistreatment; third, an 'operational' definition which gives measurable outcomes of those elements; fourth, a separation of the outcome of the phenomenon from the cause. Within this approach, Johnson's intrinsic definition of elder mistreatment is 'a state of self-or-other-inflicted suffering unnecessary to the maintenance of the quality of life of the older person' (1986, p. 180). Johnson then identifies the main elements of this suffering as physical, psychological, sociological, or legal circumstances, measured by their intensity (frequency and severity) and density (number of types). Finally, she focuses on the immediate causes of the suffering, neglect or abuse, which may be active (intentional) or passive (unintentional).

Fulmer and O'Malley (1987) provided a service perspective in their approach to defining abuse. In their definition all cases of abuse and neglect were described as 'inadequate care', defined as the presence of unmet needs for personal care. The needs included all basic requirements, as well as those of supportive relationships, the opportunity to define an acceptable lifestyle, and the freedom from all forms of violence. Thus, elder abuse can be defined as the 'actions of a caretaker that create unmet needs for the elderly person'. Neglect is defined as 'the

184

failure to respond adequately to established needs for care' (Fulmer and O'Malley, 1987). At present, there seems general agreement, following the work of Wolf and Pillemer (1989), for the main elements of elder mistreatment. These may be listed as follows:

1. *Physical abuse*: the infliction of physical harm, injury. Physical coercion, sexual molestation and physical restraint;
2. *Psychological abuse*: the infliction of mental anguish;
3. *Material abuse*: the illegal or improper exploitation and/or use of funds or resources;
4. *Active neglect*: the refusal or failure to undertake a caregiving obligation (including a conscious and intentional attempt to inflict physical or emotional stress on the elder);
5. *Passive neglect*: the refusal or failure to fulfil a caretaking obligation (excluding a conscious and intentional attempt to inflict physical or emotional distress on the elder).

(Wolf and Pillemer, 1989).

Glendenning (1993) concludes from his review of this area that a number of uncertainties still remain in the defining of abuse. These he identifies in terms of, first, the relationship between domestic and institutional abuse; second, the issue of whether elder abuse can be clearly differentiated from the abuse of other adults; third, the relationship between neglect and other forms of abuse. Further questions could be added to this list. In particular, there is the issue of whether we should restrict the concept to a limited range of actions (focusing, say, on physical and psychological abuse), or whether a broader focus (taking in more general social problems facing older people) is justified. Pitt (1992) makes the case for a restrictive approach, arguing for precision which will allow a quantification of the numbers of people involved and effective treatment strategies. Such a view is understandable given the slippery and evasive nature of the concept. However, the hope of containing abuse within a 'precise definition' could be illusory. No one professional group will be able to determine how abuse is defined; nor, it must be said, will there be any agreement until elders and carers are involved in the debate rather more than they are at present. Indeed, the inclusion of perspectives from older people will be essential if lasting solutions to the problem of elder abuse are to be found.

These various problems should not be taken to suggest that the concept is inherently flawed (although greater precision in its use is clearly justified). On the contrary, the position taken in this chapter is that the debate about the mistreatment of the old has been crucial for raising concerns about the quality of care for older people within domestic and institutional settings. That debate is clearly of the utmost importance and certainly justifies the place of elder mistreatment within the vocabulary of professional carers.

THE EXTENT OF ABUSE AND NEGLECT

It should be clear by now that discussions about the prevalence and incidence of abuse raise a number of difficulties. To ask how much abuse is in a given population (prevalence), and how many new cases are entering that population (incidence), is to raise questions of considerable complexity. To go back to the previous discussion: how much agreement is there on how abuse is being defined? If different agencies use different definitions then any figure produced is bound to be unreliable. Moreover, the source of information is important: are the reports from victims or are they from the records of professionals? Both raise different kinds of problems: the former issues of recall and accuracy; the latter problems of selectivity and the possibility of bias towards particular kinds of cases.

Accepting these points, there have been a limited number of prevalence studies in the US, Canada and the UK. The Boston study by Pillemer and Finkelhor (1988) involved interviews with around 2,000 older people and focused on three types of maltreatment – physical abuse, verbal aggression and neglect. Slightly more than 3 per cent of the population 65 years and older had been mistreated: twenty cases per 1,000 were physically mistreated; eleven per 1,000 were psychologically abused; and four per 1,000 were neglected. The authors estimate that if a national survey produced similar results, these numbers would represent almost a million people in the US. The survey also showed that spouse abuse was more prevalent (58 per cent) than abuse by adult children (24 per cent), that there were roughly equal numbers of male and female victims, and that economic status or age was not related to risk of abuse.

A national survey on elder abuse in Canada has been reported by Podnieks (1992). This research attempted, for the first time in Canada at a national level, to identify the prevalence and circumstances of abuse. Four categories of abuse were defined and studied: material abuse, chronic verbal aggression, physical violence, and neglect. Data were collected through a random sample telephone survey of 2,008 elderly persons living in private dwellings. The survey uncovered 80 persons who had been maltreated according to one or more of the study criteria. For the study sample, this translated into a rate of 40 mal-

186

treated elderly per 1,000 population. Material abuse emerged as the most widespread form of maltreatment in the survey, with a prevalence rate of between 19 and 33 victims per thousand. Chronic verbal aggression was the next most prevalent, affecting from 8 to 18 persons per thousand. The rate for physical violence was 3 to 9 cases per thousand, and for neglect, 2 to 6 per thousand.

Finally, the survey in Britain by Ogg and Bennett (1992) reported on results of structured interviews (through the nationwide Office of Population Censuses and Surveys omnibus survey) with almost 600 people aged 65 and over and 1,366 adult members of households in regular contact with a person of pensionable age. One in twenty older people reported some kind of abuse, but only one in fifty reported physical abuse. Although 10 per cent of adults admitted to verbal abuse, only 1 per cent acknowledged physical abuse.

All of the above studies are at least indicative of the existence of the phenomenon of abuse. On the other hand, the figures – as most of the authors of such studies admit – do need to be treated with some caution. First, questions have to be raised about the methodology of even the more rigorous research represented in the above studies. The US and Canadian work relied either wholly or in part on telephone surveys – some types of abuse may be under-reported using this type of approach. Second, some groups of older people are almost certainly under-represented in the survey – the very frail, the disadvantaged, people from minority ethnic groups. These groups may show a different pattern of abuse and neglect. Nonetheless, all three studies confirm the reality of abuse in the lives of significant numbers of older people. As Sprey and Matthews (1989) suggest, whether 3 per cent or 6 per cent or 10 per cent of all persons over 65 are abused is largely irrelevant. They argue (1989, p. 61): 'What must be known is who and where they are, and equally important, which forms of elder-elder and elder-other relationships are most likely to be associated with *what* types of mistreatment or neglect.' Following this, before reviewing some of the theories for abuse, we shall briefly consider research on the characteristics of the abused and those who abuse, as well as the issue of institutional abuse of older people.

THE CHARACTERISTICS OF THE ABUSED AND ABUSER

The Boston and Canadian prevalence studies both identified some important characteristics of abused elders. Both studies found victims to be in poor health; abused elderly were more likely to be living with someone else; and neglected elders were most likely to have no one to turn to for support. The Boston research, as already noted, reported that 58 per cent of the perpetrators were spouses. The underlying dynamic, as outlined by Pillemer and Finkelhor (1988), is that an elderly person is most likely to be abused by the person with whom he or she lives. Many more elders live with their spouses than with their children and thus many more elders are abused by spouses.

Additional information on the characteristics of abused older people is provided by the Three Model Project (of which the Boston prevalence study was one element), a detailed examination of elder abuse supported by the US National Institute on Aging. Bennett (1990) reports that in the three years of work of this project, 328 substantiated cases of abuse were assessed. The victims were more likely to be female, average age 76, living in a house with spouse or family. The abused were functionally impaired, half of them requiring supportive devices for mobility, a few were bedridden, a large majority had difficulties with some activities of daily living, and one-half had a cognitive impairment. The perpetrators tended to be sons rather than other family members, and psychological abuse tended to be the most common type, followed by physical abuse. The perpetrators were more likely to be dependent on the victims for finances. Their lives were stressful and they had health and financial problems. One-third had psychological problems and even more a history of mental illness and alcohol abuse. They tended to have unrealistic expectations of the capability of the abused elders and viewed their demands for attention as unreasonable.

The Three Model Project also included a special study of 42 physically abused elders with a similar number of non-abused elders acting as a control group. An interesting finding from this research was that the abused elderly did not appear to be in poorer health when compared with the control group. In contrast, the abusers were much more likely than the comparisons to be identified as having mental and emotional problems and as abusing alcohol.

Rosalie Wolf, summarising US research on the characteristics of abused and abuser, suggests that three different profiles have emerged:

1. Victims of physical abuse and psychological abuse tend to be physically well (reasonable activities of daily living scores) but have emotional problems. The abusers have a history of alcoholism and/or mental illness, live with the victim, and are dependent upon them financially.
2. Victims of neglect are usually very old, and mentally and physically impaired with little social support. The carer finds the victim a great source of stress.

3. Victims of financial (material) abuse tend to be unmarried with limited social contacts/networks. The abusers have financial problems sometimes traceable to a history of drug or alcohol abuse.

(cited in Bennett and Kingston, 1993)

The above profiles must be regarded as somewhat tentative in the light of what is still a very limited research base – drawn in any event almost exclusively from the US. The focus on the abuser having a history of social and emotional problems is controversial and may only be relevant for a proportion of those cases involving physical abuse. Moreover, it is important to consider those contexts which might trigger abuse and neglect. For an understanding of these it is clear that sociological as well as psychological explanations of behaviour are necessary. Finally, the research considered thus far can be most accurately described as examining abuse as it occurs in domiciliary settings. Such settings, taken on their own, might lead to the conclusion that abuse is exclusively located within families, between carers and vulnerable older people. Other settings, that are potential sites of abuse, could be ignored. It is then a relatively short step to 'solve' the problem by 'rescuing' the victim by placing him or her in a residential setting. That the family is not the sole, even the primary, location of abuse becomes clear once institutional abuse is considered in more detail.

INSTITUTIONAL ABUSE OF OLDER PEOPLE

A dominant approach in the research literature has been to apply a family violence model to the issue of elder abuse and neglect. However, one difficulty with this perspective is that it has tended to underplay concern with abuse in settings such as residential and nursing homes. This is somewhat surprising given that whilst the extent of abuse in informal settings is still very unclear, its existence within institutions has been widely documented (Townsend, 1962; Robb, 1967; Harman and Harman, 1989; Counsel and Care, 1991). Bennett and Kingston (1993) note that the spectrum of abuse and neglectful behaviours encountered in elderly care institutions is remarkably varied. Studies have considered the basic standards of privacy, the physical quality and care of life, the dehumanisation of older people in hospitals and homes, the burn-out of nursing staff, and financial fraud and exploitation.

There are a number of reasons why older people in residential settings may be at risk of abuse and neglect. These reasons may be summarised as follows:

- Older people in residential settings are a vulnerable group who may not complain even when they are abused.
- They may fear further abuse if they do complain.
- They may not be aware of their legal rights.
- They may be affected by physical and/or cognitive deterioration.
- They may be isolated from the wider community.
- There may be no effective complaints procedures within homes.

The characteristic features of abuse in residential care may focus around:

- Excessive use of restraints.
- Under- or over-prescribing of medication.
- Verbal aggression.
- Financial exploitation.
- Under-stimulation of residents.

Negative attitudes to older people may be more visible in long-term care facilities because of the greater concentration of older people in a single location. Kayser-Jones (cited in Monk, 1990) has grouped the most frequently reported complaints of abuse into four categories:

- *Infantalisation* – treating the patient/client as an irresponsible child;
- *Depersonalisation* – providing services in an assembly-line fashion, disregarding the patient's individual needs;
- *Dehumanisation* – not only ignoring elderly persons but stripping them of privacy and of their capacity to assume responsibility for their own lives;
- *Victimisation* – attacking the older person's physical and moral integrity through verbal abuse, threats, intimidation, theft, blackmail, or corporal punishments.

Although much of the evidence of actual abuse is exceptional, it is clearly not unknown. Moreover, if the definition of abuse is widened to include deprivation of the 'quality of life', then abuse in old people's homes might be considered widespread (Phillipson and Biggs, 1993).

Analysis of scandals in residential homes and the reasons why they occurred were outlined in Roger Clough's paper 'Scandals in Residential Centres: A Report for the Wagner Committee' (1988). This was an unpublished paper requested by the committee as background material. In his report, Clough describes some of the contributory causes for the breakdown in the system of care and the resulting scandals, under the following headings:

- Failure to agree within the managing agency about the purpose and tasks of the home.

- Failure to manage life in the centre in the appropriate way. When things went wrong, they were not sorted out.
- Resources – building and staff. Buildings may be deteriorating; there is often not enough staff.
- Confusion and lack of knowledge about the guidelines.
- The attitudes and behaviour of staff.
- Staff capacity and lack of training.
- Low staff morale.
- The low status subscribed to the work.
- Failure by management to see a pattern of events. They treated individual instances in isolation.

These areas can be summarised by using a model which would suggest that abuse and neglect may occur given factors related to characteristics of: (a) the home environment; (b) staff characteristics; and (c) resident characteristics.

In terms of the home setting, the factors which might be significant here include:

- *The extent of custodial orientation*: i.e. homes which fail to provide residents with opportunities to care for themselves, to take on responsibilities, or to exercise control over their situation.
- *Staff–patient ratios*: studies of nursing homes indicate higher staff–patient ratios lead to more care for each patient. In addition, it can be argued that workers in under-staffed facilities experience greater job stress, which in turn makes them more likely to maltreat residents.
- *Turnover rate*: higher rates of job turnover in residential homes have been reported to cause substantial distress for staff members which may lead in turn to patient maltreatment.
- *External management*: in social services departments the extent to which homes are integrated within (rather than isolated from) management within the department may be important in terms of both preventing and identifying cases of abuse.

The attitudes of staff in homes will invariably be conditioned by wider, social attitudes about the nature of work with older people, and particularly those with multiple needs in terms of chronic health conditions. Again, in relation to nursing homes, it has been argued that well-qualified persons do not choose to work in such settings, largely because of the low rates of pay and the lack of prestige relative to other health and social care settings. Some interesting findings from the US literature are: younger staff members are more likely than older staff

191

members to hold negative attitudes towards residents; there is some indication, again only from US studies, that excessive levels of job stress and burn-out can lead to the de-personalisation of residents (Pillemer and Moore, 1989).

Finally, in terms of the characteristics of the older persons, three areas have been identified in relation to the likelihood of being maltreated:

- *Health of residents* – with healthier patients receiving more humane treatment from staff (patients/residents with cognitive impairment may be particularly vulnerable to maltreatment).
- *Social isolation* – with those persons with the least social contacts at the greatest risk of abuse. Research suggests that maltreatment by abusers is inhibited by the presence of relatives and friends interested in the older person's welfare (this confirms the value of an advocacy scheme attached to a residential home).
- *Gender* – with some evidence that women are more likely then men to be victims of serious domestic elder abuse and that the same pattern may exist in nursing homes.

(Phillipson and Biggs 1992)

Based on the above evidence, and the reviews of this work by Pillemer (1988) and Bennett and Kingston (1993), it would now seem important to accept the view that there is a broad spectrum of mistreatment of older people, ranging from the interiors of private to those of public settings. It is invidious to select to select any one setting for particular emphasis, and we should clearly look for an approach which sees abuse as an issue which is not tied to any one context or relationship (Phillipson, 1993).

THEORETICAL PERSPECTIVES ON ELDER ABUSE

A number of explanations have been developed to account for the existence of abuse and neglect of older people. As well as focusing on different aspects of the phenomena, these theories also tend to focus on different levels of explanation – from the individual characteristics of the abused or the abuser, to the structural features of the society in which they are located. This section will review some of the key theories and will conclude with an assessment of the role of theory in the phenomena of mistreatment.

192

The situational model

This approach focuses on the way in which the dependency of the older person causes stress for the abuser. As the stress facing the carer increases, the likelihood of abuse may also increase. Phillips (1986) summarises the situational variables that have been linked with abuse as: first, elder-related factors such as physical and emotional dependency, poor health, impaired mental status, and a 'difficult' personality; second, structural factors such as emotional strains, social isolation, and environmental problems; and, third, caregiver-related factors such as life crisis, 'burn-out' or exhaustion with care-giving. This approach features prominently in early British reports on elder abuse and neglect. One such example was Eastman's (1984) study of social service staff attitudes to abuse and neglect. The actual cause of abuse was considered mainly to be stress related, with 80 per cent considering stress to be the overriding factor.

Bennett and Kingston (1993) argue that the scenario of the stressed carer has been difficult to dispute because research was not available to support any other conceptual frameworks. However, they suggest that it quickly became apparent that not all carers abused or neglected the older people they cared for, even though they experienced a significant degree of stress. This led some researchers to ask the question: what is unique about those who commit abusive acts?

The pathology model

One response has been to suggest that abuse might be linked to some degree of pathology on the part of the abuser, typically relating to their social or mental health status. As already noted, research conducted as part of the Boston study would appear to give some credence, given findings suggesting high levels of pathology on the part of the carer when compared with those in the non-abused group (see, also, Homer and Gilleard, 1990). In this perspective, the focus shifts from a an exhausted carer to that of a disturbed individual with a history of sociopathic behaviour, now involved in caring role, but lacking the skills or resources to maintain this responsibility. The idea of the abuser having a history of psychiatric and related problems is clearly important. However, it needs to be considered whether such a feature is encountered in some types of abuse more than others. We also need to learn more about those factors (situational or otherwise) which may trigger mistreatment of older people.

Exchange theory

This model draws us into considering the dynamics of family life and the possibility of abuse as a factor in the power relationships which are characteristic of social institutions such as the family (Pillemer, 1993). Exchange theory focuses on the impact of dependency on either the abused or the abuser. The theory sees interaction between people as an exchange of rewards or punishments, where individuals seek to maximise rewards or minimise punishments in their relationships. Failure to achieve a balanced exchange of rewards will, it is argued, lead to conflict. This model would suggest that abuse may be seen as a response to a breakdown in the norm of reciprocity (i.e. the notion of a balance between receiving and contributing within social relationships). Abuse may also be seen as a response by those (such as some carers) who lack power (or perceive that they do) to restore control. Where resources or alternative solutions are lacking, abuse or neglect may be one possible outcome. Wolf (1992) notes that Pillemer has suggested 'social exchange' theory as a model for intervention in which the rewards of reducing dependency on the elder and/or the costs of abusing the elder are increased. Vocational counselling, housing placement, job opportunities and financial support may be necessary to enable the child to achieve independence. Increasing the costs to the perpetrator of abusive behaviour can be accomplished by legal interventions of various kinds.

Interactionist theory

This approach, following Herbert Blumer (1969) and McCall and Simmons (1966), suggests that the way social life is organised arises from within society itself and out of the processes of interaction between its members. With this theory, mistreatment of the old would be viewed as a consequence of the interaction within either families or institutions. More specifically, the theory would predict that processes arising from social and biological ageing might change role definitions within the social groups the older person was interacting in. Such alterations might challenge hitherto stable identities causing stress within social relationships. This could be resolved by the negotiation of new self-validating identities. Alternatively, forms of psychological abuse (such as infantalisation) could emerge, possibly leading to other forms of abuse and neglect.

The implication of an interactionist perspective is that our understanding of abuse should acknowledge the way in which ageing processes affect workers and carers at a personal level. Contact with older people may be difficult (or may be avoided) because it is seen as unrewarding or reminds carers of their own ageing. This is partly because they have no direct experience of old age and therefore have to rely upon social stereotypes. As these are predominantly negative, they affect perceptions of our own future old age as a time of dependency, poor health, poverty and vulnerability, even though this may bear little relationship to the lived experience of many older people or the type of old age which they may expect.

The social construction of old age

Interactionist perspectives focus on the question of how individuals adapt and respond to old age. Critical or political economy perspectives, in contrast, examine the impact of society on the lives of older people, both within and beyond domestic settings. This model would argue that many of the problems facing older people are not the result of natural or biological processes of ageing; instead, they reflect social inequalities which limit the roles and resources open to older people. Peter Townsend (1981), for example, developed the term 'structured dependency' to refer to the way in which economic and political forces contribute to feelings of powerlessness among both older people and their carers. This approach also suggests that health and social services are involved in the marginalisation of older people. These services are seen to reinforce the dependency created through the wider social and economic system. The implication of this approach is that abuse may arise from the way in which older people come to be marginalised by society. If people are predisposed to abuse the old because of their biological dependency, the likelihood is increased through social forces which discriminate against both older people and those involved in their care. Such a perspective would suggest that the challenge to abuse must be seen as an issue of both social policy as well as individual pathology.

In terms of assessing the merit of the above theories it is probably helpful to see them as explaining different facets of the mistreatment of older people. It is almost certainly inaccurate to see these theories as mutually exclusive and researchers and practitioners will need to draw upon all of the theories identified in analysing and developing responses to mistreatment. Sprey and Matthews (1989) contest the assumption that the different theoretical perspectives are necessarily competing. They note (1989, p. 58):

'The usefulness of each explanatory approach depends on exactly what is being explained. Lines of questioning become of decisive importance in making theoretical sense of a set of events that on a surface level seem to defy meaningful categorical conceptualization. To ask why given individuals turn into abusers or exploiters, for instance, is essentially a phycological issue. To query under what conditions such persons actually abuse quite specific others requires social-psychological analysis. And to ask which attributes or familial structures may induce relations that are violent or neglect-prone is for sociologists or anthropologists to explain.'

The above argument is of considerable importance in terms of striking balance in the debate on elder abuse. Certainly, at this early stage of conceptualisation and intervention, exclusive reliance upon a particular theoretical model would be a mistake.

UNDERSTANDING ELDER ABUSE: A REVIEW OF CURRENT ISSUES

Having reviewed some of the key issues running through the debate on elder abuse, some areas for concern will now be identified. The main areas to be discussed are: elder abuse and domestic violence; the role of legislation, and perspectives on intervention.

Elder abuse and domestic violence

One current difficulty with the debate is the attempt to place elder abuse as a form of family violence (Steinmetz, 1988). This linkage has almost certainly hindered clarification of the issues involved with elder mistreatment and there is now a clear need to move on from the restrictions of this approach. It's easy to think that there may be similarities between old age abuse and child abuse. Both are about problems which result from an imbalance of power; both are about people being deprived of rights and liberties; and both are concerned with the failure to provide optimal conditions for development. But we should be careful about carrying the analogy too far. A child is assumed to require a guardian with custodial authority. In the case of adults, in contrast, we assume they are competent to make basic life decisions on their own. The danger of the child abuse analogy here is that it suggests we (the professionals) should take over decision-making for the vulnerable elderly person. This may, however, simply increase the powerlessness of the older person. It may also lead to further forms of abuse (Biggs and Phillipson, 1992).

The child abuse analogy also suggests that the older person may be in a dependent relation with the carer. However, as our review of the research suggests, this is not necessarily the case. In fact the abuser may be the dependent one, as in the case of a middle-aged adult with learning difficulties, living at home with his/her now elderly parents. The danger with the child abuse analogy in this case is that it leads to a misleading assessment of the causes of the abuse. Thus it may not be the consequence of the burden of caretaking; it may be seen, instead, as a rebellion against the position of dependency.

In the case of child abuse the concern to protect vulnerable children may lead either to residential care or a long-term foster placement. The danger here is that the innocent party (the older person) is forced to leave his or her home for a temporary placement in, for example, an older person's home. The likelihood, however, is that this becomes permanent. It may also be the case that the trauma of the move to residential care may outweigh the original impact of the abuse (see Crystal, 1986, for a detailed review of these issues).

The above considerations lead in to a more general consideration of the validity of the domestic violence analogy. Is, for example, 'elder abuse...clearly only part of a spectrum of domestic violence which affects all ages' (Department of Health, 1992)? The view taken here is that elder abuse is similar but also very different from many other forms of domestic violence. Unlike other types of violence there may not be a clear victim or perpetrator. Because most elderly adults are legally (and actually) autonomous human beings, it may be difficult to determine the precise cause of abuse acts. This leads, as Linda Phillips (1986, p. 89) has pointed out, to difficult questions for professionals working in the field:

'Is it the responsibility of an adult child to enforce rules of cleanliness on a legally competent elder when the elder does not want to be clean? What is the effect of geographic distance or filial distance on legal and moral responsibilities? Who is the victim and who is the perpetrator in situations where a legally competent elder refuses to act in this or her own interests? And perhaps even more basic than any of these is the question of how can responsibility be assigned in a society that has yet to establish clear criteria regarding the minimum material and emotional rights to which every individual in society is entitled.'

Use of the family violence model also raises problems in that it may only account for a limited amount of abuse and neglect. Sprey and Matthews (1989) make this point in the American context, where *self-neglect* is the 'modal category of those requiring adult protective services'. They go on to argue (1989, p. 55) that 'the conceptually narrow and often normative approach characteristic of the domestic-violence field is useful for the study of only a few of the many faces of elderly mistreatment. At best it may be appropriate for the analysis of verbal and physical violence between older spouses and between members of different age categories in families and kin groups. The danger of overuse of this approach is that it deflects attention from the most commonly reported type of problem, self-neglect.'

It remains unclear whether self-neglect is as important in the UK given different family and welfare support structures. However, it is certainly possible that the family violence model may only be applicable to a minority of cases of abuse. Moreover, it does not help to illuminate the other major site of potential mistreatment – in special settings such as residential homes and nursing homes.

The legal context

The issues raised by elder abuse has already led to calls for more substantial powers of intervention to protect vulnerable elders. The Law Commission has published a paper setting out what statutory powers might actually look like (Law Commission, 1993), and groups involved in the campaign on elder abuse are pressing for a review of the legal area (*Community Care*, 1 July, 1993). The question of greater legal powers does raise complex issues and brings out fundamental questions about the rights both of older people and those involved with their care. The view to be put forward here is that critical questions need to be asked about whether new legal powers are justified. It will be argued that there are, in fact, grounds for believing that such powers will be counter-productive, reducing rather than adding to the rights and freedoms of older people.

The first point to make is that there already exists substantial legislation relevant to the protection and support of vulnerable elders. This varies from service-oriented legislation such as the 1990 National Health Service and Community Care Act, to protective legislation such as the 1983 Mental Health Act. In addition, criminal legislation such as the Offences Against the Person Act 1861, the Matrimonial Homes Act 1983, and injunctions available under the Law of Tort, may also be relevant in cases of abuse (DoH, 1993; Griffiths *et al.* (1993). Given the available legislation we need to ask what prevents it from being used and would new legislation (such as specific powers aimed at the frail elderly) be any more effective? Griffiths *et al.* (1993) give three reasons for the current difficulties in implementing existing legislation. First, some legal procedures, particularly criminal prosecutions, are inappropriate in many cases of elder abuse, because the perpetrators of the abuse are themselves victims of the situation (for example, carers subject to an excessive degree of stress). Second, legal procedures are often under-utilised because of negative attitudes/lack of expertise on the part of professionals such as lawyers and social workers. Third, the notion of abuse is seldom conceptualised in legal terms. Griffiths *et al.* (1993, p. 64) argue that:

> 'according to Eastman ..., "granny bashing" can consist of physical assault, threats of physical assault, neglect, including locking a dependent in a bedroom; abandonment, either to residential or hospital care; exploitation, including appropriation of finance and property; sexual abuse; and psychological abuse. The result is a highly diffuse definition of elder abuse ... Also, according to Eastman, abuse by persons other than relatives caring for the elderly person should not be included within this analytical framework. To differentiate in this way, between caregiving relatives and other abusers, seems arbitrary and illogical, and makes little sense in terms of the law.'

It is doubtful if any of these problems would be changed – they may in fact be exacerbated – by the introduction of a new set of statutory powers. Moreover, it must also be said that new legislation would be pointless without a significant commitment of resources – both social as well as legal. Unfortunately, we already have many examples where major legislation has been introduced (such as the 1986 Disabled Persons Act), only to be rendered ineffective through the failure to commit sufficient funds for full implementation.

Many reports do of course cite the US experience of adult protective legislation, suggesting that this has given significant support to vulnerable elders (Department of Health, 1992). However, the evidence is that in the absence of supportive services, legislation can actually do more harm than good, resulting in unnecessary institutionalisation and premature separation of the older person from the caregiver. The criminalisation of abuse and neglect would seem to be a pathway to be avoided, at least judging from recent commentaries on the US experience. Formby (1992), in a review of protective services in the US, suggests that it is much more productive to treat elder abuse as a social service problem than to deal with it as a new area of criminal behaviour. Formby notes Heisler's view that by handling elder abuse as a crime, with the criminal justice system charging and prosecuting the offence, offenders (abusers) will learn that threats, coercion, and manipulation are not acceptable practices. Formby (1992, p. 128) goes on:

'This may well be true if the abuser contemplates the offense and its consequences. However, abusive and neglectful behaviour which arises out of ignorance or as a stress reaction by the caregiver would most likely not be affected by fear of apprehension and punishment. The desired intervention strategy may be more successful if focused upon educating or providing assistance to the caregiver. Furthermore, abused persons may be less likely to report their situation if they believe that caregivers will be subject to criminal sanctions ... Certainly, if the abuse and/or neglect was committed in a deliberate manner with intent to harm the victim physically, emotionally, or materially, a criminal investigation should be initiated. This could then be handled as an ordinary criminal proceeding, and the abuser dealt with through routine channels of the criminal justice system.'

Salend *et al.* (cited in Callahan, 1988), after studying elder abuse reporting statutes in sixteen states, reported that the statutes failed to ensure consistent information within or across the state, that neglect, particularly self-neglect, was more often reported than abuse, and that the number of prosecutions was relatively low. The authors warned against infantilising older persons and concluded (cited in Callahan, 1988, p. 457):

'Perhaps we should take a few steps backward in advocacy of mandatory reporting for a thorough conceptualization of what should be reported and why. In any event, more study of the effectiveness and consequences of existing elder abuse statutes would be desirable.'

Although not directly applicable, this point certainly has relevance for the debate in the UK: caution will clearly be necessary before proceeding towards developing additional statutory powers in the area of abuse and neglect.

Intervention in the field of abuse

Greater clarity will also be needed in determining more general patterns of intervention in the area of abuse. US research on this issue has identified three distinct categories of abuse, each requiring a different type of intervention (O'Malley, Everitt and Sarson, 1984). The first category consists of chronically sick elders whose needs have been neglected for a short period of time due to the exhaustion of the caregiver. The key response here will be to provide a framework of support to assist carers, the range of options including:

- developing local registers of carers
- encouraging the formation of carers' support groups
- developing services sensitive to the needs of carers from different races and cultures
- developing flexible forms of respite care
- developing collective forms of welfare rights.

The second category of abuse consists of elders with a physical or mental health illness who are not dependent on a family caregiver, despite their condition, who tend to be financially exploited and psychologically abused. The key tasks here will include: providing a range of supportive services to the older person, separating the older person from the caregiver, and/or treating the pathologies of the abuser.

The third category consists of independent older persons who experience abuse by family members who are not caregivers. In this instance, emphasis will be on treatment of the abuser rather than services to the older person.

An additional category which should be added is that of abuse and neglect in institutional settings (see above). The options here will need to include:

- The degree to which the home encourages resident participation should be assessed.
- Staffing ratios should be at a level which allows maximum stimulation of residents.
- Staff training should be carried out on the issue of abuse and neglect.
- Homes should have clear mechanisms for gathering consumer views about the quality of life inside homes.
- Advocacy schemes and charters of rights should be implemented inside homes.
- Schemes for maintaining contact with informal carers should be devised.
- The physical environment of the home should be evaluated for its effect on residents' morale.
- The extent to which individual residents are socially isolated should be monitored.

Finally, intervention will need to be guided by principles for determining the scope of intervention in the field of abuse. The following points are illustrative:

- Workers should be encouraged to be vigilant about the possibility of abuse/neglect whilst being aware of the fact that there are no clear criteria for identifying abused elders and few interventions that are totally acceptable to all the parties involved.

- Shared decision-making is essential. Sharing should be conducted both by involving a range of professional workers in developing a strategy for tackling abuse and by ensuring that workers are supported in the decisions they make about protecting vulnerable elders.
- Departments will need to develop policies which empower older people in situations where they lead marginal lives. Policies for tackling abuse must therefore be concerned with advocacy and strengthening self-care abilities in later life.
- The goal of work in the field of abuse should be ensuring that older people enjoy a life free of violence and mistreatment. This requires intervention and vigilance in a range of settings: at a macro-social level in terms of social attitudes and beliefs about older people; in the care provided by paid and unpaid carers; and in the environments of nursing and residential homes. A comprehensive policy on mistreatment will need to address these different levels of abuse if it is to be fully effective.

CONCLUSION

This chapter has tried to summarise current debates and concerns in the field of elder abuse. There is substantial evidence that abuse and neglect of older people is fast achieving the status of a social problem in the UK, and that a consistent response from health and social services professionals is beginning to emerge (Ogg and Munn-Giddens, 1993).

Attempts to define and map the extent of elder abuse indicate that it should not be seen as a single, monolithic phenomenon, but that it takes a variety of forms in different settings and in different kinds of relationships. Victims and perpetrators exhibit different characteristics depending on the nature of abuse. Moreover, it should not be thought of as exclusively a problem faced by families coping with the pressures of informal care: the issue of abuse in residential and nursing home settings should certainly be given a higher profile than is currently the case.

The relationship between community care and the development of adequate responses to elder abuse is a complex one and this chapter has attempted to alert practitioners to the danger of criminalisation that might arise in that setting. Whatever the circumstances, responses to elder abuse should be based on an understanding of the way in which older age is socially constructed. Elders, as adults with civil rights and unique life histories, should not be subject to practices and procedures

202

devised in response to a different set of issues, such as those arising from child protection work.

Developments in practice might usefully be based upon two factors, namely, the empowerment of older people and inter-generational mediation. The first of these would include starting from the older person's perception of the problem and their life-circumstances, facilitating self-care and self-help groups for abused elders, and the encouragement of collective action among older people themselves in order to challenge a climate of prejudice and misunderstanding about their needs (Bernard and Phillipson, 1991). In this context professional workers should see themselves as allies as well as advocates in the struggle to gain appropriate resources for and an understanding of elder abuse and how it arises.

Secondly, it has to be recognised that we know relatively little about the relationship between inter-generational communication, conflict and elder abuse. The codes for negotiating relationships between adult children and their parents, young practitioners and users of services for the elderly, are often poorly developed, perhaps reflecting the fact that increased numbers of older people in society is a relatively recent phenomenon. However, few would deny that misunderstanding and conflict often occur between generations, and a specific service, drawing on skills that would increase assertiveness, the understanding of family and institutional dynamics, and promote conflict resolution, would seem to be required to address some of the issues raised in this chapter.

CHAPTER EIGHT

Health Perspectives and Elder Abuse

G. C. J. Bennett*

Health care workers were first alerted to the possibility that elderly people were being physically abused in the 1970s (Baker, 1975; Burston, 1977). Despite a vociferous compaign (Eastman, 1982), the issue drifted from not only the media headlines but from professional consciousness. Elder abuse at that time had not generated the 'moral panic' needed to establish it as a potential social problem. The 1980s saw a more sustained campaign by a wider circle of interested parties – doctors (Edwards, 1982), social workers (Eastman, 1984), voluntary organisations (Tomlin, 1989) – and the first major conference (Tomlin, 1989). Health care workers quickly became aware that their US counterparts had reacted far more readily to the initial UK warnings and had progressed their understanding through research (Pillemer and Finkelhor, 1988). The difference appeared to be that in the US elder abuse became a social problem, whereas in the UK, according to Blumer's (1971) theory, it had still failed to do so.

The 1990s have been a watershed time for the recognition of the phenomenon in the UK. Homer and Gilleard's (1990) paper on abuse of the mentally frail by carers realerted a by-now primed audience. Guidelines for staff began appearing, confirming the need for practical help for health and social care workers (Association of Directors of Social Services, 1990). Despite government apathy and junior minister denials, the first large-scale tangible evidence of the problem was published in the autumn of 1992 (Ogg and Bennett, 1992). In 1993 the organisation Action on Elder Abuse was launched supported by Age Concern England. This multidisciplinary group aims to raise awareness and disseminate information on research and education and form a focus for debate on the topic. The 1990s should see elder abuse joining child abuse and domestic violence as social problems in the UK.

TYPES OF ABUSE

It is now recognised that abuse can take many forms:

- Physical
- Chronic verbal aggression
- Emotional (psychological)
- Sexual
- Deprivation of help needed in daily living
- Deprivation of or excess administration of medication
- Forced isolation
- Financial

Definitional changes such as the concept of *inadequate care* by Fulmer and O'Malley (1987) allow health and social care workers greater flexibility when assessing a given situation without having to attach the label and stigma of 'abuse'. Currently, however, the recognition of elder abuse (inadequate care) is at an extremely low level. The most commonly recognised aspect of abuse is that of physical mistreatment (though probably not the most common form of elder abuse). Even in these cases if there is no disclosure by victim or perpetrator quite dramatic features need to be present before the correct questions are asked. The symptoms and signs associated with psychological and sexual abuse are far less well authenticated than similar situations concerning children. Two major reasons may account for the anomalous situation. Any form of child abuse was considered rare even a few decades ago. The issue became a social problem following case reports in the medical and lay press of children with fractures that had occurred at different times and bruising at different stages of healing (as indicated by colour) probably caused by parental/carer violence. Sexual abuse of children was not given conscious thought by doctors and social workers. Gradually, accident and emergency units began 'seeing' the condition and the relevant professionals began the long hard learning curve to the current knowledge base. With the benefit of hindsight, research and, unfortunately, scandals, these initial assessment procedures now seem simple, naive and inaccurate. Child abuse was recognised as a social problem and solutions are being sought. This process has barely started with elder abuse.

The second reason behind the different knowledge bases between child and elder abuse is more complex. Children have well-defined and clear developmental stages. Health and social care workers dealing with normal healthy children have their own experience and numerous charts and guidelines to indicate fairly accurately what children should be achieving, and growth norms etc. Children also get seen frequently by a wide variety of people – health visitors, district nurses, GPs, teachers etc. – who all have the opportunity to spot abnormal symptoms and signs. These can range from physical pointers (failure to thrive, unexplainable skin marks, etc.) to abnormal behaviour (sudden onset of bed-wetting, undue fearfulness or precocious sexual behaviour). There is now a vast library of information available to help professionals decide what is normal and what is abnormal in a child's development progress.

DIAGNOSING ELDER ABUSE

It is an entirely different scenario when dealing with elderly people and a similar knowledge base will prove more difficult to establish. The physiological and psychological changes that occur with ageing remain poorly understood even by most health and social care workers dealing with elderly people. Gerontology, the study of ageing, is still a new science. Normal ageing is a more gradual and benign process than was originally thought. It involves a slow and almost imperceptible decline from maturity (30-40!) onwards in most of the body processes. Muscle strength and power, lung and heart functions all gradually decline, but a normal fit 80-year-old is mobile, continent and intellectually the match of anyone younger (usually from the benefit of experience). This is in marked contrast to the generally held view concerning elderly people – i.e., the period of a second childhood, intellectually frail, falling repeatedly, incontinent and immobile. This scenario does occur but is the result of disease, i.e., abnormal not normal ageing.

The distinction between what is normal ageing and what is disease is crucial to the formation of an adequate knowledge base in the field of recognition and assessment of possible cases of abuse/inadequate care. The dilemma for social workers can be illustrated by highlighting a few areas. As we age our skin changes, but the changes due to ageing are at the microscopic level. Most people, however, equate ageing skin with wrinkles, warts and 'liver spots'. This is not normal ageing. These changes are due to ultraviolet light (sunlight), and hence sunbathing/sunlight exposure hastens these processes, causing more wrinkles to occur than would otherwise have been the case (i.e. via family genetics). Wrinkles, however, are only a cosmetic problem; other changes have a potentially much more serious outcome. Ultraviolet light exposure is implicated in the increased occurrence of skin tumours. These tumours can be benign (solar keratosis) or malignant. Basal cell carcinomas are usually small (they get bigger if untreated), occur on the face, have a pearly edge with blood vessels (telangiectasia) and are easily cured by minor surgery or radiotherapy. Malignant melanomas are pigmented skin cancers which, if not caught early, when superficial, can be fatal.

In most elderly people (women especially) the unavoidable exposure of their skin to the sun (forearms and legs) results in the skin becoming thinner. The underlying supporting tissue (collagen) acts as a scaffold for the blood vessels just under the skin surface and this too is affected. It supports the vessels less well, so that minor trauma (e.g. a knock) can cause a vessel to break, leaving a bruise (purpura). The mechanism for clearing away the blood is less effective as we age and hence such bruises persist for long periods. The situation is made more complex by some elderly people being more affected than others. A small group go on to develop the *transparent skin syndrome,* where the skin becomes paper thin. This means that the skin can bruise and even break on normal handling, i.e., touching or dressing. The result can look appalling and suspicious. It also means that bruising in elderly people is not a straightforward issue and cannot always be used as a definitive sign in possible elder abuse cases.

Falls and incontinence of urine are two conditions that occur more frequently in elderly people. Neither are part of normal ageing and are a signalling of an underlying disease process. Investigation will hopefully result in a disease process being found and treated, and for the majority of people alleviation if not cure of the problem. In the few cases where help is not curative other coping strategies can be organised. If the connection between falls, incontinence and illness is not made, the resulting injuries, bruises and evidence of poor hygiene can lead to the mistaken assumption of abuse/inadequate care. The physiological changes that occur in ageing and disease will thus have great bearing on the recognition and assessment procedures. Physical signs should be interpreted with caution until the knowledge base is built up as a result of experience and research. The assessment procedure for a possibly abused elderly person must be as holistic as possible. The time-honoured approach of history-taking and physical examination is modified to gain as much information as possible. In the US, health care professionals working in the field are far more confident of their recognition and assessment criteria than their counterparts in the UK. Alerting features for the doctor have been outlined by Cochran and Petrose (1987). These include a discrepancy between the history and the observed injury, inappropriate injuries (fractures in a bedbound individual), conflicting stories, vague explanations or denial. There may be bizarre or inappropriate explanations, or insistence from a client that an injury is severe when no injury exists (presumably as a way of getting professional help). A long delay in reporting the injury is also suspicious. An explanation of an elderly person being 'accident prone' should be cause for added attention, as should evidence of previous injuries, untreated old injuries or multiple injuries, especially if at various stages of healing. Repeat attendances of clients to accident and emergency departments from the same institutions should also trigger concern.

RAISING AWARENESS OF ELDER ABUSE

Awareness raising in members of the medical profession is one of the next crucial steps. These gatekeeper roles (recognition and then alerting the appropriate system) are shared by doctors working in accident and emergency departments and general practitioners. There is as yet no research work to indicate how well informed junior and senior doctors are concerning even the potential diagnosis of elder abuse. The author has a submission to an august research body to do just that. It would entail questionnaire evaluation of all grades of doctor in all specialties that had contact with elderly people. I suspect a very low level of awareness but hopefully a willingness to learn via education packages, books, videos etc. The knowledge base will need to begin during the medical undergraduate education programme and then form part of postgraduate updates.

US doctors are also being alerted to injuries in areas usually covered by clothing, injuries consistent with the shape of a weapon or bruising/laceration on the lips (from forced feeding or gagging). Whiplash injuries can occur from shaking, and sexual abuse can result in laceration, bruising or bleeding of the rectum and or genitalia (see also below). Fractures in the usually immobile, alopecia (hair loss) and bleeding from hair pulling are other suspicious signs. Conditions for which it is difficult to establish causation include malnutrition, dehydration, weight loss and pressure-sore formation. A history of previous physical abuse and previous suicide attempts should also alert the assessor.

Fulmer and O'Malley (1987) list the manifestations of inadequate care that should alert health and social care professionals:

- Abrasions
- Lacerations
- Contusions
- Burns
- Freezing

- Dehydration
- Malnutrition
- Inappropriate clothing
- Poor hygiene
- Over-sedation

- Depression
- Fractures
- Sprains
- Decubiti (pressure sores)
- Dislocations

- Over/under-medication
- Untreated medical problems
- Failure to meet legal obligations
- Behaviour that endangers client or others

Fulmer and O'Malley also list physical indicators of abuse not shared with neglect:

Unexplained bruises and welts:
Face, lips and mouth, torso, back, buttocks, thighs, in various stages of healing. Clustered, forming regular patterns reflecting shape of article used (cord, buckle) on several different surface areas. Lesions which regularly appear after absence, weekend or holiday.

Unexplained burns:
Cigar, cigarette, especially on soles, palms, back or buttocks. Immersion burns (sock-like on feet, glove-like on hands, doughnut-shaped on buttocks or genitalia) patterned like electric burner, iron etc. Rope burns on arms, legs, neck or torso.

Unexplained fractures:
To skull, nose, facial structure, in various stages of healing. Multiple or spiral fractures.

Unexplained lacerations or abrasions:
To mouth, lips, gums or eye. To external genitalia.

Sexual abuse:
Difficulty in walking or sitting, torn, stained or bloody undercloth-ing, pain or itching in the genital area, bruises or bleeding in the external genitalia, vaginal or anal areas. Venereal disease.

The most common presentations of inadequate care usually involve combinations of symptoms and signs, e.g. poor nutrition, poorly controlled medical problems, frequent falls and confusion. Thus the general practitioner, district nurse, health visitor or casualty officer may be the first people to be presented with the diagnostic dilemma. Less often legal services, the police or social services become involved because of financial abuse or housing problems. The presence of one or more of the listed manifestations of inadequate care obviously does not establish a diagnosis of abuse or neglect; the same or similar findings can occur in ill and frail elderly people as part of their acute or chronic health process. In spite of this, the presence of these symptoms or signs should alert the attending worker to the possibility of inadequate care.

Occasionally elderly people themselves report the abuse. This can happen when they have formed a close enough relationship with someone to divulge their worries. If the situation seems to warrant it then the history-taking should be expanded and specific questions asked. This will involve enquiring about theft or misappropriation of resources, about possible enforced social isolation or confinement. The client will need to be asked about any threats or coercion, the use of restraints, being locked up, any episodes of battering, sexual abuse, threats of punishment or the withholding of food, clothing or privileges to enforce behaviour.

SEXUAL ABUSE

The knowledge base on child abuse was built upon the early reports of physical violence and neglect. Research and investigation increased the spectrum of knowledge to include emotional abuse, and then, to apparent disbelief and shock, child sexual abuse was 'discovered'. Although not yet a social problem in the same sociological terms the knowledge base on elder abuse is building upon physical, emotional and financial abuse reports and research. The concept of elder sexual abuse is as shocking as its counterpart with children, yet health and social care workers are now identifying cases of elder sexual abuse by family members or other carers. Malcolm Holt, a social worker in Northumberland, is researching this issue and liaising closely with an acknowledged expert in the US, Holly Ramsey-Klawsnik.

Dependent elderly people who rely upon others for care appear to be especially vulnerable to sexual assault, as it appears not to be their physical attributes but rather the powerlessness and vulnerability which attract a sexual offender to a particular victim. Dependent elderly people, particularly those with speech, mobility or other limitations, are very attractive as potential sexual abuse victims. Research studies of elder sexual abuse are few. In one involving 52 cases of suspected sexual abuse, 60 per cent of the victims were dependent on care (Ramsey-Klawsnik, 1993). Almost all the victims were women and almost all the offenders men. Over 30 per cent of the offenders were husbands caring for their dependent wives, forcing themselves sexually without consent. Almost 30 per cent of the offenders were grown sons who sexually assaulted their elderly mothers.

Other offenders included brothers, grandsons, lodgers and non-related caregivers. The most common sexual assault was vaginal rape and in one-third of the cases repeated vaginal rape was suspected. Most of the cases were identified by specialist workers after they had been called in to assist elderly people who had suffered other forms of abuse by carers.

Ramsey-Klawsnik (1993) offers guidelines to workers who may be involved in interviewing elderly people about possible sexual abuse:

- Become educated about elder sexual abuse; it makes interviewing easier.
- Be aware of the symptoms and signs – especially if a 'cluster' of cases occurs.
- Interview the elderly person privately unless it is indicated that a 'trusted other' be present.
- Allow the person to have as much control over the interview as possible (choosing the place, seating arrangements etc.).
- Treat the person with respect – for instance, calling the person by their surname, e.g. Mrs Jones.
- Don't take notes during the interview (wait until immediately after).
- Build rapport with non-threatening conversation and other methods before asking questions about possible sexual abuse.
- Proceed slowly and carefully using speech and language appropriate to the person and situation.
- Ask questions singly and remind the person they can refuse one or all of the questions.
- Phrase questions in a non-leading, non-suggestive manner which (if subsequently necessary) will not legally compromise the results of the interview. It is appropriate and necessary to ask direct questions.
- If a person discloses that they have been sexually abused, remain calm, thank them and ask them to tell you more about it. Assure them that you will work to help their future safety from further sexual assault.
- Do not share your own emotions with your client.
- Ask clarifying questions (when and where and for how long and what form of sex abuse activities). Identify anyone else involved.
- When appropriate use non-verbal means of communication such as anatomical dolls and anatomical drawings to elicit details of the abuse. This can be very helpful to those elderly people who suffer speech and language impairments, as well as those who can communicate but are too embarrassed to use words to describe their assault(s).
- Tell the victims that they are not alone, that this form of abuse happens to other older people. Explain that it is not their fault, they did not cause it.
- Refrain from expressing judgement towards the offender.

- Make a plan for the elder person's safety, encouraging decision-making. Document all findings with a complete report.
- If the person denies sexual abuse but clinical evidence suggests the contrary, embarrassment or fear may be the cause. Give some relevant information, reassure and explain your concerns indicating that you plan to return later to give him/her another opportunity to talk to you.

Ramsey-Klawsnik (1993) also lists the myths surrounding sexual abuse in an effort to ensure better understanding of the problem:

Myths about victims
1. Only females are sexually abused.
2. Sexual assault occurs primarily in the lower socio-economic groups.
3. If the victim is not afraid or terrified of an abuse they have not been hurt by the assault.
4. Disclosure then retraction indicates initial lying. After disclosure the story is easier to repeat; if not, then the victim is lying.
5. The victim of one episode of sexual abuse is not likely to allow this to happen again by the same person or by anyone else.
6. When incest occurs all family members are responsible (even the victim).
7. All child victims of sexual abuse are at high risk of becoming abusers in the future.
8. Victims 'get over' sexual abuse victimisation by forgetting about it.
9. Physical attributes and sexual desirability attract a sexual offender to a particular situation.

Myths about offenders
1. Only males sexually abuse dependent others.
2. An individual who adamantly and strenuously denies alleged sexual abuse and even willingly seeks services to 'prove' innocence must be innocent.
3. Individuals who sexually abuse others have stopped engaging in consenting sexual relationships. One can know whether or not an individual could possibly sexually abuse by the individual's displayed behaviour and personality.
4. Individuals who rape do so to achieve sexual gratification.

Myths about activities
1. Sexual assault by a stranger is more traumatic than sexual abuse by a known and trusted other.
2. Sexual abuse activities which are non-violent will do no lasting harm to the victim.

212

3. Once an abuser is under supervision of the court or other authority, the chances of continued sexual abuse become very small.

Myths about professional services
1. Most professional service providers (clinicians, psychiatrists, nurses, psychologists, social workers, therapists, etc.) are trained to assess and treat sexual abuse.
2. Families receiving mental health and or social work and other services cannot hide sexual abuse from the professional.
3. Psychological testing will reveal whether or not an individual has been sexually abused.
4. Medical examination of the victim will usually reveal evidence of sexual abuse.

The sexual abuse continuum developed by Ramsey-Klawsnik (1993) delineates the range and types of sexually abusive behaviour. It was developed from extensive experience interviewing child and adult victims of sexual violence. The continuum presents the activities typically described by victims listed in rank order from (generally) the least to the most severe in terms of degree of violence and trauma to the victim. Sexual abuse often begins with activities in the less severe range and escalates over time to more severe types of abuse. To constitute sexual abuse the victim would have been forced, tricked, threatened or otherwise coerced into the sexual contact against his or her will and without consent.

ASSESSMENT

Many different interview techniques are available. All usually require meetings over a period of time and hence the information-gaining procedure can be very time-consuming. One interview technique involves the five P's:

Privacy   (Interview the client in a private area, e.g. special interview room. Interview the carer separately.)

Pacing   (Neither client nor carer should be rushed. The assessor should appear to have plenty of time for the task, no telephone or other interruptions, being prepared for emotionally disturbing periods requiring brief breaks to regain composure.)

Planning   (A set list of questions and procedures for the assessor to work through.)

Pitch   (A steady voice tone and attitude to impart trust and confidence.)

Punctuality   (When meeting clients at home or with a prearranged interview in an institution – an indication to the client that they are 'worthy' of professional time and punctuality.)

Locally produced guidelines and policies may help with interview techniques. In the US, the achievement of a disclosure is assuming major importance as an 'issue' in some welfare establishments. Social work and counselling interview techniques are being superseded by adversarial ones taught by ex-police/government instructors. The focus of the interview becomes disclosure at all costs using verbal and nonverbal (body language etc.) communication techniques. The focus of attention is usually the suspected perpetrator, and with legal issues so predominant in the US system it is hardly surprising that professional interviewing is becoming a training and legal battlefield.

Quinn and Tomita (1986) describe the importance of enquiring about a typical day. This naturally leads into a verbal assessment of the client's ability to perform activities of daily living. This may need to be very detailed, giving both client and carer an opportunity to describe their perceived and actual difficulties. This task may be best performed by an experienced worker using one useful tool, The Cost of Care Index (Kosberg and Cairl, 1986).

This index gives a numerical indication of the amount of 'stress' a carer might be under. It may prove a useful preventive tool when assessing in a predictive way a certain client–carer relationship, i.e. prior to hospital discharge. Quinn and Tomita (1986) also describe the need to explore the client's expectations about care, getting information on recent crises in the family as well as the sensitive areas of alcohol problems, drug use/abuse, illnesses and behaviour problems within the household or family members.

The client's current mental status should always be ascertained before detailed questioning begins (see below). This will have to be explained, as mentally competent people can get irritated by having their memory assessed. Failure to assess memory can lead to great difficulties later. Where there seems to be an indication of some unusual circumstances then more in-depth questions should follow, tact and accuracy and a non-leading approach being paramount.

The most sensitive area for questioning is that of actual abusive episodes detailing verbal, physical and other incidents. Specific questions relating to the episodes may need to be asked for greater clarification. Interviewing the caregiver is another emotionally demanding situation. Many people rely on the use of a formal protocol – an *aide-mémoire* to formalise the interview situation.

214

SCREENING INSTRUMENTS

Formal protocols (screening instruments) for use in suspected cases of elder abuse are being developed in the US. They can be very lengthy to complete but are thus thorough and provide detailed information on which to base reports regarding alleged abuse/inadequate care. One such tool is the Elder Assessment Instrument (EAI) (Fulmer, 1984). The EAI has eight sections and is designed and arranged to elicit symptoms and signs by health care professionals, the total forming a small booklet:

Section 1 – consists of demographic data (age, sex, address, next of kin). It also includes an assessment of the client's mental state.

Section 2 – is concerned with a general assessment – hygiene, nutrition, skin integrity and clothing (with ranges from 'very good' to 'very poor').

Section 3 – involves a physical assessment of bruises, contractures, pressure sores, lacerations etc. (with ranges of 'definite evidence' through to 'no evidence'). Other screening instruments include in this section a human-figure chart (back-and-front) so that accurate location of marks/bruises can be made with estimations of dates of bruises etc. In many formats the use of photographs (with written consent) is encouraged.

Section 4 – involves an assessment of the elderly person's usual lifestyle specifically enquiring about medication, ambulation, continence, feeding, hygiene, finances and family involvement (with ranges of 'totally independent' or 'totally dependent').

Section 5 – is a social assessment identifying interactions between client and family, friends and other caregivers. It involves detailed knowledge of social support systems and the client's ability to express needs and participate in daily activities (often relying on observational skills). A financial assessment is also made.

Section 6 – is the medical assessment often backed up by laboratory and radiological test results. It can involve assessment of alcohol/substance abuse, dehydration, fractures, excess medication etc. (again ranging from 'definite evidence' to 'no evidence').

Section 7 – summarises the evidence and states whether there is proof of either financial/possession abuse, physical, psychological abuse or neglect.

Section 8 – looks at the outcome, i.e., referral to the elder abuse assessment team (US concept) or to lawyer, police, etc. It also provides comment and follow-up.

The EAI is proving a useful tool in the US by providing a detailed and standardised assessment of elderly people suspected of being abused/inadequately cared for. The evaluation of such screening instruments (modified for a UK population) is urgently needed.

MENTAL STATE ASSESSMENT

From what has been said previously the gathering of information from the client especially is vital. The recollection of painful memories and events is always difficult but legal requirements will necessitate dates, timing, and descriptions. This information and evidence gathering must be sound and for the benefit of all as accurate and precise as possible. It is therefore imperative that the mental state of the client be assessed early in the information-gathering proceedings. This clarifies the situation by protecting both client and assessor. It also prevents problems later in any judicial process.

Ageism in its widest sense is all-pervasive in our society including the medical and legal professions. Elderly people are expected to be 'muddled' or 'confused' and the term 'demented' is banded about loosely. The fact that over 80 per cent of all elderly people are completely mentally competent has escaped most professional and lay attention. The remaining 20 per cent may have some deficiencies but there will be a range of loss and many 'confused' elderly people will have degrees of competency in certain areas. This very difficult situation has recently been reviewed by the Law Commission and the new rulings will hopefully clarify the legal position. The elderly mentally infirm form one of the most difficult diagnostic, treatment and research areas in all health care. The label/term 'dementia' is used so inappropriately in most cases that it should be abandoned. The terms 'acute confusion' and 'chronic confusion' are much more accurate and less stigmatising.

Acute confusion

This is the term best used to describe the form of confusion otherwise known as 'delirium'. It can occur over minutes or hours or have a slower onset presenting over time (up to three months). The person is usually disorientated in time and place and may look unwell, flushed or sweating. They are intermittently drowsy and often have visual hallucinations. Speech may be slurred and they may be unsteady on their feet. In younger people the stimulus to produce this effect has to be severe, e.g. malaria. In elderly people almost any disease state can cause it but characteristic conditions include urinary tract infections, pneumonia heart attacks and small stokes. Drug side-effects are another common cause. Once the acute confusional state is correctly recognised as an illness and not due to old age then a cause has to be found and correct care and treatment given. This may take a period of time but most cases of acute confusion are fully reversible.

Chronic confusion

This is more complicated in that two sub-groups can be identified – reversible and non-reversible (the dementias). Chronic confusion by definition has been present for at least three months and usually a lot longer.

The reversible causes are extremely important as they account for about 10 per cent of cases and if not diagnosed a mistaken label of 'dementia' is given. Conditions such as hypothyroidism (underactivity of the thyroid gland) and syphilis (a venereal disease) can present as chronic confusion states. An important diagnosis to exclude is depression – sometimes termed pseudo-dementia. Depression is a very common psychiatric illness in elderly people and in some the symptoms can mimic dementia. Some brain tumours, e.g. meningioma, are benign and can be surgically removed.

The irreversible causes are more common and most can be diagnosed from the history. The two most common conditions are Alzheimer's disease and multi-infarct dementia. Alzheimer's disease is a condition of slow onset with a gradual decline in numerous faculties. The most obvious loss is in short-term memory, though many other aspects of brain function are affected, e.g. numeracy skills, judgement, personality etc. The disease often has a slowly progressive course but in a minority it appears to be aggressive and the mental decline is accompanied by physical ill-health and death occurs within a few years. In multi-infarct dementia there is a period of sharp decline in mental and often physical health associated with 'minor' strokes. The brain is usually affected in a more haphazard way but, again, memory is still a major area for loss of function. The two conditions can prove to be difficult to distinguish in some people though a CT brain scan may show up the infarcts (areas of furred-up blood vessels resulting in lack of blood and an area of tissue death). A definitive diagnosis may only be made post-mortem.

The two conditions account for about 10 per cent of 'dementia' in the over-65s and 20 per cent in the over-80s. To complicate matters those with chronic confusion can develop intercurrent illness (such as infections) and so become acutely worse, the so-called acute-on-chronic confusional state. It is obvious therefore that confusional states in elderly people are potentially difficult areas for making firm diagnoses and predictions. What is clear, however, is that the word 'dementia' should not be applied until after a vigorous medical history and examination.

ASSESSMENT

It is because of these difficulties that some areas in the UK have developed an assessment process often called a *memory clinic*. This usually involves a clinician, psychiatrist and a clinical psychologist as its core members, though they are usually assisted by nurses, social workers and therapists. The client is given a thorough medical history and examination and the psychiatrist assesses for depression and other mental health problems. The clinical psychologist uses various tests to examine the client's memory processes to see if a deficiency exists and how severe the impairment. Some clinics have an 'open-access' policy; others receive referrals from GPs and other health care professionals. This system ensures that all the reversible causes of confusion are looked for and treated if possible.

A client's current mental status should always be ascertained before detailed questions concerning other aspects are obtained. This is to identify the mentally frail/compromised client early, not to dismiss their account of events but to put it into perspective and to allow more time for repetition etc. No two people with chronic confusion are alike and some objective assessment of their mental state is necessary to try and identify the areas of greatest 'loss'.

One quick screening test is the simple 'mental test score' or abbreviated mental test (Hodgkinson, 1972). This consists of ten questions which test short and long-term memory, orientation and numeracy. It is a rather crude assessment and a low score by itself does not imply a permanent impairment. Its value lies in its repetition over time when a rising score indicates a resolving acute confusion whereas a persistently low score may indicate a more chronic confusional state. All clients should be informed sensitively and politely that it is necessary to test their memory. The clients most upset by testing often have a memory loss that they are aware of and have been trying to cover up. The ten

questions below should be written down, as most assessors only remember nine:

Name
Age
Date of birth
Date and time of day
Address
Name of Prime Minister
Date of First World War
Place
Remember an address five minutes later
Count back from 20 to 1

This assessment may indicate an obvious problem, and further
history-taking must be interpreted with caution. A more detailed evaluation of memory, etc. is provided by performing a 'mini-mental state'
test which involves 20 questions (Folstein, 1975). Workers in this area
should become conversant with the different aspects of 'confusion' and
its assessment. Many clients may need the experienced skills of a
memory-clinic approach or at least the opinion of a psychogeriatrician.

A poor score on a mental test does not equate with a blanket lack of
capacity to consent or mean that a person is totally lacking in judgement concerning certain situations. It is a difficult area, however, where
medicine, law, ethics, morality and professional experience overlap. It
is useful to compare the two approaches adopted by the UK and the
US. In the UK the balance of assessment is weighted towards the professional experience with the sparse legal framework kept in the background. A list of the possible legal aspects that may form part of an
individual case are as follows:

Mental Health Act 1983
Guardianship
Section 47 of the National Assistance Act (1948)
Court of Protection
Power of Attorney (Enduring)
Agency
The Chronically Sick and Disabled Persons Acts
The Living Will (Advance Directive)

The amount of legislation pertaining to elderly people, and the
elderly mentally frail especially, is small. This leaves a large 'grey' area
of care where professionals are expected to act in the person's 'best interests'. The concepts of competence and judgement are alien to most

health care workers who through lack of legislative guidance are forced into crude assessment procedures where a statement of whether a person is 'demented' or not forms the basis of a professional decision.

In the US the pendulum has swung the other way, with legal issues dominating the area:

Mandatory Reporting Laws (for elder abuse)
Competency hearings
Durable Powers of Attorney (in health care)
The Living Will (advance directive)

At the moment there is no major evidence that a state system heavily influenced by governmental process (US) is providing better overall 'care' of its vulnerable elderly (Folstein *et al.*, 1975). It is probable that a combination of the two systems – i.e. professional expertise allowed to assess a situation but backed up by some pertinent legislation – is the correct approach.

The elderly mentally frail need a detailed social and medical assessment in advance of potential crisis situations such as suspected abuse/inadequate care, so that if such a situation does occur, valuable time is not taken up in investigating the whole picture. The actual episode can be put into some kind of context, helpful for the professionals concerned. The degree to which the cognitive impairment (e.g., Alzheimer's disease) affects judgement and consent needs to be assessed and recorded. This may obviously vary for different issues – a person may be considered able to express a wish and make decisions over some home care issues, accepting home-help and meals on wheels but refusing a day centre. However they may be considered incapable of more complex decisions such as personal payment of bills.

Numerous professionals and carers may be involved in this assessment and ongoing care process. Decisions involving compulsory placement (for whatever reason) are some of the most difficult. Except at times of extreme emergency these decisions should never be rushed. The client's views and wishes are crucial but when circumstances dictate these may have to be overruled. Experience has shown that the more time spent in explaining why a move has to occur the better the long-term outcome. Despite a client's mental (and often physical) frailty repeated attempts to reassure, visits to meet new staff/carers and see new accommodation can decrease the undoubted morbidity (illness) and mortality (death) associated with moving, the so-called translocation effect.

The medical and health perspectives concerning elder abuse are at a critical stage. The physical and psychological manifestations of abuse/inadequate care will gradually become incorporated into the medical knowledge base (as has happened with child abuse) and greater diagnostic expertise will develop. In the meantime the possibility of abuse should be borne in mind by health and social care workers when dealing with elderly people.

The abuse of elderly people will prove to be another area where multi-professional assessment will come to the fore. Doctors will have a crucial but limited role in the diagnosis of physical or sexual abuse. Disclosure, however, or the picking up of important physical, psychological or social parameters will probably fall onto the other members of the health care team, namely nurses, physiotherapists, occupational therapists, district nurses, health visitors, community psychiatrist nurses and social workers. To be successful for the client, assessments and interventions must remain multi-professional with the commitment to joint working and a sharing of knowledge and skill. The way forward is through research and the continued role of education for all the health care team.

*The author is extremely grateful to Dr Holly Ramsey-Klawsnik for permission to reproduce some of her work.

CHAPTER NINE

Social Perspectives on Elder Abuse

Bridget Penhale and Paul Kingston

INTRODUCTION

Elder abuse has had something of a chequered history in the United Kingdom. The abuse of older people is not a new phenomenon; indeed, researchers have outlined documentary evidence in the US of the existence of such abuse in earlier times (Steinmetz, 1990; Kosberg, 1983). It is highly likely that similar evidence exists in relation to the UK for the discerning researcher to uncover. What is more problematic, however, is the extent to which, in recent times, the phenomenon of elder abuse has been recognised as a social issue worthy of attention and concern, and by whom. It is these aspects, and the more recent history of the topic, which are perhaps of greater interest and relevance here. The chapter will present the recent history of elder abuse in the UK and then move to a general consideration of the construction of social problems from the available literature. An attempt is made to compare the extent of the 'fit' between elder abuse and social problem construction in order to determine whether elder abuse can at present be properly considered to be a social problem in its own right, and the reasons for this situation. Possible future directions are then suggested. The second part of the chapter aims to take some of the issues raised further. A fuller consideration of marginalisation and elder abuse will be followed by such pertinent issues as empowerment and intervention strategies.

HISTORICAL BACKGROUND

It is not possible here to provide an adequate historical analysis of elder abuse in the UK in previous centuries, however interesting such an endeavour might be. Instead we are discussing late twentieth-century elder abuse in the private domain–in the domestic setting rather than in the wider sphere of public institutions. Our focus is on abuse which is perpetrated by (informal) carers, usually (but not always) members of the older person's family. As in other western countries, recognition of the abuse of older people occurred subsequent to the identification of child abuse and spouse abuse (domestic violence). In the United Kingdom, child abuse was 'discovered' as a problem in need of attention from the 1970s onwards, following a number of inquiries after well-publicised child deaths. Domestic violence in a wider sense was identified as a social problem in the decade of the 1980s, although a number of pressure groups (Women's Aid, Rape Crisis Centres) had been working for some years lobbying to increase awareness of the issues involved and to promote the need for social policy reform. The parallel situation in the United States in terms of timescale was of the identification of child abuse as a problem in need of attention from the 1960s onwards; and a similar recognition of spouse abuse in the 1970s. Elder abuse was determined as a social problem in the US from the late 1970s, with investigations to examine the nature of the problem and enquiries which included a Senate Committee Hearing in 1980. Such endeavours led to the pressure for social policy and legislative reform which was prevalent throughout the 1980s.

Developments in the field of familial violence can thus be seen to occur in the UK on average some ten years after similar developments in the US. In relation to elder abuse in the UK, the earliest mentions of the phenomenon in recent years can be credited to Drs Baker and Burston who both published material in medical journals in 1975 highlighting situations referred to by the terms 'granny battering' and 'granny bashing' (see Bennett and Kingston, 1993, p. 4, for an overview of terminology). These early UK reports prompted researchers in America to investigate the phenomenon of elder abuse in order to determine the extent of the problem. The UK experience was very different, however. There was something of an hiatus from the mid-1970s to the early 1980s, when the next surge of interest developed, largely spearheaded by the voluntary organisation Age Concern. A national conference was held, and two publications commissioned by the group – a review of the literature available at that time (Cloke, 1983) and a book concerning the re-named phenomenon of 'old age abuse' (Eastman, 1984). Various local initiatives were also held, including study and training days to raise awareness of the issues involved in the abuse of older people.

This momentum was not continued, and despite attempts by professionals at local levels, there was another lull in the process from a national perspective. This was clearly not assisted by the refusal of government to recognise or take any action on the associated issues. In the autumn of 1988, however, there was another attempt on the part of professionals working with older people to promote awareness of the phenomenon. The British Geriatrics Society (BGS) held a national conference to press the case for work to commence on trying to determine the nature of the problem from a UK perspective. This conference was reported by Tomlin (1989). In addition, a need was identified for the development of guidelines for professionals working in this area and to this end a working party of concerned organisations was set up to produce practice guidelines (Age Concern, *et al.*, 1990).

Since that time there have been continued and fairly consistent developments concerning the promotion of awareness about the phenomenon. There has been a steady trickle of conferences held at both local and national levels and an ever-increasing number of publications. In 1990, Age Concern Institute of Gerontology was commissioned by the Department of Health to conduct a study to establish a picture of what was known about the topic (McCreadie, 1991). At the same time the Council of Europe also set up a working group in order to discover what was happening from a European perspective (Council of Europe, 1992). Some small research projects have been completed since 1989 in different locations in the UK on a number of different aspects of the phenomenon and the results were reported (Homer and Gilleard, 1990; Kingston, 1990; Hildrew, 1991; Penhale, 1993a). Research on such issues as financial abuse and the sexual abuse of elderly people has recently been carried out (see papers by Rowe and Holt respectively in the UK guest-edited 1993 autumn edition of the *Journal of Elder Abuse and Neglect*) and a prevalence study is also now available (Ogg and Bennett, 1992). Major publications are also increasing in the field (Bennett and Kingston, 1993; Phillipson and Biggs, 1992; DeCalmer and Glendenning, 1993; Pritchard, 1992). Further substantial journal publications are available (Penhale, 1992a; Penhale, 1993b; McCreadie and Tinker, 1993; Ogg and Munn-Giddings, 1993; Kingston and Penhale, 1994; Kingston and Phillipson, 1994). A national organisation, Action on Elder Abuse, for professionals concerned about the problem has also been established. One of the principal aims of the organisation is to co-ordinate available information about elder abuse and to act as a clearing house for the dissemination of this information. The mission statement expresses the organisation's aims:

'To prevent abuse in old age by promoting changes in policy and practice through raising awareness, education, promoting research and the collection and dissemination of information.'

(Action on Elder Abuse, June 1993)

These aims may well be pursued in conjunction with groups recently established and connected with the abuse of vulnerable adults from other areas of speciality, such as learning disabilities (NAPSAC). In effect, since 1988, the developments, albeit slow, have continued. Included in these developments is increased attention from the media. Such developments largely reflect the efforts of a small (but steadily increasing) number of committed professionals from the fields of health and social welfare. The most recent responses from government spokespersons will be referred to later. Successive governments have been questioned at intervals since 1982 as to whether elder abuse was perceived by them as a problem. All have declined to identify the issue as in need of attention other than to state that professionals could determine their own local solutions if, indeed, any were necessary. The Department of Health has had some involvement, in commissioning the McCreadie study (1991) and by following up with their own small research project concerning responses to elder abuse by two social services departments in London (SSI, 1992). As an adjunct to this project, stage 2 of the enterprise comprised a number of inter-professional workshops held in the early part of 1992 in various locations. There has been further involvement (stage 3 of the project) in attempting to establish standards for good practice for social service/health authority departments involved in elder abuse (publication July 1993, referred to later in the chapter). Additionally the Law Commission has been considering the related set of issues concerning Mentally Incapacitated Adults and Decision-Making and the necessity or otherwise for legislative changes which would include the protection of incapacitated adults who are vulnerable and require 'proper safeguards ... against exploitation, neglect, and physical, sexual or psychological abuse' (Law Commission, 1991, p. 110).

The consultation process concerning these issues has, of necessity, been somewhat lengthy given the range of client groups involved within the spectrum of mental incapacity. The proposals for change suggested by the Law Commission have been recently published and are subject to a further period of consultation (Law Commission, 1993). Following this somewhat simplistic description of recent events within the field of elder abuse, it is necessary to move to an examination from a sociological perspective of the processes involved in the construction

225

of social problems. It will then be possible to establish the extent of the fit (or otherwise) of recent events within the field to determine whether elder abuse can properly be considered a social problem.

SOCIAL PROBLEM CONSTRUCTION

In the early 1970s, Blumer developed a thesis that considered how a re-definition of a social problem was determined by a process of collective definition (Blumer, 1971). Traditionally, sociologists had viewed social problems as existing as an independent set of objective conditions (or social arrangements) within society. Using a rather different and original approach, Blumer expounded the theory of the developmental stages of social problems. In this treatise, the process (of collective definition) consisted of a number of distinct phases which determined whether social problems arise, become legitimated and addressed in social policy terms. These phases are as follows:

- Emergence of a social problem
- Legitimation of the problem
- Mobilisation of action
- Formation of official action plan
- Implementation of the official plan

In addition, there is no guarantee that a particular social problem will necessarily be resolved by the implementation of a set of social policies designed to alleviate it. For Blumer, it is the whole process which is important. It is this which is vital in determining whether the issue is perceived, recognised and considered by the society in which it occurs; how it is considered, and what is done, in terms of action, to resolve or re-define the problem. As Blumer stated, 'Social problems have their being, their career, and their fate in this process' (Blumer, 1971, p. 305). Further explanation of each of these stages will be given later in this chapter when considering the situation pertaining to elder abuse (and whether elder abuse can be considered as a social problem).

Subsequent to the work by Blumer, further work, from a social constructionist perspective, has appeared describing the process of the development of social problems. Within this framework, social issues are constructed as social problems by a process of 'claims-making activities'. The most notable proponents of such analyses are Gusfield (1984), Schneider (1985), Spector and Kitsuse (1977) and Best (1989). Such models as have been developed tend to focus on the activities of 'claims-makers' who, as Best noted, are active in 'drawing attention to a problem' (p. 139). For Best, this process usually draws to a close at a point when a policy to deal with the problem has been devised by officials. Claims-makers are not neutral participants in these processes but, in Best's view, act to both create and promote claims and tend to be interested parties. Although some claims-makers may have personal experience of the particular problems which is being promoted, there are, equally, claims-makers who are professional experts who become involved in the delineation of problems (doctors, lawyers, scientists). Claims-makers are not always outsiders, however, and there may well be the involvement of pressure groups/activists and also officials in such processes. With regard to the situation as it has developed in America since the mid-1970s, an applied approach seems to have been the focus for much of the research into elder abuse. Such applied perspectives (in research terms) tend to concentrate on the problem areas of society, with the proposed outcome being policies and/or strategies to resolve such problems that have been defined. As Gusfield suggested:

'Professional social problems solvers supply leadership in the construction of a problem, its theory of explanation and its policies to alleviate the problem.'

(Gusfield, 1982, p. 6).

The strong message conveyed from such an applied focus is that these problems cannot be resolved without the intervention of 'troubled people professionals' such as social workers, counsellors, and service providers (Gusfield, 1982). Following on from these social constructionist perspectives there have been several analyses from the North American viewpoint to consider the development of elder abuse as a social problem. Baumann, in a well-argued chapter, explored the US field with an analysis of the research rhetoric used within the discourse, followed by an investigation of the role played by gerontologists (and other researchers) in defining elder abuse as a social problem in need of resolution (Baumann, 1989).

The Canadian perspective has been ably covered by Leroux and Petrunik who examined the development of elder abuse as a social problem using Blumer's categorisation of the stages of social problem development outlined above (Leroux and Petrunik, 1990). Various methodological techniques were used by them, including telephone interviews with key officials (at local, provincial and federal government levels); personal interviews with representatives of organisations for elderly people and analyses of reports and periodicals. The aim of this data collection and the analyses was to determine the factors behind the emergence of elder abuse as a problem in Canada. To follow the process of social problem construction which will be adopted here, it is necessary to move to an examination of the situation from a UK perspective. The process of development of elder abuse as a social problem in the UK will be considered using Blumer's (1971) categorisation together with some suggestions as to why this should be the case.

ELDER ABUSE IN THE UK

From an examination of the background and recent historical information previously described, it is evident that elder abuse has had a somewhat difficult time in terms of its emergence and legitimation as a social problem.

Emergence

The earliest mention of elder abuse in recent literature is credited to Burston in the *British Medical Journal* (1975). In America, the earliest subsequent mention is Steinmetz (1978), whereas in the UK we must look to Cloke's *Review*, published in 1983 (Cloke, 1983) and to Eastman (1984) for further serious mention of the topic. These and subsequent papers produced by a small number of professionals appear to have begun to raise awareness of the issue. No awareness appears to have existed prior to this. As Blumer stated:

> 'A social problem does not exist for a society until it is recognized by that society to exist.'

> (Blumer, 1971, pp. 301–2)

If the problem is not acknowledged or perceived as existing by society, it simply is not present (as a problem). There appears to be a number of factors which have contributed to the emergence of elder abuse as a social problem in need of attention. Leroux and Petrunik (1990) identified three main factors, from a Canadian perspective, which can equally be applied to the UK experience. The first of these is the inclusion of elder abuse as an aspect of the wider spectrum of family violence. Here, elderly people are viewed as possible victims of a particular form of domestic violence. It is important to acknowledge that the notion of family violence first developed following the public and professional concern which was raised with the 'discovery' of child abuse (see, for example, Kempe and Kempe, 1978). The level of concern which this issue generated then prepared the field for further 'discoveries' within the domain of family violence, namely violence against women and, subsequent to this, abuse of elderly people. Straus, writing in 1974, suggested that the emergence of family violence as a set of linked social problems related very much to an increased awareness by society of issues surrounding violence in general terms. This was followed by the development of the feminist movement and the development in sociological terms of the conflict view of society (which effectively challenged the consensus model which was dominant at that time). Although Straus wrote from a US perspective, clearly there are parallels which can be drawn from the UK experience several years later. Parton has developed an interesting treatise on what he terms the 'moral panic' surrounding child abuse in the UK; its recognition as a social problem and the political reasons for this (Parton, 1985). Such moral panic clearly has not followed the 'discovery' in the UK of either spouse abuse or elder abuse; however, different reasons for this situation might pertain to these particular types of family violence.

A further factor in the emergence of elder abuse as a social problem is related to prevalent societal views concerning later life and old age. Elderly people are increasingly viewed as dependent and a burden on the rest of society by virtue of their age. Old age is frequently viewed in a negative light by other members of society. Indeed, as Wilkes indicated, "even the very word 'old' has negative and derogatory connotations for many people" (Wilkes, 1981).

The social context in which elder abuse occurs is thus of prime importance; abuse is not just a consequence of family or even individual pathology. Individual experiences of abuse must rather be considered in the wider social context in which they take place. That elder abuse exists may indeed be related to such negative stereotypes of old age. As Pagelow suggested:

'Elderly persons are abused by a society that considers them worthless because they are no longer capable of economic productivity.'

(Pagelow, 1984, p. 372)

Ageism may in some respects even encourage abusive situations as it detracts from any influence that the elderly person may have and could lead to relationships which further adversely affect the power of the older person to either protect themselves or to prevent abuse from occurring. Work by gerontologists in the UK in the 1980s encompassed such notions as 'structured dependency' (Townsend, 1981) and the 'social construction of old age' (Walker, 1980). Within such theories,

229

social inequalities in later life are affected by economic conditions. Dependency occurs from interaction with the wider, oppressive social system. Older people are marginalised from the rest of society by virtue of their age and the master status of old age (within which age becomes the principal factor in characterisation of the person). If abuse occurs because of dependency situations of victims (and abusers), then the likelihood of abuse arising may increase due to the marginalisation of older people and their carers by a predominantly ageist society. Currently held ideologies about old age and ageing may create environments which encourage the development and perpetuation of abusive situations (Penhale, 1992b). This situation may perhaps account for some of the apparent lack of 'moral panic' concerning elder abuse. An additional dimension to this situation, as Leroux and Petrunik commented, is as follows:

> 'The view of old age as a social problem sets the stage for the call for social action concerning problems arising out of old age.'

> (Leroux and Petrunik, 1990, p. 653)

It is evident that elder abuse can be viewed as one such legitimate area of concern within the master state of old age. A view of elderly people as frail, dependent and vulnerable (if not incompetent, which appears in much of the writing about elder abuse, may not assist, however, in attempting to counter the negative assumptions and views of our ageist society. Salend et al., from a US perspective, cautioned against the development of particular procedures (in particular mandatory reporting laws) for elderly people on the grounds that such 'special treatment' might accentuate existing tendencies to infantilise older people (Salend et al., 1984). As Baumann noted, the reason that elder abuse was readily accorded social problem status in the US may link with the traditional focus of research interest concerning older people in that country: a focus on the problem areas surrounding ageing (Baumann, 1989). The view of elderly people as potential victims may in part be a result of this focus on dependency and vulnerability. Although in the UK elder abuse does not yet appear to have achieved the full status of a social problem, the same trends may perhaps be observed in terms of the negative view of age which such abuse tends to promulgate and debates now developing as to whether practice guidelines and procedures should focus specifically on older people, or rather focus on all vulnerable adults.

A third factor in the emergence of elder abuse relates to an increasing societal concern about crime and older people, and in particular elderly people as victims of crime. The stereotypical view is of elderly people as potential victims/prime targets of crime and in particular crimes of violence, with much media attention (particularly in tabloid newspapers) being given to the reporting of such incidents. Elderly people are continuously urged to exercise caution in order to protect themselves. Victimisation of elderly people has been an area of interest to criminologists in recent years; voluntary organisations have developed expertise in assisting older people with security arrangements for their accommodation (e.g. campaigns for the provision and installation of door-chains). From this consideration of these areas of social concern; the development of concern about family violence; the social construction of old age as a time of problems/difficulties; and an increased concern about the victimisation of older people, it is possible to perceive reasons for the emergence of elder abuse as a specific social problem in the UK since the mid-1970s. The fact is that the emergence has taken place over a lengthy period, and some of the possible reasons for this state of affairs will be discussed later. It is necessary in the following section to move to a consideration of the degree of legitimation (or otherwise) of the problem.

Legitimation

In order for any social problem to develop as an acknowledged problem, it requires a reasonable degree of public legitimation rather than solely an amount (however well developed and extensive) of concern by professionals. To have achieved status in terms of location on a 'professional agenda' is not sufficient in and of itself. As Blumer stated:

'a social problem must acquire social endorsement if it is to be taken seriously and to move forward in its career.'

(Blumer, 1971, p. 303)

A certain amount of 'respectability' is necessary, which means that the issue is then given consideration within the normally recognised areas in which public discussion of issues takes place. These arenas are generally agreed within our society to consist of the press and wider media; the church and other civic organisations; government offices and parliament. Following the initial stage of identification and recognition occurring through the processes of emergence, a social problem must achieve public legitimation or die as an issue. With regard to elder abuse, it is possible that the issue has acquired a place within the setting of professional agendas without necessarily achieving full legitimation in a public sense. Concerned professionals promote a particular view and awareness of the issues that concern them at any one time. The status of elder abuse in the UK at this time in terms of its legitimacy as a social problem would appear to lie with professionals; there is little by way of wider public support of it as an issue requiring attention. In recent years (effectively since 1988) a number of interest groups in the voluntary and public service domains of health and social welfare agencies have become concerned although the wider public audience has yet to be convinced.

PROFESSIONAL INTEREST AND INVOLVEMENT

The earliest group of concerned professionals, pioneers in the field, consisted of a very small number of individuals (for example, Baker, Burston, Hocking and Eastman). Others who then became involved in this field subsequently formed part of a group of first-wave innovators; committed and concerned individuals. Those professionals who were concerned about and were active in the field within this group comprised a slightly larger number, perhaps twelve to fifteen in total. These people, from a variety of professional backgrounds (e.g. health, social work and gerontology) can in some senses be regarded as the 'claims-makers' who promoted the cause of elder abuse and gained its inclusion on professional agendas. The core of this group has largely continued with commitment to the issue and formed the steering committee of the national organisation which has recently been established, Action on Elder Abuse. The names of the individuals are familiar within the UK context through conferences and publications: Bennett; Kingston; Homer; Ogg; Pritchard; Rowe; Holt; McCreadie; Penhale. Beyond this group are a further discreet group of professionals (and academics) who have some concern with and commitment to the issue but who also have wider concerns in their respective fields – for example, Greengross; Stevenson; Tinker and Phillipson. It is also possible, more recently, to discern the development of a second wave of innovators, a potentially much larger group who wish to assist in taking the issues further. One of the aims of the national organisation Action on Elder Abuse is to provide a forum particularly for professionals and their organisations rather than the general public: it will be interesting to discover what the professional membership of the organisation will be. In addition there have been calls from professional groups such as BASW (British Association of Social Workers) and BGS (British Geriatrics Society) together with Age Concern who have

232

demanded the development of guidelines for good practice (Age Concern *et al.*, 1990) as have the Association of Directors of Social Services (ADSS, 1991).

MEDIA ATTENTION

The media concerned with professionals and their interests have picked up on the issue since 1992, and there have been regular articles appearing in the 'popular' professional magazines such as *Geriatric Medicine, Nursing Times* and *Community Care*, including from April to July 1993 a campaign on the topic in the latter magazine. There has also been an increasing amount of research-based work published in the field (see above for details). Other forms of communications media have not yet developed at the same pace, perhaps due to the lack of public legitimation of the issue as a social problem. There have been a number of radio programmes/interviews with concerned professionals, usually locally based rather than given any prominence on the national networks.

In terms of television coverage, some attention has been gained, particularly in conjunction with items about caring responsibilities and the associated difficulties. There have been two documentary programmes screened since 1988; the first half-hour programme by the BBC, shown in late 1989, focused largely on carer stress and related abuse to this issue. The second programme was made by an independent production company for Channel 4 and screened in late 1992. This programme received a wider coverage than previously, particularly from the national newspapers, but tended to sensationalise the issues somewhat. Extracts from interviews with 'victims' were used to illustrate the factual material. The results of questions asked as part of the Office of Population Census and Surveys 'Omnibus Survey' (Ogg and Bennett, 1992) were revealed with an attempt to project these results to the wider population figures in order to determine likely prevalence. This latter aspect was not wholly successful as figures such as the projected 'three million elderly people at risk of abuse' tend to have little real meaning for individuals because it is too big to warrant any lasting credibility. An attempt was made, however, to widen the issues out from the somewhat narrow focus of carer stress to include such aspects as financial abuse and abuse arising from neglect. This Channel 4 programme was updated to take account of the legislative changes surrounding the NHS and Community Care Act 1990, which came into effect in April 1993. The programme was shown in late May 1993 and included an interview with the Junior Minister of Health, Tim Yeo, who stated that guidelines for local authorities would be forthcoming over the summer.

These were the Social Services Inspectorate guidelines published in July 1993 which still did not mandate Local Authority Social Services Departments to produce guidelines for such work (SSI, 1993).

CIVIC ORGANISATIONS

There is no evidence at present to suggest that elder abuse has attained recognition beyond the sphere of professional agendas and the limited media attention described in the previous section. Although some voluntary organisations concerned with older people have developed an interest in the topic (for example, Age Concern, Counsel and Care, and Help the Aged) there is as yet no lobby of elderly people specifically concerned about abuse. Organisations representing carers have indicated some concern about the issue and associated problems of carer stress but their lobby is fairly clearly directed towards their prime focus, that is, carers. Other civic groups do not appear to have developed a widespread interest in the issues. In terms of claims-making activities, in general, it is large groups who are more effective in pressing and pursuing their claims (Spector and Kitsuse, 1987). Groups with a wide and large membership, more resources available to them and greater levels of organisation tend to be most effective in this respect. Elder abuse would appear to have remained at a rather localized level of awareness and action because there has not to date been any unified national lobby pressing for change.

From the above outline, it would appear that to date there has been some progress by various concerned individuals and groups towards achieving public recognition and legitimation of elder abuse as a social problem. This progress commenced in 1989, speeding up slightly during 1992.

It is necessary now to consider Blumer's third stage in the development of social problems: mobilisation of action from the UK perspective.

MOBILISATION OF ACTION

Following the successful completion of the initial stages of recognition and legitimation by a society, a further developmental stage is reached, that of mobilisation of action. As Blumer suggests, the topic

'becomes the object of discussion, of controversy, of differing depictions and diverse claims.'

(Blumer, 1971, p. 303)

234

Wide-scale public debate and discussion occurs, through meetings (both formal and informal); the various media channels; and within the political and thus legislative arenas. The society mobilises itself for action concerning the particular problem in question. In many senses, the UK experience suggests that elder abuse is currently at this stage in the total process. It has already been suggested that in the last four years there have been increasing developments in terms of both the emergence and recognition of the problem and a degree of public legitimation of elder abuse. Various groups, mentioned already, have in recent years called for increased awareness and action concerning elder abuse. Such pleas effectively constitute the beginning of the mobilisation of action phase.

Approaches to the government to act to alleviate the problem also constitute mobilisation of action. Up until September 1993 successive governments had declined to make any commitment to act in terms of legislation or guidance concerning the problem (except for the SSI contribution). Apart from the activities of the Department of Health, which have been described in the first section, repeated questions of Ministers of Health in Parliament about elder abuse between 1981 and 1992 had failed to produce any concrete action. There had even been a number of public statements to the media to this effect. In June 1991, Virginia Bottomley (then Junior Minister of Health) was interviewed on a late night current affairs programme. In response to a question concerning elder abuse, her reply was: 'I don't frankly think that abuse of elderly is a major issue, thank goodness, in our society' (*Newsnight*, BBC, 4 June 1991). Additionally, it was stated that legislative change to alleviate the problem was not required. By the autumn of 1992, Bottomley's junior minister, Tim Yeo, made a statement to the producers of the *Dispatches* programme that in a small number of instances, carers were unable to cope with the stress involved and this resulted in abuse. The shift in these two statements appears rather minimal, given the time-scale involved (some 15 months). Further statements by Yeo in the revised programme in May 1993 did not suggest any major change in the governmental view of the problem. As Leroux and Petrunik comment, it is usually at this mobilisation of action stage that 'government determines whether the issue will fulfil its potential as a social problem warranting an official response' (Leroux and Petrunik, 1990, p. 657).

However, in retrospect, this political intervention by Tim Yeo can be seen as a real turning point, almost a 'U' turn when considered alongside Mrs Bottomley's earlier comments. When the SSI Guidelines were published in 1993 the new Junior Health Minister John Bowis wrote the foreword.

ACTION ON ELDER ABUSE

In September 1993 the first International Symposium on Elder Abuse took place in North Staffordshire with two of the most eminent American academics in this field, Professor Karl Pillemer and Professor Rosalie Wolf. The media attention for the conference was unprecedented. The following day in London, Action on Elder Abuse was formally launched. Professor Pillemer, Professor Wolf, Dr. Gerry Bennett, Sally Greengross and Ginny Jenkins all spoke about the organisation. However, political legitimation was finally achieved when John Bowis, Junior Health Minister, formally launched the organisation.

Elder abuse in the UK appears at present to be in the mobilisation of action stage, hovering on the periphery of the stage of 'formation of an official plan of action' (Blumer, 1971, p. 304). From this point, it is possible that the issue may fail to achieve any status as a social problem and thus merely fade away into obscurity. Equally, however, it is possible that continued and sustained calls for action and a more united approach to this (amongst the various groups concerned with the issue) may indeed force the government to act beyond its good practice guidelines. It is worth looking briefly at the final two stages of Blumer's taxonomy in order to try and determine whether elder abuse in the UK will continue to develop as a social problem or not.

FORMATION AND IMPLEMENTATION OF AN OFFICIAL PLAN OF ACTION

The final two stages in Blumer's developmental model consist of the creation of official plans to deal with the problem and their implementation. As Blumer indicated, this plan reflects 'the decision of a society as to how it will act with regard to the given problem' (Blumer, 1971, p. 304).

The formation of the plan is usually a process of negotiation and compromise; of re-defining and re-working of the societal view of the problem. The resulting official action plan therefore represents the official societal definition of the problem and its relevant dimensions. It includes the view of how that society is likely to act in order to resolve the problem. Social policy guidance and legislation may well be the outcome of implementation of the action plan. The implementation stage is rarely entirely trouble-free: action plans are often modified and re-worked during this period. For Blumer, this represents a further stage of definition and the chance that additional action plans will be created and subsequently executed. From the UK perspective, it is apparent that despite the increasing amount of publications and reports, including research findings, and copious recommendations/calls for action since 1988, this has not resulted in the development of action plans (on an official, government basis) or specific policy initiatives concerning elder abuse. The only action so far has been *ad hoc* local policy initiatives based on local policy formulation, many of these policies being designed in isolation from most of the leading players in Social and Health Policy provision. (For an example of good practice, see 'Health Authority and Social Service Co-operation', in Bennett and Kingston, 1993.)

There is a now a relatively large amount of policy concerned with child abuse, including more recently child sexual abuse. To a lesser extent, the 1980's have seen the development of action and policy concerning violence against women, particularly in the domestic setting; little has been developed as yet with regard to elder abuse. Elder abuse now appears to be recognised as a problem in need of attention by professionals concerned with older people and by organisations with a similar focus. Governmental response has so far been very limited. There are a number of factors contributing to this situation. In particular, it is likely that the little information on the incidence and prevalence of elder abuse from research and definitional difficulties are prominent within these. Clearly the fact that there is no standardised definition as to what constitutes abuse is problematic; indeed there are conflicts and disagreements as to the proper frame of reference for the study of elder abuse. It has been argued elsewhere that different definitions may well be required for different groups: researchers; policy-makers; practitioners; and that this may not matter a great deal (Bennett and Kingston, 1993). This situation has clearly not assisted in the developmental process of the construction of elder abuse as a social problem.

MARGINALISATION AND ELDER ABUSE

The next part of this chapter aims to look very briefly at the situation pertaining to elder abuse as a distinct example of marginalisation of older people. The implications for policies concerned with community care also need to be raised and acknowledged within this context. The social context within which elder abuse occurs is of prime importance, yet has to date to be adequately examined in this country. Elder abuse is not just a consequence of family or individual pathology. Rather, individual experiences of abuse need to be seen in the context in which they occur. In addition to a likelihood of increased health problems and frailty with age there are negative views of old age. The existence of abuse may be related to such negative stereotypes which somehow make such situations permissible since they restrict the influence that older people may have in society and could lead to behaviours and relationships which further diminish their power. The well-developed theories surrounding the 'social construction of old age' (Walker, 1980) and of 'structured dependency in later life' (Townsend, 1981) can also be considered in connection with elder abuse. Within such theories, economic conditions contribute to the social inequalities experienced by many older people and their carers. Dependency develops through interaction with the wider, oppressive social system. Elder abuse could be seen as arising from the way in which the wider marginalisation of older people occurs. If a certain amount of abuse occurs due to the dependency of the older person, then the likelihood of abuse occurring may increase due to the oppression and discrimination faced by older people and their carers from an ageist society. The current predominant societal ideologies about old age and growing older may create an environment which encourages the development and perpetuation of certain forms of abuse and neglect.

In addition to wider social and political forces which influence whether abuse occurs there are two further factors: the poverty and isolation of many older people and their carers (the economic dimension) and inadequate provision of community care for frail elderly people. These would seem to provide a further push towards marginalisation and strongly suggest that both care and abuse are inextricably linked to the wider context of oppression and life on the edges of society. Inadequate community care due to under-developed services, under-resourcing, inadequate systems of support and insufficient attention to providing real choice for those using the services, coupled with a failure to address the problems in the wider social system, may well mean that the incidence of elder abuse will continue to rise in forthcoming years. Community care should not be seen as the panacea for such problems. Phillipson (1992) proposes that policies to address elder abuse should develop within the context of empowerment and advocacy for those people 'leading marginal lives'. For him the emphasis concentrates on enabling people to live free from abuse and mistreatment (including neglect) and on the promotion of abilities for self-care in later life. There is a view espoused by Norman (1985) in relation to ethnic-minority elders that to grow old in a non-native country is to be subject to triple jeopardy. It is also tentatively suggested here (in the absence of hard data from research in the UK) in connection with elder abuse. To be old in the UK is to be marginalised (single jeopardy); to be old and abused is to be marginalised (double jeopardy); to be old and abused and female is to be marginalised (triple jeopardy). Women, as the largest group of the population of older people (Arber and Ginn, 1991), are more likely to be subject to abuse and neglect and to live in situations where abuse occurs. Their ability to avoid or resolve such situations may be limited by the poverty which faces many people in later life and thus restricts available choices about where and how to live and with whom. It is hoped that the validity of this assertion will be more fully tested by future research into the phenomenon over the next few years.

Having considered the social construction of elder abuse it is important to finally clarify the authors' position within the constructionist perspective. This is clearly necessary to justify the use of terms like 'legitimation' and 'claims-makers' used throughout this text. Manthorpe (1993) has coined the term 'elder abuse enterprise' (to plagiarise Estes's 'aging enterprise': Estes, 1979) to describe what could be construed as a deliberate attempt to construct a problem with vested interests for the service providers *vis-à-vis* the elders who are the victims of abuse. Manthorpe makes the point that elders themselves have not had any say in the definition of what is or is not abusive behaviour. These are important points that need urgent clarification. Indeed, not only have elders themselves been excluded from the debate, but leading pressure groups have had little to say thus far. This omission shows signs of being rectified in the near future with groups like Action on Elder Abuse wishing to bring a more representative forum together. It is therefore essential that debates focusing on how elder abuse is managed should concentrate upon the requirements of the elders and their carers. When policies are formulated to intervene in cases of elder abuse and neglect it will be necessary to question whether they are being designed with the best interests of elders to the fore.

It is important to avoid what Estes calls the 'aging enterprise', a term she uses not only to portray how elderly people are 'processed and treated as a commodity' but, just as important, how policy formulation can

> 'tend to segregate the aged, often with the poor, as a special class within society. Based on the concept that the aged are in need of services, these policies are often of more benefit to providers of service (physicians, hospitals, banks, mortgage insurance companies) than they are to the aged.'

> Estes (1979)

239

With this caveat in mind the response to elder abuse must be framed with the views of the abused and abuser being taken into consideration. The vested interests of service providers should have no part in the construction of elder abuse and neglect as a social problem. The sole justification in using Blumer's taxonomy is not to construct a social problem, but to try and understand why elder abuse has remained marginal in the UK and become a major social problem in the US. These insights should allow professionals time to think through a balanced and elder-orientated response, not a knee-jerk reaction.

INTERVENTIONS

Intervention strategies in cases of elder abuse and neglect are also in the development stage in the UK. Practitioners have in the past had only the standard interventions available to them, namely respite care for the abused, and in the most severe cases professionals have resorted to continuing care facilities for the elder victim. These strategies have been inadequate in the past and will not be the solution of the future. It is perhaps pertinent to even question the conceptual base that will underpin the intervention strategy. It has been argued elsewhere (Bennett and Kingston, 1993) that a framework for intervention can be based on three differing frameworks:

- a response based on the child abuse framework
- a response based on the spouse abuse framework
- a response unique to elder abuse

We agree with Bennett and Kingston's view that a response should be based on the unique phenomena of elder abuse, which has little in common with child abuse and some similarities with spouse abuse (see concluding chapter). Finkelhor and Pillemer (1984) have explored whether elder abuse deserves to be classified as a distinct form of abuse (separate from adult abuse) and, if so, should interventions be unique to this group. Critiques of this view (Crystal, 1986; Callahan, 1986) suggest that existing services could be utilised and that the elderly have more pressing problems than abuse. It is clearly the case that other forms of abuse exist, in the form of structured dependency (Townsend, 1986), marginalisation (Penhale, 1992b) and poverty (Walker, 1986). However, to suggest that existing resources, already overstretched in its attempt to deal with marginalisation and poverty, could possibly also be utilised to cope with abuse and neglect is hard to believe even within an adequately funded welfare state. The case is therefore argued that elder abuse and neglect does 'constitute a distinct category of abuse worthy of special attention' (Finkelhor and Pillemer, 1984). They suggest three reasons to justify this position:

- Older people are vulnerable to abuse because of increased frailty.
- Older people are vulnerable because of devalued social status.
- Existing social and health provision is provided with specialist services to elders.

However, it is possible to use concepts like autonomy and empowerment and individual choice which have led the way forward in the field of spouse abuse. Nevertheless, difficulties with autonomy, empowerment and choice are encountered when the victim of abuse cannot make decisions for themselves, for example individuals whose mental capacity is diminished. In situations where the victim cannot make decisions, advocates can be used to decide which options the victim would have wished given full mental competence. The debate surrounding legislation and elder abuse also appears to be 'hotting up'. The Law Commission paper (1993) suggests that 'removal of a frail, elderly person to an institutional setting' may be sometimes necessary. The Alzheimer's Disease Society's *Position Paper on Prevention of Elder Abuse* (1993) clearly takes the view that statutory changes are unnecessary:

'the society opposes those proposals from the Law Commission to create a statutory framework around failure to care, and to give social workers additional powers to enter peoples homes.'

Alzheimer's Disease Society (1993)

They further suggest that:

'Removal of a frail elderly person to an institutional setting may be abusive in itself and may even hasten death.'

There is research evidence to support this view. Crystal (1986) in a well-argued chapter suggests that legislative changes in the form of mandatory reporting laws in the US have not helped elderly people. On the contrary, studies have found that 60 per cent of those individuals receiving medical care (short-term) because of reports of abuse do not return home, perhaps a remedy worse than the cause (Faulkner, 1982). Furthermore, Blenkner's (1971) study which followed two groups of vulnerable elderly clients, of which one group received existing community services and the second an intensive case-management programme, found high levels of nursing home placement in the second group. These nursing home placements resulted in higher mortality rates associated with institutional placement.

It should also be noted that institutions are not free from abuse (for a more encompassing discussion, see 'Institutional Abuse' in Bennett and Kingston, 1993; Phillipson and Biggs, this text, Chapter 7). A scenario can be envisaged where an elderly victim of abuse is removed from a situation which she is not happy with, but wishes to tolerate, only to be placed in an institution where she is professionally abused. Perhaps a change of emphasis is required, with the abuser leaving the caring situation temporarily. This type of intervention strategy would require a professional carer to take over the short-term requirements for the abused elder, whilst interventions are considered for the abuser. This could take the form of education or counselling, perhaps even agreement that caring is beyond the skills of the carer and alternative care is clearly required. In certain situations legislation may be used to increase the costs of abuse. Pillemer suggests that 'being arrested ... would greatly outweigh the rewards obtained from abusive behaviour' (Pillemer and Suitor, 1990).

Clearly this legislative debate will continue and is necessary in order that a balanced framework is developed for the future. Lessons from the US should also help to frame the debate and there does appear to be a consensus view that mandatory reporting followed by investigation has not been effective thus far in the US. We need to be sure that if the law is changed in the UK it balances the rights of individuals against the perceived danger they may find themselves in. For competent elders the same rights, freedoms and preferences afforded to younger adults who are victims of abuse will allow them to choose if and when they wish professionals to become involved in their personal difficulties.

Beyond the legal framework the pragmatic realities for professionals mean that they will need to face the complex difficulties of abuse on an increasing number of occasions. Cases of abuse will increase; whether this is because of demographic and service provision changes or because of the increasing profile of elder abuse as a social problem remains to be seen. It has been suggested (Bennett and Kingston, 1993) that the demographic changes allied to social and health policy changes will pressure more carers to cope in situations where perhaps they should not have been asked to care. It is also the case that when a social problem emerges more people are aware of the issues and then report suspected cases. This may in fact happen with elder abuse, and therefore public education about the phenomenon of elder abuse is one effective empowering tool.

It is true to say that responses to elder abuse and neglect are in a rather crude and formative developmental stage for several reasons. Firstly UK research is noticeable by its absence, therefore even understanding the problem is difficult. Service delivery by the social service departments is resource-led not needs-led (although there is evidence that this is changing). Finally we are an ageist society and therefore a change in attitude by both society and professionals is required. However, it will not help to be pessimistic; research is beginning to untangle the complexities of abuse in later life, as it did with child and spouse abuse in preceding decades. Organisations are beginning to address the issues of elder abuse with comments, policies and education. Articles are appearing almost weekly on the issue and the momentum is increasing. A knowledge base is therefore developing. Service provision (Social and Health) is moving towards care-management with the implication of a needs-led intervention which will clearly be required with the complexities of elder abuse. Addressing the problems of ageism in society will not be quite so easy; it is the responsibility of all professionals to advocate for their elderly clients in order that they can live life free from all forms of abuse.

CONCLUSION

To summarise, elder abuse in the UK has, effectively since 1988, emerged as a social problem, acquired some public and political legitimation and seen energy on the part of professionals and concerned organisations to mobilise action. The formation and implementation of an official action plan (including legislation and specific policies) has not really occurred. This is particularly evident at a national and governmental level where the response has been limited and cautious so far. The pressure and lobbying for recognition and reform has to date come largely from professional 'claims-makers' from the fields of health and social care. This has been somewhat fragmented and lacking in direction, having developed in a rather 'ad hoc' way. It is also comparatively recent in origin, in effect since 1989. There may yet be further divisions. Kingston (1993) notes a tendency towards exclusivity and potential marginalisation of elder abuse by the medical profession. Until now there has not been any evidence of widescale public support of the issue, nor the development of an effective lobby by elderly people themselves. This may be a key (if not the determining) factor in the future of elder abuse as a social problem.

Elder abuse seems to be at a stage in its development where it may either succeed or fail as a social problem. If the momentum since 1989 does not continue or even recedes, it will fail to achieve prominence on the agenda of government and will probably become a 'non-issue' once more. Should the momentum continue or even increase, then elder abuse is likely to succeed in its attempt to gain full status as a social problem. At this point it is not possible to accurately predict the future course of events. Given the demographic trends and attendant implications, it is possible that elder abuse might become more prevalent and achieve further legitimation and mobilisation of action. This is also possible as an outcome of the current reforms concerning 'community care' and care-management in the UK which were implemented in April 1993. If such reforms are not adequately resourced then pressures on caregivers will increase and the incidence of elder abuse may rise sharply (Bennett and Kingston, 1993; Penhale, 1992b). Such a scenario might then necessitate action on the part of government. From this perspective, however, it is too early to fully analyse the construction of elder abuse as a social problem, as it is 'in process' and at a comparatively early point. It will be necessary to revisit this arena again in future, probably at several different points in time, in order to check on the progress, or otherwise, of the development of elder abuse as a social problem. At such points it might be profitable to employ further techniques such as a content analysis of newspapers/journals, direct approaches to government departments and interviews with relevant claims-makers, policy-makers and politicians. It is also crucial to seek the views of elders; as Callahan has suggested, 'abuse, like beauty, is in the eye of the beholder' (Callahan, 1986).

Elder abuse is in some respects currently at a critical juncture in its career and development as a social problem. Its progress requires monitoring, if not nurturing, over the next few years with the final outcome of the process still awaited.

Similarities, Differences and Synthesis

Bridget Penhale and Paul Kingston

This chapter has a number of different but related aims. It is necessary to provide some synthesis of the book as a whole and to present some of the crucial issues for the reader. As a precursor to this, it would seem both necessary and appropriate to consider in some depth the similarities and differences between the different types of family violence. For convenience the principal focus will be on elder abuse and to compare and contrast this with both child abuse and with spouse/adult abuse in more general terms. Some concluding comments are then offered.

SIMILARITIES OF ELDER ABUSE WITH OTHER FORMS OF FAMILY VIOLENCE

It is apparent that many agencies attempting to deal with elder abuse have looked for guidance to the experiences learned from colleagues in the child abuse/child protection arena. Indeed, following the 'discovery' of elder abuse in the United States in the late 1970s it would seem that in many areas it was claimed by experts in family violence. The reasons for this were logical. Elder abuse has certain characteristics in common with other forms of family violence and it is worth considering these similarities before moving on to consider why the comparisons may not be entirely appropriate.

When considering the wider situation, it is evident that the ideological and the methodological debates within elder abuse have, in the main, paralleled those which occurred in the child protection arena, and to a lesser extent the area of domestic violence between adults (spouse abuse). To date there has been very little thought regarding the most appropriate conceptual model which might be relevant within elder abuse;

many, if not most of the research studies until now have drawn on concepts more widely applicable within the field of family violence more generally (and in particular child abuse and spouse abuse).

The theoretical frameworks which have been developed to investigate the possible causes of abuse are similar, as attempts have been made to apply the models proposed for other forms of familial violence to elder abuse. Somewhat uncritical assumptions have been made that the theoretical frameworks and explanations from both psychological and sociological disciplines are comparable and transferable between and across different forms of abuse.

These frameworks include such theories as family dynamics/ transgenerational violence; exchange theories; stress theories (either internal or external stress for the family and/or the individuals concerned, or a combination of these); theories which propose individual psychopathology, usually of the abuser, as being crucial in the genesis of abuse; and also theories which look at the dependency and powerlessness of the victim of abuse, as being important in terms of the causation of abusive situations.

Family violence is currently conceptualised and accepted as that violence which occurs within 'familial situations' and is perpetrated against powerless and otherwise vulnerable people (Finkelhor, 1983). This broad framework certainly includes elder abuse, perhaps in particular because of the vulnerability of many older people (more on this aspect later).

There would also seem to be strong similarities in the characteristics of those individuals who commit abusive acts. Research has indicated that such people often have alcohol and/or drug misuse problems or histories of psychiatric or personality difficulties and associated relationship problems (Pillemer and Wolf, 1986). There are also rather more tentative suggestions that those who perpetrate elder abuse are likely, as in other forms of domestic violence, to have been subjected to abuse within the family setting at earlier stages of their lives (Pillemer and Suitor, 1988).

With regard to what is known about risk factors for elder abuse, some of these would seem to be similar to those found in other forms of familial violence. In particular, conditions of extreme stress (both internal and external) within families, of social isolation and poverty appear to be common within all forms of domestic violence.

The effects of different forms of abuse on victims also appear to show areas of correspondence (even allowing for individual differences in terms of reactions to abuse). Such effects include attitudes of self-blame and stigma; a lowering of self-esteem and reduction in the general

246

coping skills of the person. Other effects of note may be depression, sleep disturbances, a sense of isolation and despair and an increase in feelings of dependence. These can be seen in victims of virtually all forms of familial violence (although not in every situation) and may well relate to such structural issues as the inequalities of power within relationships which may lead to the development of abusive situations.

Within the differing forms of family violence, difficulties have been encountered in terms of establishing appropriate strategies of intervention. There is a societal stigma surrounding abuse (of all types) and this will in all probability lead to a reluctance on the part of those involved in abusive situations to accept or to seek assistance in their predicament. Victims are not infrequently both intimidated by and fearful of their abusers. Their powerless positions (and the associated perception of this) can make it difficult to empower them sufficiently to leave or change an abusive situation. In addition, within some abusive situations, there are levels of attachment and affection which the parties concerned do not necessarily wish to alter.

It may be difficult to reach a point where the existence of abuse is readily acknowledged by all parties; even gaining appropriate levels of access can be very hard for professionals to achieve on a sustained and consistent basis. The continued delivery of services and monitoring the safety of individuals may also be problematic in association with this. To achieve a successful and lasting outcome to a protection plan can require a great deal of effort and commitment from all concerned in the process.

SIMILARITIES WITH CHILD ABUSE

Within the area of family violence, elder abuse has been compared to child abuse more often than spouse abuse. This would seem to be due to the level of similarities which can be found between the two forms of abuse. It is perhaps also due to the increased attention and priority given to child protection within health and welfare agencies. It is worth exploring these in a little more depth, before considering the differences between the two types of abuse.

In its most extreme forms, elder abuse involves physical violence and physical harm to the victim – as also occurs in child and spouse abuse. In both child and elder abuse, there is most commonly abuse of a dependent person by a caregiver (usually a member of the family). In both types of situation, the dependent person may well be a source of stress (emotional, physical, financial) to the caregiver; the pressures on caregivers may be the same, with abuse being a desperate response to a situation which is, has become or is likely to become intolerable.

Additionally, the families in which elder and child abuse occur have been found to be more socially isolated and having fewer financial and social resources available to them than 'ordinary families' (Pillemer and Wolf, 1986). Familial roles seem to be distorted and disturbed within both types of abusive families and clarity of roles becomes less distinct or even obscured (Korbin *et al.*, 1989). There is some evidence, also, that the dynamics of role reversal (Steele, 1980) and 'generational inversion' (Steinmetz and Amsden, 1983) appear to operate within some abusive situations.

Apart from these general similarities, four specific areas of correspondence between child and elder abuse can be observed. The first is the increasing amount of evidence surrounding the transmission of violent responses between generations (Rathbone-McCuan, 1980; Steinmetz, 1983), so that a person who has been abused in the past, perhaps in childhood, is more likely to act abusively when adult (Pillemer and Suitor, 1988). In particular, if the abuse was perpetrated by the now-elderly parent, then a reversed cycle of violence may be established, perhaps with some suggestions of revenge as an underlying motive for the abuse of the elderly person (Steinmetz, 1981). In addition, since elderly people are often infantilised within society, the positions of vulnerable elderly people and children are quite easily equated by some people.

On occasion, professionals working with elders may act somewhat paternalistically (perhaps quite unwittingly) in their efforts to protect the individual from further harm. If these actions deny elders full involvement and participation in decision-making about their futures then the status accorded to the person is similar to that of children. It is also possible that assumptions can be made about what is best for individuals without involving them in the process. It can be difficult for professionals, whose training revolves around assistance and change to improve situations, to be fully comfortable with the notion of self-determination for elders. Professionals may require assistance to empower individuals to take their own decisions.

A second area of similarity is seen in the reasons given by some perpetrators as to why abuse occurred. It is apparent that a certain amount of abuse may arise because previous attempts to control behaviour which is perceived as difficult or problematic by the carer (of children or dependent adults) have not had the desired effect. Escalation of abuse in this way seems to occur in both child protection and elder abuse. Straus *et al.* (1980) suggested that young children and adolescents are more likely to be abused because of more non-compliant behaviours at these potentially difficult developmental stages.

Elderly people who are not used to accepting the authority of their adult children or willing to comply with their demands may be subject to the same sort of risks. Certain behaviours in children (refusing to eat; toileting accidents; crying) may be perceived and interpreted by carers as defiant and difficult and can be very stressful. Similar behaviours in frail dependent elderly people are often not anticipated or expected by carers and may be equally or even more problematic for carers to deal with. In both child and elder abuse, continuing negative interactions may escalate into abuse over time (Anetzberger, 1987; Kadushin and Martin, 1981). So, just as the abusing parent of a child could say 's/he misbehaved once too often', an adult child said of his abuse of his mother 'she made me want to hit her' (by her behaviour).

Third, within child abuse, as it is currently understood, the phenomenon which occurs most often is male violence, largely physical in nature, directed towards female children (Birchall, 1989). A parallel situation prevails in elder abuse, where the majority of victims are also female. With regard to the gender of those who abuse, many of the early studies reported that abusers were also more likely to be female, usually relatives. Further analysis of this data, which separated physical abuse from neglect, discovered a statistically significant sex difference, in that men were more likely to use physical violence and women neglectful acts (Miller and Dodder, 1989). However, these researchers also proposed that given that categories of reported neglect were very high in the studies they analysed, this also went some way towards explaining why it had appeared that the perpetrators of abuse were mostly female. Again, further research may help to clarify this position in future.

Finally, both child abuse and elder abuse occur in a society which is reluctant to admit that familial violence exists. The societal views concerning the family, and associated myths about 'happy families' (which have not been supported by historical and research evidence, as indicated by Steinmetz, 1990), affects all forms of familial violence. The element of taboo within society to accept that any abuse exists is still strong in many areas, including some professional arenas. Parton's work on child abuse and the stages of recognition of the problem as a problem, may be pertinent in this context and may assist in determining the lack of 'moral panic' surrounding elder abuse (Parton, 1985).

DIFFERENCES BETWEEN ELDER ABUSE AND CHILD ABUSE

Despite the similarities, there are some important differences between the two forms of abuse, and these should not be overlooked. The differences between elder abuse and child abuse occur on a number of different levels, at both macro (societal) and micro (individual) levels. The way that these systems interact suggests that it is imperative not to overlook the nature and extent of these differences when considering elder abuse. In particular, this aspect is important when dealing with individual situations of elder abuse. More work is needed to examine the extent of the applicability and 'fit' of the family violence model to situations of elder abuse.

Societal aspects

There does not appear to be any cultural or societal precedent which accounts for elder abuse. Whilst the use of force as a corrective is viewed by many as acceptable in terms of child rearing, a similar act towards an elderly person would be considered to be a violation of rights, if not an actual assault (Korbin *et al.*, 1989). This may mean that those who abuse elderly people are less likely to admit to the abuse.

Societal expectations and attitudes towards young and old people also come into the arena here. It is likely that children are viewed as far more vulnerable and in need of protection than older people who are stereotypically seen, in western society, as being burdensome. Child abuse is thus considered by many to be the greater crime. Largely due to the fact that recognition and intervention in child abuse situations has been with us now for several decades, statutory agencies are far more aware of the problems of child abuse. This means that when possible symptoms are present in a family setting with young children, professionals are more likely to suspect abuse, and also that child abuse is accorded a higher priority than elder abuse in such agencies. The latter situation is, of course, due also to the legislative and statutory responsibilities held in relation to children and the dearth of such systems for the protection of elderly people.

Within the wider sphere of societal views and attitudes, it is apparent that with regard to child care, there are fairly well established notions as to what constitutes 'good parenting' and concepts which include parents being both 'good' and 'bad'. By contrast, there is very limited general knowledge as to what adequate and appropriate care of elderly people might consist of; and most carers are perceived as being 'good'. In addition, whilst the concept of the nuclear family is well developed for 'young families' with children, there is very little precedent for the familial care of very dependent elders by their elderly children (due to the demographic changes of the latter part of this century).

It is also necessary to remember that the social situations of children and elderly people are in fact quite different. Elderly people, as adults, have far more legal, economic and emotional independence than is possible for children. This also includes the right to refuse offers of assistance and intervention by professionals. Older people are generally acknowledged as responsible and independent individuals who can take their own decisions. The economic independence of many elderly people may, however, make them vulnerable to a type of exploitation and abuse which is rarely seen in other forms of family violence.

In addition, parents have a clearly defined legal responsibility for their children (which has been restated within the principles of the Children Act 1989). The majority of children live with their parents and there is an implicit assumption that generally this is the best arrangement for individuals. In contrast to this, in the UK, adult children do not generally have a legal responsibility towards their parents although a presumption of moral duty (to care) might still exist. Most older people do not live with their children; the expectation that they should do so may be seen to be diminishing in this latter part of the century. This is due in part to demographic changes, to increasing numbers of women in employment in mid-life, and to changes in the structures of the family (increased divorce rate, single-parenthood, etc.), which may lead to families, in particular women, being less available to care for elderly relatives. Children and older people can thus be seen, at a structural level, to be in differing relationships from their abusers.

The child-abuse/family-violence model may not entirely fit the realities of the experience of elder abuse due to societal expectations about the nature of the relationships between the abused and the abuser which seem current within that model. Phillips (1989) has explored these issues and suggests that elder abuse has very distinctive qualities which distinguish it from models proposed for child abuse. Phillips has identified four distinct expectations:

1. The expectation that abuse causes visible harm. If this is not evident, then the situation is 'tolerable'.
2. The expectation that both victims and abusers are readily identifiable within abusive situations.
3 The expectation that victims are not involved in arousing the abusive behaviour (i.e. the victim is innocent).
4. The expectation that the abuser is wholly motivated by malevolent intent.

From what is known about elder abuse, the realities would seem to challenge the above expectations, albeit to differing degrees. It is not possible to explore these more fully here, but in any case the analysis adopted by Phillips is not unproblematic with regard to child abuse, so caution is clearly advisable in this instance.

A further difference may be seen in terms of the institutions which can be utilised for the protection of those who are victims of abuse. Apart from the differences in legal remedies which are specifically available to protect children or elders, there are also differences in general approach. There is a widely held view, even amongst professionals, that families with young children should be kept together. Institutional care for children is regarded as generally 'sub-standard', undesirable and very much a last resort. In any case it is rarely seen as a permanent solution. There may be a lack of real permanent alternatives for children and families.

The situation for elders is very different. There are a large number of institutions for older people (residential and nursing homes). These are generally seen as appropriate to meet the needs of frail and dependent elders and are socially accepted to the extent that public funding is available to support the placement of older people in such facilities. The majority of such placements are seen as permanent solutions; rehabilitation (to the community) is rarely considered as viable. Although there is some evidence to suggest that at least some professionals view admission to institutional care as a 'last resort' in situations of elder abuse (SSI, 1992), it is also apparent that abuse in the form of institutionalised ageism exists even within statutory agencies charged with the welfare of older people, let alone in the sphere of the wider public (Jack, 1992).

With regard to the professional sphere, Riley (1993) indicates the following additional differences between elder abuse and child abuse. She notes that discrepancies are apparent in the amounts of knowledge and understanding by (senior) managers of child abuse and elder abuse. Whilst primary health care may be well developed in terms of provision for child health care, the same cannot be said for elderly people. The strong research effort in the area of child abuse has to date not been matched in the field of elder abuse. Finally, Riley indicates that the numbers of qualified staff working in the field of child abuse is not readily apparent in service provision for elders where high numbers of unqualified/minimally trained staff are routinely employed (Riley, 1993).

Individual aspects

A number of significant differences in the aetiology of abuse can be discerned at the level of the individual. Firstly, the root causes of the abuse may be quite different. Many victims of elder abuse are mentally and/or physically frail and dependent, while abused children, although dependent, do not necessarily have any disability (although children with a disabling condition have been found to be at greater risk of abuse).

From research into elder abuse in the US, it would seem that there are different characteristics of victims depending on the type of abuse which is apparent. To expand slightly, from considering the US research over the past two decades, Wolf (1989) suggests that elders who are subject to neglect appear to fit the characteristics as presented above, and are a source of extreme stress to their caregiver. Those elders who are physically or psychologically abused are less likely to be physically dependent but may have emotional difficulties. This group of elders usually live with their abuser who is dependent on them financially. Elders who are victims of financial abuse are also less dependent on physical care from relatives and more likely to be unmarried and to live alone (but in comparatively isolated situations) (Wolf, 1989, cited in Bennett and Kingston, 1993).

Secondly, the abuse of elderly people can be much more difficult to detect. Elderly people do not lead such public lives and there may be a lack of contact with external agencies, or, indeed, with anyone other than the abuser. They do not attend school or have routine medical examinations. Bennett (1990) has reminded us that whilst with young children there are well-established developmental norms and standards (and any undue deviation from these may result in an investigation), with elderly people the situation is far more complex. Both the differing extent and presentation of acute and chronic illnesses in old age contributes to the absence of established comparative norms. It can be very difficult to establish, medically, for example, the difference between an accidental fall and a deliberate injury (see Homer and Gilleard, 1990). Thus medical definitions of what constitutes abuse can be misleading as it is generally difficult for doctors to be categorical about many situations which are presented to them.

A third area of difference occurs in that with most children (and most child abuse) it is possible for parents or caregivers to envisage a time when the dependency and any associated stress will not prevail and the child will attain full independence. The care of elderly people generally stands in absolute contrast to this; as people grow older they are likely to become more dependent and to place more demands on the carer. It is not always possible for a carer to foresee an outcome which is satisfactory, or to have an idea of the timescale involved. The death of the dependent person may be only a partial solution if the carer is left with unresolved guilt and remorse.

Fourthly, many of the carers of elderly people may themselves be elderly and have poor health and/or disabilities (Lau and Kosberg, 1979). It is not uncommon, given recent demographic trends, to find carers in their 70s caring for parents in their 90s, many of whom may be in better health than their children and who may outlive them. What is also apparent is that in many situations of elder abuse it may not be possible to provide an absolute distinction between the victim and the abuser. The abuser may also in some respects be a victim. It is necessary to acknowledge that at least some elder abuse is dual-direction in nature (McCreadie, 1991); the elderly person may either respond to or perhaps even provoke the abuse. Research by Homer and Gilleard (1990) seems to confirm this tendency. This phenomenon is referred to by Froggatt (1990) as 'old age abuse' who suggests that the term be specifically used for those situations where the elder abuses the carer. Additionally, Froggatt proposes that:

'In families where there is a predisposition to violence, especially where an adult was abused as a child by the parent, the concept of elder abuse offers a further example of the violence extended in that family towards the least powerful members.'

(Froggatt, 1990, p. 49)

Whilst the views presented by Froggatt are not widely accepted or in current usage, it is clear that some attempt to distinguish between differing types of elder abuse may be necessary and is attempted by Froggatt. An alternative view is of a continuum of elder abuse representing the range of abusive situations and behaviours which can occur in later life, with a number of differing victims, abusers and circumstances relating to distinctive types of abuse. Further work on this aspect may be fruitful in attempting to provide clarity in this area.

In view of these undoubtedly complex and difficult situations, as Phillipson states:

'it is important to avoid a model which presents abuse solely as a conflict between older people and inadequate carers. Abuse of older people is almost certainly more complex than this.'

(Phillipson, 1993a)

It is clear that victims of child abuse may not directly initiate the abuse to the same extent.

In situations involving child abuse, the relationships are often comparatively recent in origin, whereas elder abuse usually involves relationships of many years' duration. Abusive situations may arise as results of very long-standing difficulties within a relationship (Fulmer and O'Malley, 1987). In addition, situations appear to arise quite frequently in which the abuse is not between adult child as caregiver and the elder as dependent victim, but where the abuser is the dependent party. The abuse may be a reaction to the state of dependency (financial and/or emotional) rather than a reaction, albeit an extreme one, to the stress of caregiving (Pillemer and Wolf, 1986).

COMPARISON WITH SPOUSE ABUSE

Elder abuse is much less commonly compared with spouse abuse and associated problems of domestic violence. This is somewhat surprising, as the comparison can be a useful one, and in any case it is apparent within some situations of elder abuse that the predominant dynamic is that of spouse abuse (or abuse between partners) which is occurring in later life. It is evident too that the phenomenon of spouse abuse is quite widespread within western society (see, for example, Straus *et al.*, 1980 and chapters by Johnson, Pahl and Lloyd in this volume).

It is clear also that although in some situations the violence stops (often due to separation or divorce), in others the violent and abusive relationship continues into old age. In some of these situations the violence may actually worsen with age; the effects may in fact be more severe, although this can on occasion be due to increased frailty and vulnerability on the part of the victim.

Abusive situations between partners may begin in later life due to changes in the relationship which are not expected or planned for. The effects of illness, disability or other related trauma on relationships are not always easy to gauge or to anticipate. A relationship which has always been problematic if not actually abusive may deteriorate into abuse if unwanted and unexpected limitations and pressures are suddenly thrust upon a couple. Such situations appear particularly likely to arise with certain medical conditions: the effects of illnesses such as strokes, dementia and Parkinson's Disease may be very difficult for partners to deal with.

This may be evident in those situations where spouses are suddenly thrust into a caring role which they are not prepared for and are ill-equipped to deal with – physically, practically, or emotionally. Whilst some people adapt to the requirements of the caring role there are others who fail the transition but who may not be able to opt out of caring in any way. This may perhaps in part be due to their own feelings of duty, obligation or guilt or to wider expectations of them, either real or perceived (Qureshi and Walker, 1989).

Even where the caring role may not, to the objective and dispassionate external observer, appear to be either highly onerous or arduous, if the carer perceives the situation as very stressful for them this may be an important indicator of potential abuse (Steinmetz, 1990). If the spouse as carer then fails to receive sufficient support to alleviate the stress to reduce it to a manageable level for them, then abuse may develop even where none existed before.

Deteriorating health, both physical and psychological; thwarted hopes, expectations and plans; a diminution in capacities to function and manage; an increase in vulnerability and dependence may all contribute to the development or continuation of abusive situations within intimate relationships in old age. A lack of understanding and knowledge about the effects of an illness or disability, particularly where this is of a progressive nature, may also be of relevance.

The issues surrounding caring, dependency and abuse are of importance and will require further detailed examination and analysis in coming years. As Phillipson urges, it is essential that unpaid carers should not be marginalised by a process of criminalisation of abuse (Phillipson, 1993). The potential for conflict between carers and professionals needs to be kept to a minimum. This is likely to be assisted by a view which encompasses the wider structural factors that can precipitate abuse (inadequate resources, financial inequalities and so forth) and avoids blame which is centred on carers.

By the same token, however, it is also important to avoid according all carers an especial status as 'victim' (of circumstance) and absolving them of responsibility within the complex and sensitive area of the dynamics of abusive familial situations. Some of the work already conducted on caring and dependency (Kahana and Young, 1990; Nolan, 1993) may assist in clarification of some of these issues; additional work in this area is also likely to be necessary with regard to abuse.

In a well-publicised random sample study in the Boston area of America, Pillemer and Finkelhor (1988) found that within their sample 3.2 per cent of elderly people could be expected to be either experiencing abuse or be at risk of abuse. The highest levels of abuse discovered by the survey were between spouses/partners. Considering all types of abuse, the abuser was a spouse in 58 per cent situations, compared to the abuser being a child (or other individual) in 42 per cent of the cases. If physical abuse alone was looked at, 60 per cent of situations were of spouse abuse (Pillemer and Finkelhor, 1988).

It is important to note that this was a telephone survey: therefore it is quite likely that those who might be considered the most vulnerable and at risk (those who are very frail, either physically, mentally, or both) did not participate. Of note also in this context was the finding that more men than women were reported as victims (1:1.6 wives to husbands as victim ratio). However, when women were abused they appeared subject to more severe forms of abuse. To establish the real significance of such findings will require further research effort.

However, even where the abusive situation is not between spouses in later life, the overall situation within which elder abuse occurs may be more similar to spouse abuse and domestic violence than to that which occurs in child abuse. The individuals involved are usually adults who are independent, but linked through familial relationships of emotional (if not blood) ties. Shared living arrangements between the parties are usually because of choice (although some might argue more on grounds of moral obligation than absolute freedom of choice and action). The elder also generally has far more social, economic and psychological independence than that which would be afforded to a child.

It is important, too, not to infantilise either elders or women who experience abuse, or to reduce their situations to those which are based purely on dependence and an equivalent status to those of children. Elderly people and younger women who are abused are adults and should be accorded full legal status and rights as citizens. Assistance may be required in enabling them to make full use of this, but the principles of self-determination and autonomy should remain paramount. It is necessary to acknowledge that the sexual abuse of adults with learning disabilities, which is beginning to be identified in the UK (NAPSAC, 1993), may present some difficulties in terms of the extent to which victims can be wholly self-determining, but the principles should be essentially the same within such situations. The extent of the comparison and of the possible implications which derive from this have not yet been adequately or sufficiently explored.

A further potentially useful set of comparisons can be drawn in terms of consideration of strategies of intervention. Within the sphere of domestic violence, successful use has been made of self-help groups to provide mutual support for victims. This is now being adapted and the potential utility for elderly being tested out in the US (Wolf, 1993). In addition, awareness or consciousness raising has been an important tool within domestic violence more generally, to assert the right of women to live their lives free from violence or the threat of violence. Campaigns such as that launched in the early part of 1994 entitled 'Zero Tolerance' (see Lloyd, this volume) are useful in promoting the issues concerning domestic violence and might be adapted to future campaigns concerning elders who are or who have been subject to abuse.

A link might also be fruitfully made when considering the use of refuges or 'safe houses' for women who have experienced abuse. The major provider of 'Battered Women's Refuges' (as they were originally named), Women's Aid, has indicated that they do not discriminate on grounds of age and that their services are equally available for older women who have been subject to abuse. However, it may be unlikely for a number of different but interrelated reasons that an older women would choose to use such a resource. The development of safe houses for elders who have been victims of abuse might have much to commend it as it is based on a very different set of assumptions than the currently predominant model of institutional care as appropriate for elders who have been abused (see Cabness, 1989, and Gomez, 1991 for commentary on the situation in the US).

Specifically, the notion that such accommodation should be provided on a temporary basis, to allow the individual some space and a safe environment in which to properly consider the available options before moving on, is preferable to the somewhat paternalistic and disempowering views surrounding much existing institutional care for older people. The differences in attitude and philosophical underpinnings associated with this approach might well make this a more attractive option for older people and is already being developed in the US (Breckmann and Adelman, 1988).

The final area of comparison surrounds the sphere of legal powers which may be used in connection with domestic violence. Despite a traditional reluctance on the part of the police and legal profession to become involved and intervene in situations of family violence (and in particular the arena of violence towards younger women), this situation is now altering. As the earlier chapters on adult abuse have clearly demonstrated, the police in particular have become somewhat more pro-active and the establishment of Domestic Violence Units (or as in some places the more aptly named Family Protection Units) is clearly assisting in this process. Future developments in the law relating to mentally incapacitated (and other vulnerable) adults may also have some bearing on such situations.

The use of legal sanctions such as injunctions for older people to prevent or alleviate abusive situations is an important corollary to this. Recent practice experience suggests that there is an increasing willingness to consider and assist older people to make use of the legal remedies available to them and to advise them accordingly. Whilst wholly appropriate use of the law to provide solutions to abusive situations may be difficult to achieve due to constraints, its use should not be precluded in a paternalistic attempt to protect older people from the rigours of court appearances and the like. Older people need rather to be assisted and empowered to make full use of the law which might serve to protect them.

It is apparent, however, that the extent of the comparison between elder abuse and domestic violence in more general terms has yet to be fully tested out in terms of the true nature of the correspondence and the limits to this. Some of the reasons for this may rest in the very different origins of the two movements: elder abuse being largely driven by a professional lobby (see Penhale and Kingston, this volume) whilst the domestic violence movement is very much political in origin with a background in feminism (Wolf, 1993, comments on this in connection with the USA, but a similar situation exists in the UK: see relevant chapters, 4–6, in this volume). Further examination of an empirical nature concerning the exact nature of the similarities and differences is clearly required in future in this area in order to provide some clarity.

CONCLUDING COMMENTS

From the above discussion it is clear that elder abuse can be usefully compared to other forms of family violence, although the exact extent of the correspondence is not yet totally clear. It is possible that unless this is approached with a certain amount of caution, inappropriate assumptions and reactions (in terms of policy development, for example) could result.

It would seem to date that there is a real risk that the parallels with child abuse may have been overstated and the importance of the differences between the two has not been fully recognised. An uncritical application of the child abuse model, in terms of intervention as well as within the theoretical sphere, could lead to misleading approaches which would disadvantage and disempower the elders they were ostensibly designed to assist.

As suggested earlier, much elder abuse does not easily fit the child abuse model as it currently exists. In a practice setting in particular, when developing interventive strategies and policy responses, what would seem advisable is for there to be careful consideration of those aspects of child protection work ('best practice') most likely to be of use and benefit within elder abuse and other forms of family violence. Guidance from government for concerned professionals in this respect might well be an appropriate development in future.

It is equally apparent, as indicated above, that the extent of the comparison with the wider sphere of domestic violence has not been fully developed. That it is appropriate to begin to do so lies in the evident parallels: that of independent adults living together for a number of different but inter-related reasons. In addition, much elder abuse would appear to concern abuse between partners in later life (including situations of domestic violence of many years, standing). To take such an approach avoids any risk of infantilisation; it also allows for an examination of any inter-dependency which may be required to analyse adequately the dynamics of abusive situations.

This book is valuable in bringing to the reader, in one volume, a readily accessible and wide-ranging view of the different types of family violence and the responses made by the caring professions. What is evident to the reader is the breadth and range of knowledge which is available and some of the different perspectives between the professionals involved. This is due in part to the differing status accorded to child abuse, domestic violence and elder abuse within society, and the differing lengths of time that each has been identified as a problem in need of solutions.

As Hallett reminds us, child abuse has been the focus of attention for some twenty years in this country; the knowledge base is thus quite extensive and strategies of intervention well developed, as indicated by both Wheeler in her chapter on the health professional's role and Ogg and Dickens in their examination of some of the effects of the Children Act 1989. Domestic violence is not a new phenomenon, but as Johnson robustly indicates it is only in the last decade that the issue has been taken seriously as one which warrants attention from any quarter. Pahl and Lloyd then look at the issue from the perspective of the health and social work responses respectively. Pahl's contribution is of particular note due to the eloquence of some respondents during interview.

Elder abuse, however is the comparative infant, with scant regard being effectively paid to the issue until the last few years. This is not to suggest, however, that it is a new phenomenon. It is rather that the set of related issues have not been deemed to merit significant attention until recent years. Recent texts from the American perspective take the set of issues around family violence to a point of examining controversies (Gelles and Loseke, 1993). This text is the first of its type to look at the field from a British perspective; it is a little premature to consider fully the aspects of family violence about which controversies exist.

All the authors have certain commonalities between them, despite their different fields of concern. The first of these is that none of them condones violence and all appear to consider that there should be limits on what is considered acceptable behaviour. As Browne states, '... both the law and social policy attempt to distinguish between socially

acceptable "normal" violence and unacceptable "abusive" violence ...'
(Browne, 1989).

A further area of similarity between contributors would seem to be the view that family violence is an appropriate field of concern, that it is, moreover, a legitimate area for concern by the general public. What is undoubtedly an area of private distress is perceived as an appropriate arena for public concern and action. There is a distinction to be made between what might be a suitable field for academic and scientific study and what should be primarily the focus of social and political concern and change. That the wider field of familial violence is deemed to merit attention, albeit of different sorts and different degrees, does not appear to be in question, however.

Another area of commonality is that all parties seem to be in accord that the fields of concern are frequently changing as additional types of abuse are identified and become the focus of attention (ritualistic and sexual abuse of children; date rape and sexual abuse of learning-disabled adults; sexual abuse of elders, to name some recent examples). These examples serve to illustrate the complexity and scope of the fields of enquiry and the seemingly ever-changing nature of family violence.

The final area of correspondence which it is necessary to highlight concerns what might be termed the principles of intervention within the different forms of family violence. For all areas, these generally reflect issues surrounding attempts to redress the imbalances of power which arise and exist within abusive situations. Thus professionals working in child and adult protection (including the protection of elders) are exhorted to work in partnership and participation with individuals to resolve difficulties. The current emphases are firmly stated as being to enable and to empower those individuals who are disadvantaged and disempowered by abusive situations. It is crucial to avoid blaming the victim (whether the victim is seen as abused or abuser) and creating or perpetuating guilt and stigma. The overall objective is to assist and enable individuals to live lives free from abuse, neglect and exploitation.

Family violence is a complex and sensitive area which places heavy demands on those who are concerned to deal with the problem and to find solutions to it, or to deal effectively with the aftermath of its occurrence. To find appropriate and meaningful strategies of intervention is likely to remain the challenge to the caring professions for many years to come. That there is commitment to do so is apparent within the caring professions as a whole; the indications are also evident within this current volume.

Aberdeen District Council (1990) *Violent Marriages in the Aberdeen Area: A Report for the Women's and Equal Opportunities Committee.* Aberdeen.

Adams, D. (1988) Feminist-based interventions for battering men. In L. Caesar and K. Hamberger (eds), *Therapeutic Interventions with Batterers: Theory and Practice.* New York: Springer.

ADSS (1991) *Adults at Risk: Guidance for Directors of Social Services.* Stockport, Social Services Division, Metropolitan Borough of Stockport.

Age Concern *et al.* (1990) *Abuse of Elderly People: Guidelines for Action.* London: Age Concern.

Aggleton, P. (1990) *Health.* London: Routledge.

Ajdukovic, M. (1993) The condition of refugees in Europe – mental health problems of displaced children. Paper presented to 4th European Conference on Child Abuse and Neglect, Padua, Italy.

Alzheimer's Disease Society (1993) *Position Paper on Prevention of Elder Abuse.* London: Alzheimer's Disease Society.

American Association for Protecting Children (1986) *Highlights of Official Child Abuse and Neglect Reporting 1984.* Denver: American Humane Association.

Ammerman, R. T. and Hersen, M. (1990) *Treatment of Family Violence: A Sourcebook.* Chichester: John Wiley.

Andrews, B. (1987) *Violence in Normal Families.* Paper presented at Marriage Research Centre Conference, London.

Andrews, B. and Brown, G. (1988) Marital violence in the community: a biographical approach. *British Journal of Psychiatry*, 153, pp. 305–12.

Anetzberger, G. J. (1987) *The Etiology of Elder Abuse by Adult Offspring.* Springfield, Illinois: Chas. Thomas.

Appleton, J. V. (1993) An exploratory study of the health visitor's role in identifying and working with vulnerable families in relation to child protection. Unpublished MSc thesis, Kings College, London University.

Araji, S. and Finkelhor, D. (1986) Abusers: a review of the research. In D. Finkelhor *et al.* (eds), *A Sourcebook on Child Sexual Abuse.* London: Sage Publications.

Arber, S. and Ginn, J. (1991) *Gender and Later Life.* London: Sage.

ARC/NAPSAC (1993) *It Could Never Happen Here.* Nottingham: NAPSAC.

Ashurst, D. and Hall, Z. (1989) *Understanding Women in Distress.* London: Routledge.

Atherton, C. (1991) *Client Participation in Child Protection Procedures and Conferences: Research Findings*. London: Family Rights Group.

Avon County Council and Department of Health (1989) *'Sukina' – An Evaluation of the Circumstances Leading to her Death*. London: Department of Health.

Baker, A. A. (1975) Granny Battering. *Modern Geriatrics*, 5 (8) pp. 20–4, 54–5.

Baker, A. and Duncan, S. (1985) Child sexual abuse: a study of prevalence in Great Britain. *Child Abuse and Neglect*, 9, pp. 457–67.

Barker, W. (1990) Practical and ethical doubts about screening for child abuse. *Health Visitor*, 63 (1) pp. 14–17.

Baumann, E. (1989) Research rhetoric and the social construction of elder abuse. In J. Best (ed.), *Images of Issues: Typifying Contemporary Problems*. New York: Aldine de Gruyter.

Beagley, J. (1987) Do gender issues illuminate your practice? *Social Work Today*, 16 February.

Beauchamp, T. L. and Childress, J. F. (1989) *Principles of Biomedical Ethics*, 3rd edn. New York: Oxford University Press.

Belsky, J. (1978) Three theoretical models of child abuse: a critical review. *Child Abuse and Neglect*, 2, pp. 37–49.

Bennett, G. (1990) Action on elder abuse in the '90s: new definition will help. *Geriatric Medicine* (April) pp. 53–4.

Bennett, G. (1990) Shifting emphasis from abused to abuser. *Geriatric Medicine* (May) pp. 45–7.

Bennet, G. and Kingston, P. (1993) *Elder Abuse: Concepts, theories and interventions*. London: Chapman & Hall.

Berliner, L. (1991) Treating the effects of sexual assault. In K. Murray and D. Gough (eds), *Intervening in Child Sexual Abuse*. Edinburgh: Scottish Academic Press.

Bernard, M. and Phillipson, C. (1991) Self-care and health in old age. In S. Redfern (ed.), *Nursing Elderly People*. Edinburgh: Churchill Livingstone.

Best, J. (1989) *Images of Issues: Typifying Contemporary Social Problems*. New York: Aldine de Gruyter.

Biggs, S. (1993) *Understanding Ageing*. Milton Keynes: Open University Press.

Binney, V., Harkell, G. and Nixon, J. (1981) *Leaving Violent Men: A Study of Refuges and Housing for Battered Women*. Bristol: Women's Aid Federation England.

Birchall, E. (1989) The frequency of child abuse – what do we really know? In O. Stevenson (ed.), *Child Abuse: Public Policy and Professional Practice*. London: Harvester Wheatsheaf.

Birchall, E. (1992) *Working Together in Child Protection: A Survey of the Experience and Perceptions of Six Key Professions*. Report to the Department of Health, Stirling: University of Stirling.

Blagg, H., Hughes, A. and Wattam, C. (1989) Introduction: discovering a child centered approach. In H. Blagg, A. Hughes and C. Wattam (eds), *Child Sexual Abuse: Listening, Hearing and Validating the Experiences of Children*. NSPCC.

Blenkner, M. (1971) A research and demonstration project of protective services. *Social Casework*, 52, pp. 483–99.

Block, M. R. and Sinott, J. D. (1979) *The Battered Elder Syndrome: An Exploratory Study.* College Park University of Maryland Centre on Ageing.

Blumer, H. (1969) *Symbolic Interactionism.* Englewood Cliffs, NJ: Prentice Hall.

Blumer, H. (1971) Social problems as collective behaviour. *Social Problems,* 18 (3) pp. 298–306.

Bookin, D. and Dunkle, R. E. (1985) Elder abuse: issues for the practitioner. *Social Casework,* 66 (1) (January) pp. 3–12.

Bookin, D. and Dunkle, R. E. (1989) Assessment problems in cases of elder abuse. In R. Filinson and S. R. Ingman (eds), *Elder Abuse: Practice and Policy.* New York: Human Sciences Press Inc.

Borkowski, M., Murch, M. and Walker, V. (1983) *Marital Violence: The Community Response.* London: Tavistock Press.

Bourlet, A. (1990) *Police Intervention in Marital Violence.* Buckingham: Open University Press.

Bowder, B. (1979) The wives who ask for it. *Community Care,* 1 (March).

Bowker, L. (1983) *Beating Wife Beating.* Lexington, Mass: Lexington Books.

Bowker, L., Arbitell, M. and McFerron, J. (1988) On the relationship between wife beating and child abuse. In K. Yllo and M. Bograd (eds), *Feminist Perspectives on Wife Abuse,* Beverly Hills: Sage.

Braye, S. and Preston-Shoot, M. (1993) Empowerment and partnership in mental health: towards a different relationship practice. *Journal of Social Work Practice,* 7 (2) pp. 115–28.

Breckman, R. S. and Adelman, R. D. (1988) *Strategies for Helping Victims of Elder Mistreatment.* Newbury Park: Sage.

Brown, H. and Craft, A. (1989) *Thinking the Unthinkable: Papers on Sexual Abuse and People with Learning Difficulties.* London: FPA Education Unit.

Browne, K. (1988) The nature of child abuse and neglect: an overview. In K. Browne, C. Davies and P. Stratton (eds), *Early Prediction and Prevention of Child Abuse.* Chichester: Wiley.

Browne, K. (1989) Family violence: elder and spouse abuse. In K. Howells and C. R. Hollin (eds), *Clinical Approaches to Violence.* London: John Wiley.

Burman, M. and Lloyd. S. (1993) *Specialist Police Units for the Investigation of Violent Crimes Against Women and Children in Scotland,* Central Research Unit Papers. Edinburgh: The Scottish Office.

Burston, G. R. (1975) Granny battering. *British Medical Journal,* 3 (6) p. 592.

Burston, G. (1977) Do your elderly patients lie in fear of being battered? *Modern Geriatrics,* 7(5) pp. 54–50.

Cabness, J. (1989) The emergency shelter: a model for building the esteem of abused elders. *Journal of Elder Abuse and Neglect,* 1 (2) pp. 71–82.

Caffey, J. (1946) Multiple fractures in the long bones of infants suffering from chronic subdural hematoma. *American Journal of Roentology,* 56, pp. 163–73.

Callahan, J. J. (1982) Elder abuse programming: will it help the elderly? *Urban and Social Change Review,* 15, pp. 15–19.

Callahan, J. J. (1986) Guest editors perspective. *Pride Institute Journal of Long Term Home Health Care,* 5. p. 3.

Callahan, D. (1988) Elder abuse: some questions for policymakers. *The Gerontologist,* 28, (4) pp. 453–8.

Campbell, B. (1988) *Unofficial Secrets – Child Sexual Abuse: The Cleveland Case.* London: Virago Press.

Campbell, B. (1993) Home alone with a murderer. *The Independent*, 16 June.

Campbell, J. and Humphreys, J. (1993) *Nursing Care of Survivors of Family Violence*. London: Mosby.

Carlson, B. E. (1977) Battered women and their assailants. *Social Work*, 22, pp. 455–60.

Carty, A. and Mair, J. (1990) Some post-modern perspectives on law and society. *Journal of Law and Society*, 17 (4) pp. 395–410.

Central Council for Education and Training in Southwark (1989) *Regulations for The Programmes Leading to the Diploma in Social Work* (DSW). London: CCETSW.

Chadwick, R. and Tadd, W. (1992) *Ethics and Nursing Practice*. London: Macmillan.

Chambers, G. and Millar, A. (1983) *Investigating Sexual Assault*. Edinburgh: HMSO.

Chaplain, J. (1988) *Feminist Counselling in Action*. London: Sage.

Children Act Advisory Committee (1993) *Annual Report 1992–93*. London: Lord Chancellor's Department.

Childwatch (1986) Unpublished manuscript. London: Childwatch.

Christopherson, J. (1989) European child abuse management systems. In O. Stevenson (ed.), *Child Abuse: Public Policy and Professional Practice*. London: Harvester Wheatsheaf.

CIBA Foundation (1984) *Child Sexual Abuse Within the Family*. London: Tavistock.

City of Aberdeen District Council (1991) *Violent Marriages in the Aberdeen Area*. Report for Women's and Equal Opportunities Committee, Aberdeen.

Cleveland County Council and National Children's Bureau (1993) *Investigation into Inter-Agency Practice Following Cleveland Area Child Protection Committee's Report Concerning the Death of Toni Dales*. Cleveland.

Cleveland Refuge and Aid for Women and Children (1988) *Private Violence: Public Shame*. London: Women's Aid Federation, England.

Clifton, J. (1985) Refuges and self-help. In N. Johnson (ed.), *Marital Violence*. London: Routledge & Kegan Paul.

Cloke, C. (1983) *Old Age Abuse in the Domestic Setting: A Review*. Mitcham: Age Concern.

Cloke, C. and Naish, J. (1992) Introduction: the politics of child protection work. In C. Cloke and J. Naish (eds), *Key Issues in Child Protection for Health Visitors and Nurses*. London: Longman.

Clyde, J. J. (1992) *The Report of the Inquiry into the Removal of Children from Orkney in February 1991*. Edinburgh: HMSO.

Cobbe, F. P. (1878) Wife torture in England. *Contemporary Review* (April) pp. 55–87.

Cochran, C. and Petrose, S. (1987) Elder abuse. The physician's role in identification and prevention. *Illinois Medical Journal*, 171, pp. 241–6.

Commonwealth Department of Community Services and Health (1989) *National Women: Advancing Women's Health in Australia*. Canberra: Australian Government Publications.

Conte, J. and Berliner, L. (1988) The impact of sexual abuse on children: empirical findings. In L. Walker (ed.), *Handbook of Sexual Abuse of Children: Assessment and Treatment Issues*. New York: Springer.

Convention of Scottish Local Authorities (COSLA) (1991) *Women and Violence. Report of Working Party*. Edinburgh.

Cooper, D. M. (1993) *Child Abuse Revisited, Children Society and Social Work*. Buckingham: Open University Press.

Cosis Brown, H. (1992) Lesbians, the state and social work practice. In M. Langan and L. Day (eds), *Women, Oppression and Social Work*. London: Routledge. pp. 201–20.

Council of Europe (1992) *Violence Against Elderly People*. Strasbourg: Council of Europe.

Counsel and Care (1991) *Not Such Private Places*. London: Counsel and Care.

Creighton, S. (1980) *Child Victims of Physical Abuse, 1976*. London: NSPCC.

Creighton, S. (1984) *Trends in Child Abuse*. London: NSPCC.

Creighton, S. (1985) *Child Abuse Deaths*, Information briefing no. 5. London: NSPCC.

Creighton, S. (1992) *Child Abuse Trends in England and Wales, 1988–1990*. London: NSPCC.

Creighton, S. and Owtram, P. (1977) *Child Victims of Physical Abuse*. London: NSPCC.

Creighton, S. and Noyes, P. (1989) *Child Abuse Trends in England and Wales, 1983–1987*. London: NSPCC.

Crittenden, P. (1988) Family and dyadic patterns of functioning in maltreating families. In K. Browne, C. Davies and P. Stratton (eds), *Early Prediction and Prevention of Child Abuse*. Chichester: Wiley.

Croft, S. (1986) Women, caring and the recasting of need – a feminist reappraisal. *Critical Social Policy*, 16, pp. 23–9.

Crystal, S. (1986) Social policy and elder abuse. In K. A. Pillemer and R. S. Wolf (eds), *Elder Abuse: Conflict in the Family*. Dover, Mass.: Auburn House.

Dalley, G. (1988) *Ideologies of Caring: Rethinking Community Collectivism*. London: Macmillan.

Davies, G., Wilson, C. and Williams, G. (1993) *The Effects of the Criminal Justice Act on Children* (Department of Psychology, University of Leicester). Paper presented to the Cumberland Lodge Conference 'Working together for children's welfare: Child protection and the criminal law', 6–8 September 1993.

DeCalmer, P. and Glendenning, F. (eds) (1993) *The Mistreatment of Elderly People*. London: Sage.

Department of Health (1988) *Protecting Children: A Guide for Social Workers Undertaking a Comprehensive Assessment*. London: HMSO.

Department of Health (1989a) *The Children Act: An Introductory Guide for the NHS*. Department of Health.

Department of Health (1989b) *An Introduction to the Children Act (1989)*. London: HMSO.

Department of Health (1989c) *Caring for People: Community Care in the Next Decade and Beyond*, Cm 849. London: HMSO.

Department of Health (1990) *The Care of Children: Principles and Practice in Regulations and Guidance*. London: HMSO.

Department of Health (1991a) *Children Act 1989. Guidance and Regulations: Volume 1, Court Orders*. London: HMSO.

266

Department of Health (1991b) *Patterns and Outcomes in Child Placement: Messages from Current Research and their Implications*. London: HMSO.

Department of Health (1991c) *Working Together under the Children Act 1939: A Guide to Arrangements for Inter-Agency Cooperation for the Protection of Children from Abuse*. London: HMSO.

Department of Health (1991d) *Child Abuse: A Study of Inquiry Reports, 1980–1939*. London: HMSO.

Department of Health (1992a) *Child Protection: Guidance for Senior Nurses, Health Visitors and Midwives*. London: HMSO.

Department of Health (1992b) *The Children Act, A Training and Study Pack for NHS Personnel Workbook*. London: HMSO.

Department of Health (1993a) *Children Act Report 1992*. London: HMSO.

Department of Health (1993b) *Children and Young People on Child Protection Registers Year Ending 31 March 1992*. London: Department of Health.

Department of Health, Department of Social Security, Welsh Office and Scottish Office (1989) *Caring for People*, Cm 849. London: HMSO.

Department of Health, Scottish Home and Health Department, Welsh Office and Northern Ireland Office (1989) *Working for Patients*, Cm 555. London: HMSO.

Department of Health/Social Services Inspectorate (1992) *Confronting Elder Abuse: An SSI London Region Survey*. London: HMSO.

Department of Health/Social Services Inspectorate (1993) *No Longer Afraid: The Safeguard of Older People in Domestic Settings*. London: HMSO.

Department of Health and Social Security (1974) *Report of the Committee of Inquiry into the Care and Supervision Provided in Relation to Maria Colwell*. London: HMSO.

Department of Health and Social Security (1982) *Child Abuse: A Study of Inquiry Reports 1973–1981*. London: HMSO.

Department of Health and Social Security (DHSS) (1985a) *Review of Child Care Law: Report to Ministers of an Inter-Departmental Working Party*. London: HMSO.

Department of Health and Social Security (DHSS) (1985b) *Social Work Decisions in Child Care*. London: HMSO.

Department of Health and Social Security (DHSS) (1986) *Working Together: A Draft Guide to Arrangements for Inter-Agency Cooperation for the Protection of Children from Abuse*. London: HMSO.

Department of Health and Social Security (DHSS) (1987) *The Law on Child Care and Family Services*, White Paper, Cm 62. London: HMSO.

Department of Health and Social Security (DHSS) (1988)*Working Together: A Guide to Arrangements for Inter-Agency Cooperation for the Protection of Children from Abuse*. London: HMSO.

Dickie, D. (1989) *Domestic Violence Probation Project*. Paper to Conference on Domestic Violence Offenders: A New Perspective. Edinburgh.

Dimond, B. (1990) *Legal Aspects of Nursing*. Englewood Clifts, NJ.: Prentice-Hall.

Dingwall, R. (1989) Predicting child abuse and neglect. In O. Stevenson (ed.), *Child Abuse: Public Policy and Professional Practice*. London: Harvester Wheatsheaf.

Dingwall, R., Eekelaar, J. and Murray, T. (1983) *The Protection of Children.* Oxford: Basil Blackwell.

Dobash, R. E. and Dobash, R. P. (1980) *Violence against Wives.* London: Open Books.

Dobash, R. E. and Dobash, R. P. (1981) Community response to violence against wives: abstract justice and patriarchy. *Social Problems,* 28 (5) pp. 563–81.

Dobash, R. E. and Dobash R. P. (1984) The nature and antecedents of violent events. *British Journal of Criminology,* 24 (3) pp. 269–88.

Dobash, R. E. and Dobash, R. P. (1992) *Women, Violence and Social Change.* London: Routledge.

Dobash, R. E., Dobash, R. P. and Cavanagh, K. (1985) The contact between battered women and social and medical agencies. In J. Pahl (ed.), *Private Violence and Public Policy.* London: Routledge & Kegan Paul.

Dominelli, L. (1988) *Anti-Racist Social Work: A Challenge for White Practitioners.* London: Macmillan.

Dominelli, L. and McLeod, E. (1989) *Feminist Social Work.* London: Macmillan.

Donzelot, J. (1980) *The Policing of Families: Welfare versus the State.* London: Hutchinson.

Driver, E. and Droisen, A. (eds) (1989) *Child Sexual Abuse: Feminist Perspectives.* London: Macmillan.

Eastman, M. (1982) Granny battering: a hidden problem. *Community Care,* 27 May.

Eastman, M. (1984) *Old Age Abuse.* London: Age Concern England.

Eastman, M. (1984a) Honour thy father and thy mother. *Community Care,* 26 January, pp. 17–20.

Eastman, M. (1984b) At worst just picking up the pieces. *Community Care,* 2 February.

Eastman, M. (1989) Studying old age abuse. In J. Archer and K. Browne (eds), *Human Aggression: Naturalistic Approaches.* London: Routledge.

Eastman, M. (forthcoming). *Old Age Abuse,* 2nd edn. London: Chapman & Hall/Age Concern.

Edwards, S. (1982) Granny battering: a problem that doctors are failing to detect? *Medical News,* 14, pp. 16–18.

Edwards, S. (1985) A socio-legal evaluation of gender ideologies in domestic violence, assault and spousal homicides. *Victimology,* 10 (4) pp. 186–205.

Edwards, S. (ed.) (1986) *Gender, Sex and the Law.* London: Croom Helm.

Edwards, S. S. M. (1989) *Policing Domestic Violence.* London: Sage.

Eekelaar, J. and Dingwall, R. (1990) *The Reform of Child Care Law.* London: Tavistock/Routledge.

Eisikovitz, Z. and Edleson, J. (1989) Interviewing with men who batter: a critical review of the literature. *Social Service Review,* 63 (3) pp. 384–414.

Elmer, E. and Gregg, G. (1967) Developmental characteristics of abused children. *Pediatrics,* 40, pp. 596–602.

Estes, C. (1979) *The Aging Enterprise.* San Francisco: Jossey-Bass.

Estes, C. (1993) The ageing enterprise revisited. *The Gerontologist,* 33 pp. 299–307.

Ewles, L. and Simnett, I. (1992) *Promoting Health, A Practical Guide to Health Education,* 2nd edn. Chichester: Wiley.

Faragher, T. (1985) The police response to violence against women in the home. In J. Pahl (ed.), *Private Violence and Public Policy*. London: Routledge & Kegan Paul.

Farmer, E. and Owen, M. (1993) *Decision-Making, Intervention and Outcome in Child Protection Work*. Report to the Department of Health, Department of Social Policy, University of Bristol.

Farmer, R. and Miller, D. (1991) *Lecture Notes on Epidemiology and Public Health Medicine*, 3rd edn. Oxford: Blackwell Scientific Publications.

Faulkner, L. (1982) Mandating the reporting of suspected cases of elder abuse: an inappropriate, ineffective and ageist response to the abuse of older adults. *Family Law Quarterly*, 16 (1) pp. 69–91.

Fennell, G., Phillipson, C. and Evers, H. (1988) *The Sociology of Old Age*. Milton Keynes: Open University Press.

Ferraro, K. J. and Johnson, J. M. (1982) How women experience battering: the process of victimisation. *Social Problems*, 30 (3) pp. 325–39.

Finkelhor, D. (1983) Common features of family abuse. In D. Finkelhor, R. Gelles, G. Hotaling and M. Straus (eds), *The Dark Side of Families: Current Family Violence Research*. Beverly Hills, Ca: Sage.

Finkelhor, D. (1984) *Child Sexual Abuse: New Theory and Research*. New York: Free Press.

Finkelhor, D. (1986) *A Sourcebook on Child Sexual Abuse*. Beverley Hills: Sage.

Finkelhor, D. (1988) *Stopping Family Violence*. Newbury Park, California: Sage.

Finkelhor, D. (1991) The scope of the problem. In K. Murray and D. Gough (eds), *Intervening in Child Sexual Abuse*. Edinburgh: Scottish Academic Press.

Finkelhor, D. and Pillemer, K. A. (1984) Elder abuse and its relationship to other forms of family violence. Paper presented at the Second National Conference for Family violence Researchers, July, Durham, NH.

Finkelhor, D. and Pillemer, K. A. (1988) Elder abuse: its relationship to other forms of domestic violence. In G. T. Hotaling, D. Finkelhor, J. T. Kirkpatrick and M. A. Straus (eds), *Family Abuse and its Consequences*. Newbury Park: Sage.

Folstein, M. F., Folstein, S. E. and McHugh, P. R. (1975) Minimental method for grading the cognitive state of patients for the clinician. *Journal of Psychiatric Research*, 12, pp. 189–98.

Formby, W. A. (1992) Should elder abuse be decriminalized? A justice system perspective. *Journal of Elder Abuse and Neglect*, 4 (4) pp. 121–30.

Fox Harding, L. (1991) *Perspectives in Child Care Policy*. London: Longman.

Friend, B. (1993) RCN favours stopping active care for Bland. *Nursing Times*, 89 (6) p. 7.

Frieze, I. H. (1983) Investigating the causes and consequences of marital rape. *Signs*, 8 (3) pp. 532–53.

Froggatt, A. (1990) *Family Work with Elderly People*. London: BASW Macmillan.

Frost, N. (1992) Implementing the Children Act 1989 in a hostile climate. In P. Carter, T. Jeffs and M. K. Smith (eds), *Changing Social Work and Welfare*. Buckingham: Open University Press.

Fulmer, T. T. (1984) Elder abuse assessment tool. *Dimensions of Critical Care Nursing*, 10 (12) pp. 16–20.

269

Fulmer, T. and O'Malley, T. (1987) *Inadequate Care of the Elderly: A Health Care Perspective on Abuse and Neglect.* New York: Springer.

Furniss, T. (1984) Conflict-avoiding and conflict-regulating patterns in incest and child sexual abuse. *Acta paedopsychiat,* 50, pp. 299–313.

Garbarino, J. Kostelny, N. and Dubrow, N. (1991) *No Place To Be a Child: Growing Up in a War Zone.* New York: Lexington Books.

Gayford, J. J. (1975) Wife battering: a preliminary survey of 100 cases. *British Medical Journal* (January) pp. 194–7.

Gayford, J. J. (1976) Ten types of battered wives. *Welfare Officer,* 25 (1) pp. 5–9.

Gayford, J. J. (1978) Battered wives. In J. P. Martin (ed.), *Violence in the Family.* Chichester: John Wiley.

Gelles, R. J. (1974) *The Violent Home.* Beverly Hills: Sage.

Gelles, R. J. (1975) The social construction of child abuse. *American Journal of Orthopsychiatry,* 45 (3) (April) pp. 363–71.

Gelles, R. J. (1976) Abused wives: why do they stay? *Journal of Marriage and the Family,* (November).

Gelles, R. J. (1977) No place to go: the social dynamics of marital violence. In W. Roy (ed.), *Battered Women.* New York: Van Nostrand Reinhold.

Gelles, R. (1979) Psychopathology as cause: a critique and reformulation. In D. Gil (ed.), *Violence Against Children.* Cambridge, Mass.: Harvard University Press.

Gelles, R. (1980) Violence in the family: a review of research in the seventies. *Journal of Marriage and the Family,* 42, pp. 143–55.

Gelles, R. (1982) Problems in defining and labelling child abuse. In R. Starr (ed.), *Child Abuse Prediction: Policy Implications.* Cambridge, Mass.: Ballinger.

Gelles, R. (1983) An exchange/social control theory. In D. Finkelhor, R. Gelles, G. Hotaling and M. Straus (eds), *The Dark Side of Families.* Beverly Hills: Sage.

Gelles, R. (1987) *Family Violence,* 2nd edn, Sage Library of Social Research, No. 84. California: Sage.

Gelles, R. J. and Cornell, C. (1983) *International Perspectives on Family Violence.* Lexington: Lexington Books.

Gelles, R. J. and Cornell, C. P. (1990) *Intimate Violence in Families.* London: Sage.

Gelles, R. J. and Loseke, D. R. (1993) *Current Controversies on Family Violence.* London: Sage.

Gelles, R. and Straus, M. (1979) Violence in the American Family. *Journal of Social Issues,* 35 (2) pp. 15–39.

Gelles, R. and Straus, M. (1987) Is violence towards children increasing? *Journal of Interpersonal Violence,* 2 (2) pp. 212–22.

Gibbons, J., Conroy, S. and Bell, C. (1993) *Operation of Child Protection Registers.* Report to the Department of Health, Social Work Development Unit, University of East Anglia.

Gibson, C. H. (1991) A concept analysis of empowerment. *Journal of Advanced Nursing,* 16, pp. 354–61.

Gil, D. (1979) *Child Abuse and Violence.* New York: AMS Press.

Gil, D. (1981) The United States versus child abuse. In L. Pelton (ed.), *The Social Context of Child Abuse and Neglect.* New York: Human Services Press.

Gil, D. and Noble, J. (1979) Public knowledge, attitudes and opinions about physical abuse in the United States. In D. Gil (ed.), *Violence Against Children*. Cambridge, Mass.: Harvard University Press.

Gilardi, J. (1991) Child protection in a South London district. *Health Visitor*, 64 (7) pp. 225–7.

Gillon, R. (1986) *Philosophical Medical Ethics*. Chichester: John Wiley.

Giovannoni, J. and Becerra, R. (1979) *Defining Child Abuse*. New York: Free Press.

Glaser, D. and Frosh, S. (1988) *Child Sexual Abuse*. London: Macmillan.

Glendenning, F. (1993) What is elder abuse and neglect? In P. Decalmer and F. Glendenning (eds), *The Mistreatment of Elderly People*. London: Sage Books.

Goldner, V. (1992) Moving past our polarised debate about domestic violence. *Networker* (March/April) pp. 54–61.

Gomez, E. (1991) Clinical intervention in an emergency shelter for adult protective service clients. Paper presented to the 8th Annual Adult Protective Services Conference, San Antonio, USA.

Gondolf, E. W. (1985) Anger and oppression in men who batter: empirical and feminist perspectives and their implications for research. *Victimology*, 10, pp. 311–24.

Gondolf, E. W. (1988) *Battered Women as Survivors*. Lexington: Lexington Books.

Gordon, L. (1989) *Heroes of Their Own Lives: The Politics and History of Family Violence*. London: Virago.

Gough, D. (1992) Survey of Scottish child protection registers 1990–1991. In Directors of Social Work in Scotland, *Child Protection Policy Practice and Procedure*. Edinburgh: HMSO.

Graham, B. (1991) *The Facts about Child Sexual Abuse*. London: Cassell Educational Ltd.

Grampian Regional Council (1993) Child Care Staffing Issues – Aberdeen City Division; Establishments of Post of Project Officer 'Violence in the Family Project'. Reports to Social Work Committee, Aberdeen, August.

Griffiths, A., Roberts, G. and Williams, J. (1993) Elder abuse and the law. In P. Decalmer and F. Glendenning (eds), *The Mistreatment of Elderly People*. London: Sage Books.

Gusfield, J. (1982) Deviance in the welfare state: the alcoholism profession and the entitlement of stigma. In M. Lewis (ed.), *Research in Social Problems and Public Policy*. Greenwich, CT: JA1.

Gusfield, J. (1984) On the side: practical action and social constructivism in social problems theory. In J. Schneider and J. Kitsuse (eds), *Studies in the Sociology of Social Problems*. Norwood, N.J.: Ablex.

Hadley, S. (1992) Working with battered women in the emergency department: a model program. *Journal of Emergency Nursing*, 18 (1) pp. 18–23.

Hall, L. and Lloyd, S. (1993) *Surviving Child Sexual Abuse. A Handbook for Helping Women to Challenge their Past*. London: Falmer Press.

Hall, M. (1975) A view from the accident and emergency department. In A. W. Franklin (ed.), *Concerning Child abuse*.

Hallett, C. (1989) Child abuse inquiries and public policy. In O. Stevenson (ed.), *Child Abuse: Public Policy and Professional Practice*. London: Harvester Wheatsheaf.

Hallett, C. (1993) *Working Together in Child Protection – a Case Study in Interagency Coordination*. Report to the Department of Health, University of Stirling, Stirling.

Hallett, C. and Stevenson, O. (1980) *Child Abuse: Aspects of Interprofessional Co-Operation*. London: George Allen & Unwin.

Hammersmith and Fulham Borough (1988) *'What Support?' Domestic Violence Project. Summary of Final Report*. Polytechnic of North London.

Hampton, R. and Newberger, E. (1988) Child abuse incidence and reporting by hospitals: significance of class and race. In G. Hotaling, D. Finkelhor, J. Kirkpatrick and M. Straus (eds), *Coping with Family Violence: Research and Policy Perspectives*. Newbury Park: Sage, pp. 212–21.

Hanmer, J. and Maynard, M. (eds) (1985) *Women, Violence and Social Control*. London: Macmillan.

Hanmer, J. and Saunders, S. (1983) Blowing the cover of the protective male. A community study of violence to women. In E. Gamarnakow *et al.* (eds), *The Public and the Private: Social Patterns of Gender Relations*. London: Heinemann.

Hanmer, J. and Saunders, S. (1984) *Well-Founded Fear*. London: Hutchinson.

Hanmer, J. and Saunders, S. (1987) *Women, Violence and Crime Prevention*. Bradford: University of Bradford.

Hanmer, J. and Statham, D. (1988) *Women and Social Work. Towards a Woman-Centred Practice*. London: Macmillan.

Harding, L. F. (1991) *Perspectives In Child Care Policy*. London: Longman.

Harman, H. and Harman, S. (1989) *No Place Like Home*. London: HMSO.

Harris, R. N. and Bologh, R. W. (1985) The dark side of love: blue and white collar wife abuse. *Victimology*, 10, pp. 242–52.

Heisler, C. J. (1991) The role of the criminal justice system: elder abuse cases. *Journal of Elder Abuse and Neglect*, 3 (1), pp. 5–25.

Helton, A. (1986) *Protocol of Care for the Battered Woman*. Houston, Texas: Women's University.

Hickey, T. and Douglass, R. L. (1981) Mistreatment of the elderly in the domestic setting: an exploratory study. *American Journal of Public Health*, 71 (5) pp. 500–7.

Hildrew, M. (1991) New age problem. *Social Work Today*, 49 (22) pp. 15–17.

Hill, M. (1990) The manifest and latent lessons of child abuse enquiries. *British Journal of Social Work*, 20(3) pp. 197–214.

Hobbs, C. J. and Wynne, J. M. (1986) Buggery in childhood: a common syndrome of child abuse. *The Lancet*, 4 Oct, pp. 792–6.

Hodgkinson, H. M. (1972) Evaluation of mental test score for assessment of mental impairment in the elderly. *Age and Ageing*, 1, pp. 233–8.

Hoff, L. A. (1990) *Battered Women as Survivors*. London: Routledge.

Holt, M. (1993) Elder sexual abuse in Britain: preliminary findings. *The Journal of Elder Abuse and Neglect*, 5 (2) pp. 63–73.

Home Affairs Committee (1992) *Domestic Violence: Memoranda of Evidence*, HC 245-i. London: HMSO.

Home Office (1989) *Report of the Advisory Group on Video Evidence*. London: HMSO.

Home Office (1992) *Memorandum of Good Practice on Video-Recorded Interviews with Child Witnesses for Criminal Proceedings*. London: Home Office/DH.

Home Office, Department of Health, Department of Education and Science, Welsh Office (1991) *Working Together under the Children Act 1989*. London: HMSO.

Homer, A. and Gilleard, C. (1990) Abuse of elderly people by their carers. *British Medical Journal*, 301, pp. 1359–62.

Homer, M., Leonard, A. and Taylor, P. (1984) *Private Violence: Public Shame. A Report on the Circumstances of Women Leaving Domestic Violence in Cleveland*. Cleveland Refuge and Aid for Women and Children.

Homer, M., Leonard, A. and Taylor, P. (1985) The burden of dependency. In N. Johnson (ed.), *Marital Violence*. London: Routledge & Kegan Paul.

Horley, S. (1988) *Love and Pain: A Survival Handbook for Women*. London: Bedford Square Press.

House of Commons (1992) *The Report of the Inquiry into the Removal of Children from Orkney in February 1991*. London: HMSO.

Howitt, D. (1992) *Child Abuse Errors: When Good Intentions Go Wrong*. London: Harvester Wheatsheaf.

Hughes, B. and Mtezaka, M. (1992) Social work and older women: where have the older women gone? In M. Langan and L. Day, *Women, Oppression and Social Work*. London: Routledge, pp. 220–42.

Hugman, R. (1991) *Power in Caring Professions*. London: Macmillan.

Irvine, R. (1988) Child abuse and poverty. In S. Becker and S. MacPherson (eds), *Public Issues: Private Pain*. London: Insight.

Iwaniec, D., Herbert, M. and Sluckin, A. (1988) Helping emotionally abused children who fall to thrive. In K. Browne, C. Davies and P. Stratton (eds), *Early Prediction and Prevention of Child Abuse*. Chichester: Wiley.

Jack, R. (1992) Institutionalised elder abuse, social work and social services departments. *Baseline*, 50 (Oct.) pp. 24–7.

Jackson, H. and Nuttall, R. (1993) Clinician responses to sexual abuse allegation. *Child Abuse and Neglect*, 17, pp. 127–43.

Jaffe, P., Wolfe, D. and Wilson, S. (1990) *Children of Battered Women*. Beverley Hills: Sage Publications.

Jaffe, P., Wolfe, D., Wilson, S. and Zak, L. (1986a) Emotional and physical health problems of battered women. *Canadian Journal of Psychiatry*, 31, pp. 625–9.

Jaffe, P., Wolfe, D. A., Wilson, S. and Zak, L. (1986b) Similarities in behavioral and social maladjustment among child victims and witnesses to family violence. *American Journal of Orthopsychiatry*, 56 (1) pp. 142–6.

James, A. L. (1992) An open or shut case? Law as an autopoietic system. *Journal of Law and Society*, 19 (2) pp. 271–83.

Jehu, D. (1988) *Beyond Sexual Abuse: Therapy with Women Who Were Childhood Victims*. Chichester: John Wiley.

Jezierski, M. (1992) Guidelines for intervention by ED nurses in cases of domestic abuse. *Journal of Emergency Nursing*, 18 (1) pp. 298–300.

Johnson, N. (1985) Police, social work and medical responses to battered women. In N. Johnson, *Marital Violence*. London: Routledge & Kegan Paul.

Johnson, T. F. (1986) Critical issues in the definition of elder mistreatment. In K. Pillemer and R. Wolf (eds), *Elder Abuse: Conflict in the Family*. Dover: Auburn House.

Johnson, T. F. (1991) *Elder Mistreatment: Deciding Who Is At Risk*. New York: Greenwood Press.

Jones, A. (1989) *Domestic Violence*, Home Office Research Study, 107. London: HMSO.

Jones, T., Maclean, B. and Young, J. (1986) *The Islington Crime Survey*. Aldershot: Gower.

Kadushin, A. and Martin, J. (1981) *Child Abuse: An International Event*. New York: Columbia University Press.

Kahana, E. and Young, R. (1990) Clarifying the caregiving paradigm: challenges for the future. In D. E. Biegel and A. Blum. (eds), *Aging and Caregiving: Theory, Research and Policy*. Nebury Park, Ca.: Sage.

Kalmuss, D. S. and Straus, M. A. (1981) A wife's marital dependency and wife abuse. *Journal of Marriage and the Family* (May) pp. 277–86.

Kelly, L. (1988) *Surviving Sexual Violence*. Cambridge: Polity Press.

Kempe, C. H., Silverman, F. N., Steele, B. F., Droegemuller, W. and Silver, H. K. (1962) The battered child syndrome. *Journal of the American Medical Association*, 181, pp. 17–24.

Kempe, R. S. and Kempe, C. H. (1978) Child abuse. In J. Bruner, M. Cole and B. Lloyd (eds), *The Developing Child*. London: Fontana Open Books.

Kennedy, H. (1992) *Eve was Framed. Women and British Justice*. London: Chatto & Windus.

King, M. (1991) Child welfare within the law: the emergence of a hybrid discourse. *Journal of Law and Society*, 18 (3) pp. 303–22.

King, M. and Piper, C. (1990) *How the Law Thinks About Children*. Aldershot: Gower.

King, M. and Trowell, J. (1991) *Children's Welfare and the Law: The Limits of Legal Intervention*. London: Sage.

Kingston, P. (1990) Elder Abuse. Dissertation for MA in Gerontology, University of Keele. Unpublished.

Kingston. P. (1991) Elder abuse. In C. McCreadie (ed), *Elder Abuse: An exploratory Study*. Age Concern Institute of Gerontology. London: Kings College.

Kingston, P. A. (1993) Personal communication.

Kingston, P. and Hopwood, A. (1994) The elderly. In L. Sbaih, *Issues in Accident and Emergency Nursing*. London: Chapman & Hall.

Kingston, P. and Penhale, B. (1994) Recognition of a major problem: assessment and management of elder abuse and neglect. *Professional Nurse* (February).

Kingston, P. and Phillipson, C. (1994) Elder abuse, *British Journal of Nursing* (in press).

Kitzinger, J. and Hunt, K. (1994) *Evaluation of Edinburgh District Council's Zero Tolerance Campaign: The Full Report*. Edinburgh: Edinburgh District Council Women's Committee.

Koning, A. de (1992) Confidential doctors in the Netherlands. Paper submitted to the Ninth International Congress on Child Abuse and Neglect, Chicago, USA.

Korbin, J. E., Anetzberger, G. J. and Eckert, J. K. (1989) Elder abuse and child abuse: a consideration of similarities and differences in intergenerational family violence. *Journal of Elder Abuse and Neglect*, 1 (4) pp. 1–14.

Kosberg, J. I. (ed.) (1983) *Abuse and Maltreatment of the Elderly: Causes and Interventions*. Boston, Mass.: J. Wright.

Kosberg, J. I. and Cairl, R. (1986) The cost of care index: a case management tool for screening informal care providers. *The Gerontologist*, 26 (3) pp. 273–8.

Koss, M. P. and Cook, S. L. (1993) Facing the facts: date and acquaintance rape are significant problems for women. In R. J. Gelles and D. R. Loseke (eds), *Current Controversies on Family Violence*. London: Sage.

Kurz, D. (1993) Physical assaults by husbands: a major social problem. In R. J. Gelles and D. R. Loseke (eds), *Current Controverises on Family Violence*. London: Sage.

La Fontaine, J. (1988) *Child Sexual Abuse: An ESRC Research Briefing*. London: ESRC.

Langan, M. (1985) The unitary approach: a feminist critique. In E. Brook and A. Davis, *Women and Social Work*. London: Tavistock.

Langan, M. and Day, L. (1992) *Women, Oppression and Social Work*. London: Routledge.

Large, S. (1992) Attitudes to child sexual abuse. *Health Visitor*, 65 (9) pp. 320–2.

Lasch, C. (1977) *Haven in a Heartless World: The Family Besieged*. New York: Basic Books.

Lau, E. E. and Kosberg, J. I. (1979) Abuse of the elderly by informal care providers. *Aging*, 299, pp. 10–15.

Law Commission (1991) *Mentally Incapacitated Adults and Decision-Making: An Overview*, Consultation Paper 119. London: HMSO.

Law Commission (1992) *Domestic Violence and the Occupation of the Family Home*, Law Commission Paper 207. London: HMSO.

Law Commission (1993) *Mentally Incapacitated Adults and Decision-Making: A New Jurisdiction*, Consultation Paper 128. London: HMSO.

Lerman, L. G. (1984) Mediation of wife abuse cases: the adverse impact of informal dispute resolution on women. *Harvard Law Journal*, 7 (1) pp. 57–113.

Leroux, T. G. and Petrunik, M. (1990) The construction of elder abuse as a social problem: a Canadian perspective. *International Journal of Health Services*, 20 (4) pp. 651–63.

Lobel, K. (1986) *Naming the Violence – Speaking Out About Lesbian Battering*. New York: Seal Press.

London, J. (1978) Images of violence against women. *Victimology*, 2 (3/4) pp. 510–24.

London Borough of Brent (1985) *A Child in Trust: Report of the Panel of Inquiry Investigating the Circumstances Surrounding the Death of Jasmine Beckford*. London: London Borough of Brent.

London Borough of Greenwich (1987) *A Child in Mind: Protection of Children in a Responsible Society, Report of the Commission of Inquiry into the Circumstances Surrounding the Death of Kimberley Carlile*. London: London Borough of Greenwich.

Loney, M. (1992) Child abuse in a social context. In W. Stainton Rogers, D. Hevey, J. Roche and E. Ash (eds), *Child Abuse and Neglect: Facing the Challenge*. London: B. T. Batsford Ltd, in association with the Open University.

Lothian Regional Council (1989) *Domestic Violence Offenders: A New Perspective*. Report of Conference jointly hosted by Lothian Social Work Department and Women's Unit, Edinburgh.

Lynch, M. (1988) The consequences of child abuse. In K. Browne, C. Davies and P. Stratton (eds), *Early Prediction and Prevention of Child Abuse*. Chichester: Wiley.

Lynch, M. (1992) Child protection – have we lost our way? *Adoption and fostering*, 16 (4) pp. 15–22.

Lynch, M. and Roberts, J. (1977) Predicting child abuse. *Child Abuse and Neglect*, 1, pp. 491–2.

Lyon, C. and de Cruz, P. (1990) *Child Abuse*. Pub by Family Law and publishing imprint of Jordan & Sons Ltd, Bristol.

Maguire, S. (1988) Sorry love – violence against women in the home and the state response. *Critical Social Policy*, 23, pp. 34–46.

Mama, A. (1989a) *The Hidden Struggle: Statutory and Voluntary Sector Responses to Violence Against Black Women in the Home*. London: The Runnymede Trust.

Mama, A. (1989b) Black women and domestic violence: race, gender and state responses. *Feminist Review*, 23.

Mandt, A. (1993) The curriculum revolution in action: nursing and crisis intervention for victims of family violence. *Journal of Nursing Education*, 32 (1) pp. 44–6.

Manning, N. (ed.) (1985) *Social Problems and Welfare Ideology*. Aldershot: Gower.

Manthorpe, J. (1993) Major publications reviewed: elder abuse: concept, theories and interventions. *Action on Elder Abuse Bulletin*. London: Age Concern.

Maracek, J. and Kravetz, D. (1977) Women and mental health: a review of feminist change efforts. *Psychiatry*, 40 (4) pp. 323–29.

Marsden, D. (1978) Sociological perspectives on family violence. In J. Martin (eds), *Violence in the Family*. Chichester: John Wiley.

Martin, D. (1976) *Battered Wives*. San Francisco: Glide Publications.

Masson, J. (1992) Implementing change for children: action at the centre and local reaction. *Journal of Law and Society*, 19 (3) pp. 320–38.

Maynard, M. (1985) The response of social workers to domestic violence. In J. Pahl (ed.), *Private Violence and Public Policy*. London: Routledge & Kegan Paul.

Maynard, M. (1993) Violence towards women. In D. Richardson and V. Robinson (eds), *Introducing Women's Studies*. London: Macmillan.

McCall, G. J. and Simmons, J. L. (1966) *Identities and Interactions*. New York: Free Press.

McCreadie, C. (1991) *Elder Abuse: An Exploratory Study*. London: Age Concern Institute of Gerontology.

McCreadie, C. and Tinker, A. (1993) Review: abuse of elderly people in the domestic setting: a UK perspective. *Age and Ageing*, 22, pp. 65–9.

McIlwaine, G. (1989) Women victims of domestic violence. *British Medical Journal*, 299, pp. 995–6.

McLaren, Lady (1909) *The Women's Charter of Rights and Liberties*. London: Grosvenor.

McLeer, S. and Anwar, R. (1989) A study of battered women presenting in an emergency department. *American Journal of Public Health*, 79 (1) pp. 65–6.

McLeod, M. and Saraga, E. (1988) Challenging the orthodoxy in family secrets. *Feminist Review*, 28, pp. 16–55.

McMahon, B. (1992) Incest: the family context. Understanding and detecting childhood sexual abuse. *Professional Nurse*, 7 (11) pp. 701–5.

276

McMahon, R. (1991) Therapeutic nursing: theory, issues and practice. In R. McMahon and A. Pearson (eds), *Nursing as Therapy*. London: Chapman & Hall.

McMahon, R. and Pearson, A. (eds) (1991) *Nursing as Therapy*. London: Chapman & Hall.

Metropolitan Police (1986) *Report of the Working Party into Domestic Violence*. London: Metropolitan Police.

Metropolitan Police and Bexley Social Services (1987) *Child Sexual Abuse, Joint Investigative Project: Final Report*. London: HMSO.

Millar, J. (1993) Fifth of Britons now in poverty. *Times Higher*, 3rd September, p. 5.

Miller, R. B. and Dodder, R. A. (1989) The abused–abuser dyad: elder abuse in the State of Florida. In R. Filinson and S. R. Ingman (eds), *Elder Abuse: Practice and Policy*. New York: Human Sciences Press.

Millett, K. (1969) *Sexual Politics*. London: Rupert Hart-Davis.

Mills, C. Wright (1970) *The Sociological Imagination*. Harmondsworth: Penguin Books.

Monck, E., Bentovim, A., Goodall, G., Hyde, C., Lewin, R. and Sharland, E. (1992) *Child Sexual Abuse: A Descriptive and Treatment Study*. Report to the Department of Health, London: Institute of Child Health, University of London.

Monk, A. (1990) Gerontological social services: theory and practice. In A. Monk (ed.), *Handbook of Gerontological Services*. New York: Columbia University Press.

Moody, S. (1983) *Diversion from the Criminal Justice Process: A Report on the Diversion Scheme at Ayr*. Edinburgh: Scottish Office Central Research Unit Papers.

Moore, D. (1979) *Battered Women*. Beverly Hills: Sage.

Moore, J. G. (1975) Yo-yo children: victims of matrimonial violence. *Child Welfare*, 54, pp. 557–66.

Morgan, P. A. (1985) Constructing images of deviance: a look at state intervention into the problem of wife-battery. In N. Johnson (ed.), *Marital Violence*. London: Routledge & Kegan Paul.

Mullen, P., Romans-Clarkson, S., Watton, V. and Herbison, G. (1988) The impact of sexual and physical abuse on women's mental health. *The Lancet* (16 April) pp. 841–5.

Munhall, P. L. and Oiler, C. J. (1986) Language and nursing research. In P. L. Munhall and C. J. Oiler, *Nursing Research: A Qualitative Perspective*. Norwalk, CT: Appleton-Century-Crofts.

Murphy. J. E. (1988) Date abuse and forced intercourse. In G. T. Hotaling, D. Finkelhor, J. T. Kirkpatrick and M. A. Straus (eds), *Family Abuse and Its Consequences: New Directions in Research*. London: Sage.

NALGO (1991) *Responding with Authority: Local Authority Initiatives to Counter Violence Against Women*. London: National Association of Local Government Women's Committees.

Narducci, T. (1992) Race culture and child protection. In Cloke and Naish (eds), Key Issues in Child Protection for Nurses and Health Visitors. London: Layman.

Nelson, B. (1984) *Making an Issue of Child Abuse*. Chicago: Chicago University Press.

Nethercott, S. (1993) A concept for all the family. Family Centred Care. A concept analysis. *Professional Nurse*, 8 (12) pp. 794–7.

Newson, J. and Newson E. (1970) *Four Years Old in an Urban Community*. Harmondsworth: Penguin.

Newson, J. and Newson, E. (1978) *Seven Years Old in the Home Environment*. Harmondsworth: Penguin.

Ni Carthy, G. (1984) *Talking it Out. A Guide to Groups for Abused Women*. New York: Seal Press.

Nolan, M. (1993) Carer–dependent relationships. In P. Decalmer and F. Glendenning (eds), *The Mistreatment of Elderly People*. London: Sage.

Norman, A. (1985) *Triple Jeopardy: Growing Old in a Second Homeland*. London: Centre for Policy on Ageing.

NSPCC (1975) *Registers of Suspected Non-Accidental Injury: A Report on Registers Maintained in Leeds and Manchester by NSPCC Special Units*. London: NSPCC.

Ogg, J. and Bennett, G. (1992) Elder abuse in Britain. *British Medical Journal*, 305, pp. 998–9.

Ogg, J. and Munn-Giddings, C. (1993) Researching Elder Abuse. *Ageing and Society*, 13 (3) pp. 389–414.

O'Hara, M. (1993) Fistful of power. *Social Work Today*, 4 February, pp. 8–10.

Oliver, J. E. (1974) *Severely Ill-Treated Young Children in North East Wiltshire*. Oxford: Oxford Regional Health Authority.

O'Malley, H, Segars, H. and Perez, R. (1979) *Elder Abuse in Massachusetts: A Survey of Professionals and Paraprofessionals*. Boston, Mass.: Legal Research and Services for the Elderly.

O'Malley, J. A., O'Malley, H. C., Everitt, D. E. and Sarson, D. (1984) Categories of Family Mediated Abuse and Neglect of Elderly Persons. *Journal of the American Geriatrics Society*, 35 (5) pp. 362–9.

O'Malley, T., Everitt, D. E., O'Malley, H. C. and Campion, E. W. (1983) Identifying and preventing family-mediated abuse and neglect of elderly persons. *Annals of Internal Medicine*, 98, pp. 998–1005.

Orr, J. (1985) Assessing individual and family health needs. In Luker, K. and J. Orr, *Health Visiting*. London: Blackwell Scientific Publications.

Osborne, S. (1991) Programmes for batterers. Paper to conference on Confronting Male Violence, Edinburgh: Lothian Regional Council.

O'Toole, R., Turbett, P. and Nalepka, C. (1983) Theories, professional knowledge and diagnosis. In D. Finkelhor, R. Gelles, G. Hotaling and M. Straus, (eds), *The Dark Side of Families*. Beverly Hills: Sage.

Pagelow, M. D. (1981) *Woman-Battering: Victims and their Experiences*. Beverly Hills: Sage.

Pagelow, M. (1984) *Family Violence*. New York: Praeger.

Pagelow, M. D. (1985) The 'battered husband syndrome': social problem or much ado about little?. In N. Johnson (ed.), *Marital Violence*. London: Routledge & Kegan Paul.

Pahl, J. (1978) *A Refuge for Battered Women*. London: HMSO.

Pahl, J. (1979) The general practitioner and the problems of battered women. *Journal of Medical Ethics*, 5 (3) pp. 117–23.

Pahl, J. (1980) Patterns of money management within marriage. *Journal of Social Policy*, 9 (3) pp. 313–35.

Pahl, J. (1982a) Men who assault their wives: what can health visitors do to help? *Health Visitor*, 55, pp. 528–30.

Pahl, J. (1982b) The police response to marital violence. *Journal of Social Welfare Law* (November) pp. 337–43.

Pahl, J. (ed.) (1985) *Private Violence and Public Policy*. London: Routledge & Kegan Paul.

Pahl, J. (1989) *Money and Marriage*. London: Macmillan.

Parents Against Injustice (PAIN) (1992) *Child Abuse Investigations: The Families' Perspective*. Stansted: PAIN.

Parker, S. (1985) The legal background. In J. Pahl (ed.), *Private Violence and Public Policy*. London: Routledge & Kegan Paul.

Parton, N. (1985) *The Politics of Child Abuse*. London: MacMillan.

Parton, N. (1990) Taking child abuse seriously. In The Violence Against Children Study Group, *Taking Child Abuse Seriously: Contemporary Issues in Child Protection Theory and Practice*. London: Unwin Hyman.

Parton, N. (1991) *Governing the Family: Child Care, Child Protection and the State*. London: Macmillan.

Peall, C. (1992) Partnership and professional power. In C. Cloke and J. Naish (eds), *Key Issues in Child Protection for Health Visitors and Nurses*. London: Longman.

Pearson, A., Durand, I. and Punton, S. (1988) *Therapeutic Nursing: An Evaluation of an Experimental Nursing Unit in the British National Health Service*. Oxford: Burford and Oxford Nursing Development Units.

Pedrick-Cornell, C. and Gelles, R. J. (1982) Elder abuse: the status of current knowledge. *Family Relations*, 31 (July) pp. 457–65.

Pelton, L. (1981) Child abuse and neglect: the myth of classlessness. In L. Pelton (ed.), *The Social Context of Child Abuse and Neglect*. New York: Human Sciences Press.

Pence, E. and Paynar, M. (1990) *Power and Control: Tactics of Men Who Batter. An Educational Curriculum*. Duluth, Minnesota: Minnesota Programme Development.

Penhale, B. (1992a) Elder abuse: an overview. *Elders*, 1 (3) pp. 36–48.

Penhale, B. (1992b) Elder abuse and the marginalisation of elderly people: a case of triple jeopardy? Paper given at the 21st Annual Conference of the British Society of Gerontology, Canterbury.

Penhale, B. (1993a) Local authority guidelines and procedures. In *Elder Abuse: New Findings and Policy Guidelines, Proceedings of Age Concern Ageing Update Conference*. London: Age Concern Institute of Gerontology.

Penhale, B. (1993b) The abuse of elderly people: considerations for practice. *British Journal of Social Work*, 23 (2) pp. 95–112.

Pföhl, S. J. (1977) The 'discovery' of child abuse. *Social Problems*, 24 (3) pp. 310–23.

Phillips, L. R. (1983) Elder abuse – what is it? who says so? *Geriatric Nursing* (May/June) pp. 167–70.

Phillips, L. (1986) Theoretical explanations for elder abuse. In K. Pillemer and R. Wolf (eds), *Elder Abuse: Conflict in the Family*. Mass: Auburn House Publishing.

Phillips, L. R. (1989) Issues involved in identifying and intervening in elder abuse. In R. Filinson and S. R. Ingman, *Elder Abuse: Practice and Policy*. New York: Human Sciences Press.

Phillips, L. R. and Rempusheski, V. F. (1986) Making decisions about elder abuse. *Social Casework*, 67 (3) pp. 131–40.

Phillipson, C. (1982) *Capitalism and the Construction of Old Age*. London: Macmillan Books.

Phillipson, C. (1992) Confronting elder abuse. *Generations Review*, 2 (3) pp. 2–3.

Phillipson, C. (1993a) Abuse of older people: sociological perspectives. In P. Decalmer and F. Glendenning (eds), *The Mistreatment of Elderly People*. London: Sage Books.

Phillipson, C. (1993b) Elder abuse and neglect: social and policy issues. In Action on Elder Abuse Working Paper No.1: *A Report of the 1st International Symposium on Elder Abuse*. London: Action on Elder Abuse.

Phillipson, C. and Biggs, S. (1992) *Understanding Elder Abuse: A Training Manual for Helping Professions*. London: Longman.

Phillipson, J. (1992) *Practising Equality. Women, Men and Social Work*. London: Central Council for Education and Training in Social Work.

Pilkington, E. (1993) WI plea for wives driven to murder. *The Guardian*, 9 June 1993.

Pillemer, K. A. (1993) The abused offspring are dependent: abuse is caused by the deviance and dependence of abusive caregivers. In R. J. Gelles and D. R. Loseke (eds), *Current Controversies on Family Violence*. London: Sage.

Pillemer, K. A. and Finkelhor, D. (1988) The prevalence of elder abuse: a random sample survey. *The Gerontologist*, 28 (1) pp. 51–7.

Pillemer, K. A. and Moore, D. (1989) Abuse of patients in nursing homes: findings from a survey of staff. *The Gerontologist*, 29 (3), pp. 314–20.

Pillemer, K. A. and Suitor, J. (1988) Elder abuse. In V. Van Hasselt, R. Morrison, A. Belack and M. Hensen (eds), *Handbook of Family Violence*. New York: Plenum Press.

Pillemer, K. A. and Suitor, J. J. (1990) Prevention of elder abuse. In R. T. Ammerman and M. Hersen (eds), *Treatment of Family Violence*. New York: John Wiley.

Pillemer, K. A. and Wolf, S. (eds) (1986) *Elder Abuse: Conflict in the Family*. New York: Auburn House.

Pitt, B. (1992) Abusing old people. *British Medical Journal*, 305, pp. 968–9.

Pizzey, E. (1974) *Scream Quietly or the Neighbours Will Hear*. Harmondsworth: Penguin Books.

Pizzey, E. and Shapiro, J. (1982) *Prone to Violence*. London: Hamlyn.

Podnieks, E. (1992) National survey on abuse of the elderly in Canada. *Journal of Elder Abuse and Neglect*, 4, pp. 5–58.

Pritchard, J. (1992) *The Abuse of Elderly People: A Handbook for Professionals*. London: Jessica Kingsley.

Pyne, R. H. (1992) *Professional Discipline in Nursing, Midwifery and Health Visiting*, 2nd edn. Oxford: Blackwell Scientific Publications.

Quinn, M. J. and Tomita, S. K. (1986) *Elder Abuse and Neglect: Causes, Diagnosis and Intervention Strategies*. New York: Springer.

Qureshi, H. and Walker, A. (1989) *The Caring Relationship: Elderly People and their Families*. London, Macmillan.

Radbill, S. (1980) A history of child abuse and infanticide. In R. Helfer and C. Kempe (eds), *The Battered Child*, 3rd edn, pp. 3–20. Chicago: University of Chicago Press.

Ramsey-Klawsnik, H. (1991) Interviewing elders for suspected sexual abuse: guidelines and techniques. *The Journal of Elder Abuse and Neglect*, 5 (1) pp. 5–19.

Rathbone-McCuan, E. (1980) Elderly victims of family violence and neglect. *Social Casework*, 61 (5) pp. 296–304.

Rathbone-McCuan, E., Travis, A. and Voyles, B. (1983) Family Intervention: the task-centred approach. In J. I. Kosberg (ed.), *Abuse and Maltreatment of the Elderly: Causes and Interventions*. Boston, Mass.: J. Wright.

Reder, P., Duncan, S. and Gray, M. (1993) *Beyond Blame: Child Abuse Tragedies Revisited*. London: Routledge.

Reid, B. (1991) Developing and documenting a qualitative methodology. *Journal of Advanced Nursing*, 16, pp. 544–51.

Research Team (1990) *Child Sexual abuse in Northern Ireland*. Antrim: Greystone Books.

Richards, M. (1975) Non-accidental injury to children in an ecological perspective. In Department of Health and Social Security, *Non-Accidental Injury to Children: proceedings of a conference*. London: HMSO.

Riddoch, L. (1994) Zero tolerance: the second wave. *Harpies and Quines*, 12, pp. 8–11.

Riley, P. (1993) Differences between child and adult abuse. In Social Services Inspectorate, *No Longer Afraid: The Safeguard of Older People in Domestic Settings*. London: HMSO.

Robb, B. (1967) *Sans Everything*. London: Nelson.

Roberts, J. (1988) Why are some families more vulnerable to child abuse? In K. Browne, C. Davies and P. Stratton (eds), *Early Prediction and Prevention of Child Abuse*. Chichester: Wiley.

Roberts, J. and Taylor, C. (1993) Sexually abused children and young people speak out. In L. Waterhouse (ed.), *Child Abuse and Child Abusers*. London: Jessica Kingsley.

Rojek, C., Peacock, G. and Collins, S. (1988) *Social Work and Received Ideas*. London: Routledge.

Roy, M. (1982) Four thousand partners in violence: a trend analysis. In M. Roy (ed.), *The Abusive Partner*. New York: Van Nostrand Reinhold.

Rumbold, G. (1993) *Ethics in Nursing Practice*, 2nd edn. London: Balliere Tindall.

Russell, D. (1982) *Rape in Marriage*. New York: Collier Books.

Sacks, O. (1985) *The Man Who Mistook His Wife for a Hat*. London: Picador, pub by Pan Books.

Salend, E., Kane, R., Satz, M. and Pynoos, J. (1984) Elder abuse reporting: limitations of statutes. *The Gerontologist*, 24 (1) pp. 61–9.

Salvage, J. (1990) The theory and practice of the new nursing. Occasional paper. *Nursing Times*, 86 (4) pp. 42–5.

Salvage, J. (1992) The new nursing: empowering patients or empowering nurses? In Robinson *et al.* (eds), *Policy Issues in Nursing*. Milton Keynes: Open University Press.

Saunders, A. (1993) *Women's Aid Refuges: Adult Reflections on the Experience of Childhood in a Refuge*. MA dissertation, Department of Social Work, University of Sussex.

Schechter, S. (1982) *Women and Male Violence*. Boston: South End Press.

Schneider, J. (1985) Social problems theory: the constructionist view. *Annual Review of Sociology*, 11, pp. 209–29.

Scottish Women's Aid (1989) *Women Talking to Women – A Women's Aid Approach to Counselling*. Edinburgh: Scottish Women's Aid.

Scottish Women's Aid (undated) *Working With Asian Women*. Scottish Women's Aid Training, Edinburgh.

Scottish Women's Aid (1992) *Annual Report*, Edinburgh.

Seccombe, W. (1993) *The Decline of the Working Class Family*. London: Verso Books.

Secretary of State for Social Services (1988) *Report of the Inquiry into Child Abuse in Cleveland 1987*, Cm 412. London: HMSO.

Seedhouse, D. (1986) *Health: The Foundations for Achievement*. Chichester: John Wiley.

Seedhouse, D. (1988) *Ethics the Heart of Health Care*. Chichester: John Wiley.

Select Committee on Violence in Marriage (1975) *First Report*. London: HMSO.

Shemmings, D. (1991). *Family Participation in Child Protection Conferences: 2 – Report of a Pilot Project in Lewisham Social Services Department*. Norwich: University of East Anglia.

Shephard, J. and Farrington, D. (1993) Assault as a public health problem. *Journal of the Royal Society of Medicine*, 86, pp. 89–92.

Sherman, L. W. and Berk, R. A. (1984) The specific deterrent effects of arrest for domestic assault. *American Sociological Review*, 49, pp. 261–72.

Sinclair, D. (1985) *Understanding Wife Assault*. Toronto: Ontario Government Bookstore.

Skelton, R. (1994) Nursing and empowerment: concepts and strategies. *Journal of Advanced Nursing*, 19, pp. 415–23.

Smith, L. J. F. (1989) *Domestic Violence: An Overview of the Literature*, Home Office Research Study no. 107. London: HMSO.

Smith, M., Goodman, C., Heverin, A., Nobes, G., Poland, G. and Upton, P. (forthcoming) *Parental Control Within the Family*. London: Thomas Coram Research Unit.

Smith, S., Baker, D., Buchan, A. and Bodiwala, G. (1992) Adult domestic violence. *Health Trends*, 24 (3) pp. 97–9.

Snell, J., Rosenwald, R. and Robey, A. (1964) The wifebeater's wife. *Archives of General Psychiatry*, 11, pp. 107–12.

Social Services Inspectorate (SSI) (1992) *Court Orders Study: A Study of Local Authority Decision Making About Public Law Court Applications*. London: Department of Health.

Social Work Services Group (1992) *Child Protection in Scotland – Management Information Joint Steering Group Report*. Edinburgh: Scottish Office.

Sonkin, D. J. and Durphy, M. (1989) *Learning to Live Without Violence*. New York: Volcano Press.

Spector, M. and Kitsuse, J. (1977) *Constructing Social Problems*. Menlo Park, CA: Cummings.

Spinetta, J. and Rigler, D. (1972) The child abusing parent: a psychological review. *Psychological Bulletin*, 77, pp. 296–304.

Sprey, J. and Matthews, S. (1989) The perils of drawing implications from research: the case of elder mistreatment. In R. Filinson and S. Ingman (eds), *Elder Abuse: Policy and Practice*. New York: Human Sciences Press.

Staffordshire County Council (1991). *The Pindown Experience and the Protection of Children: The Report of the Staffordshire Child Care Enquiry.* Staffordshire County Council.

Stainton Rogers, W. and Roche, J. (1992) Putting it all together: The Children's Act 1989. In C. Cloke and J. Naish (eds), *Key Issues in Child Protection for Health Visitors and Nurses.* London: Longman.

Stanko, E. (1985) *Intimate Intrusions: Women's Experience of Male Violence.* London: Routledge & Kegan Paul.

Stark, E. and Flitcraft, A. (1985) Woman-battering, child abuse and social heredity: what is the relationship? In N. Johnson, *Marital Violence.* London: Routledge & Kegan Paul.

Stark, E., Flitcraft, A. and Frazier, W. (1979) Medicine and patriarchal violence. *International Journal of Health Services,* 9 (3) pp. 461–93.

Stearns, P. (1986) Old age family conflict: the perspective of the past. In K. A. Pillemer and R. S. Wolf (eds), *Elder Abuse: Conflict in the Family.* Dover, MA: Auburn House Press.

Steele, B. and Pollock, C. (1968) A psychiatric study of parents who abuse infants and small children. In R. Helfer and C. H. Kempe (eds), *The Battered Child.* Chicago: Chicago University Press.

Steele, R. F. (1980) Psychodynamic factors in child abuse. In C. H. Kempe and R. E. Helfer (eds), *The Battered Child,* 3rd edn. Chicago: University of Chicago Press.

Steinmetz, S. K. (1977) Wifebeating, husbandbeating – a comparison of the use of physical violence between spouses to resolve marital fights. In M. Roy (ed.), *Battered Women.* New York: Van Nostrand Reinhold.

Steinmetz, S. K. (1978a) The battered husband syndrome. *Victimology,* 2 (3/4) pp. 499–509.

Steinmetz, S. K. (1978b) Battered parents. *Society,* 15 (5) pp. 54–5.

Steinmetz, S. K. (1981) Elder abuse. *Aging* (Jan–Feb) pp. 315–16, 6–10.

Steinmetz, S. K. (1983) Dependency, stress and violence between middle-aged caregivers and their elderly relatives. In J. I. Kosberg (ed.), *Abuse and Maltreatment of the Elderly: Causes and Interventions.* Boston, Mass.: J. Wright.

Steinmetz, S. K. (1988) *Duty Bound: Elder Abuse and Family Care.* London: Sage.

Steinmetz, S. K. (1990) Elder abuse: myth and reality. In T. H. Brubaker (ed.), *Family Relationships in Later Life,* 2nd edn. Newbury Park, Ca.: Sage.

Steinmetz, S. K. and Amsden, G. (1983) Dependent elders, family stress and abuse. In T. H. Brubaker (ed.), *Family Relationships in Later Life.* Beverly Hills: Sage.

Steinmetz, S. K. and Straus, M. A. (1974) *Violence in the Family.* New York: Harper & Row.

Straus, M. A. (1974) Foreword. In R. J. Gelles (ed.), *The Violent Home.* Beverly Hills, Ca.: Sage.

Straus, M. A. (1980a) A sociological perspective on the causes of family violence. In M. R. Green (ed.), *Violence and the Family.* Boulder, Col.: Westview Press.

Straus, M. A. (1980b) Victims and aggressors in marital violence. *American Behavioral Scientist,* 23 (5) pp. 681–704.

Straus, M. A. (1983) Ordinary violence, child abuse and wife-beating: what do they have in common? In D. Finkelhor *et al.* (eds), *The Dark Side of Families*. Beverly Hills: Sage.

Straus, M. A. (1987) Social Stratification, Social bonds and wife beating in the United States, Paper presented to the American Society of Criminology, Montreal, November. Cited in Smith, L. J. F. (1989) *Domestic Violence: An Overview of the Literature,* Home Office Research Study no. 107. London: HMSO.

Straus, M. A. (1993) Physical assaults by wives: a major social problem. In R. J. Gelles and D. R. Loseke (eds), *Current Controversies on Family Violence*. London: Sage.

Straus, M. A. and Gelles, R. (1986) Societal change and change in family violence, 1975 to 1985, as revealed in two national surveys. *Journal of Marriage and the Family*, 48, pp. 465–79.

Straus, M. A., Gelles, R. A. and Steinmetz, S. K. (1980) *Behind Closed Doors: Violence in the American Family*. Garden City, NY: Anchor Books.

Straus, M. A. and Hotaling, G. T. (1979) *The Social Causes of Husband–Wife Violence*. Minneapolis: University of Minnesota Press.

Sweet, J. and Resick, P. (1979) The maltreatment of children: a review of theories and research. *Journal of Social Issues*, 35 (2) pp. 40–59.

Tallman, I. (1976) *Passion, Action and Politics*. San Francisco: Freeman.

Tardieu, A. (1857) *Étude médico-légale sur les attentats aux moeurs*. Paris.

Tardieu, A. (1860) Étude médico-légale sur les services et mauvais traitements exerces sur des enfants. *Annales d'hygiene publique de medicine legale*, 13, pp. 361–98.

Taylor, C. and Campbell. V. (1994) *Evaluation of Joint Social Work/Police Investigation Team*. Research Report, Social Work Research Centre, University of Stirling, Stirling.

Taylor, S. (1992) How prevalent is it? In W. Stainton Rogers, D. Hevey, J. Roche and E. Ash (eds), *Child Abuse and Neglect: Facing the Challenge*, 2nd edn. London: B. T. Batsford Ltd, in association with the Open University.

Taylor, S. and Tilley, N. (1989) Health visitors and child protection: conflict, contradictions and ethical dilemmas. *Health Visitor*, 62 (9) pp. 273–5.

Taylor, S. and Tilley, N. (1990) Interagency conflict in child abuse work – reducing tensions between social workers and health visitors. *Adoption and Fostering*, 14 (4) pp. 13–17.

Thomson, P. (1992) Parents at case conferences – a legal advisor's viewpoint. *The Journal of Child Law*, January, pp. 15–18.

Tomlin, S. (1989) *Abuse of Elderly People: An Unnecessary and Preventable Problem*, Public Information Report. London: British Geriatrics Society.

Townsend, P. (1962) *The Last Refuge*. London: Routledge.

Townsend, P. (1981) The structured dependency of the elderly: creation of social policy in the twentieth century. *Ageing and Social Policy*, 1 (1) pp. 5–28.

Townsend, P. (1986) Ageism and social policy. In C. Phillipson and A. Walker, *Ageing and Social Policy*. Gower: Aldershot.

Townsend, P. and Wedderburn, D. (1965) *The Aged in the Welfare State*. London: Bell.

Trowell, J. (1992) Does interprofessional care matter in child protection? *Journal of Interprofessional Care*, 6 (2) pp. 103–7.

Tschudin, V. (1992) *Ethics in Nursing: The Caring Relationship*, 2nd edn. London: Butterworth Heinemann.

UKCC (United Kingdom Central Council for Nursing, Midwifery and Health Visiting) (1987) *Confidentiality: A Framework to Assist Individual Professional Judgement.*

UKCC (United Kingdom Central Council for Nursing, Midwifery and Health Visiting) (1992) The *Code of Professional Conduct*, 3rd edn. UKCC.

United Nations (1989) *Violence against Women in the Family*. Vienna: Centre for Social Development and Humanitarian Affairs, United Nations.

United States Congress House Select Committee on Aging (1980) *Elder Abuse: The Hidden Problem*. Washington DC: Government Printing Office.

Victim Support (1992) *Domestic Violence. Report of a National Inter-agency Working Party*. London: Victim Support.

Wagner, G. (1988) *Residential Care: A Positive Choice*. London: National Institute of Social Work/HMSO.

Walker, A. (1980) The social creation of poverty and dependency in old age. *Journal of Social Policy*, 9, pp. 45–75.

Walker, A. (1981) Towards a political economy of old age. *Ageing and Society*, 1 (1) pp. 73–94.

Walker, A. (1986) Pensions and the production of poverty in old age. In C. Phillipson and A. Walker, *Ageing and Social Policy*. Gower: Aldershot.

Walker, L. E. (1978) Battered women and learned helplessness. *Victimology*, 2 (3/4) pp. 525–34.

Walker, L. E. (1979) *The Battered Woman*. New York: Harper & Row.

Walker, L. E. (1984) *The Battered Woman Syndrome*. New York: Springer.

Walker, L. E. (1985) Psychological impact of the criminalization of domestic violence on victims. *Victimology*, 10, pp. 281–300.

Walton, M. (1993) Regulation in child protection – policy failure. *British Journal of Social Work*, 23 (2), pp. 139–56.

Waters, J. (1992) 'Protecting children' and 'preventing' child abuse: or consensus of conflict. In C. Cloke and J. Naish (eds), *Key Issues in Child Protection for Health Visitors and Nurses*. London: Longman.

Watson, S. and Austerberry, H. (1986) *Housing and Homelessness. A Feminist Perspective*. London: Routledge.

Webb, C. (1992) The use of the first person in academic writing: objectivity language and gatekeeping. *Journal of Advanced Nursing*, 17, pp. 747–52.

Wheeler, S. J. (1992) Perceptions of child abuse. *Health Visitor*, 65 (9) pp. 316–19.

Widom, C. S. (1989) Does violence beget violence?: a critical examination of the literature. *Psychological Bulletin*, 106, pp. 3–28.

Wilkes, R. (1981) *Social Work with Undervalued Groups*. London: Tavistock.

Williams, F. (1992) Women with learning difficulties are women too. In M. Langan and L. Day (eds), *Women, Oppression and Social Work*. London: Routledge, pp. 149–69.

Wilson, E (1983) *What is to be Done About Violence Against Women?*. Harmondsworth: Penguin Books.

Wise, S. (1984) *Becoming a Feminist Social Worker: Studies in Sexual Politics*, University of Manchester.

Witz, A. (1992) *Professions and Patriarchy*. London: Routledge.

Wolf, R. S. (1989) Testimony before the Subcommittee of Human Services: Select Committee on Aging: US House of Representatives Hearings on Elder Abuse. In G. Bennett and P. Kingston, *Elder Abuse: Concepts, Theories and Interventions*. London: Chapman & Hall.

Wolf, R. (1992) Victimization of the elderly: elder abuse and neglect. *Reviews in Clinical Gerontology*, 2, pp. 269–76.

Wolf, R. S. (1993) Responding to elder abuse in the USA. In Action on Elder Abuse Working Paper No. 1: *A Report on the Proceedings of the 1st International Symposium on Elder Abuse*. London: Action on Elder Abuse.

Wolf, R. S. and Pillemer, K. A. (1984) *Working with Abused Elders: Assessment, Advocacy and Intervention*. Worcester, Mass.: University of Massachusetts Medical Centre.

Wolf, R. S. and Pillemer, K. A. (1989) *Helping Elderly Victims: The Reality of Elder Abuse*. New York: Columbia University Press.

Wolfe, D. A., Jaffe, P., Wilson, S. and Zak, L. (1985) Children of battered women: the relation between child behaviour, family violence and maternal stress. *Journal of Consulting and Clinical Psychology*, 55 (5) pp. 657–65.

Wolock, I. and Horowitz, B. (1984) Child maltreatment as a social problem: the neglect of neglect. *American Journal of Orthopsychiatry*, 54 (4), pp. 530–43.

Women's Aid Federation England (1991) *Women's Aid Federation Information Pack*. PO Box 391, Bristol.

Women's National Commission (1984) *Violence Against Women: Report of an ad hoc Working Group*. London: Cabinet Office

Women's Support Project (1991) *Leaving an Abusive Relationship*. Glasgow.

Woolley, P. V. Jr. and Evans, W. A. Jr. (1955) Significance of skeletal lesions in infants resembling those of traumatic origin. *Journal of the American Medical Association*, 158, pp. 539–43.

Wynne, J. (1992) The construction of child abuse in the accident and emergency department. In C. Cloke and J. Naish (eds), *Key Issues in Child Protection for Health Visitors and Nurses*. London: Longman.

289

Dobash, R. E. and Dobash, R. P. –
   cont'd
      161; learned helplessness
      115, 126, 158; politics   102,
      103, 104, 104–5, 106;
      psychotherapy   142;
      re-enactment   174; violent
      event   112
Domestic Proceedings and
   Magistrates' Courts Act (1978)
   (DPMCA)   110, 120, 121
domestic violence (spouse abuse)   2,
   9–15, 101–77, 223, 260
   accommodation   120–4
   causation theories   114–18
   children   see children
   effects   111–13, 130–1
   elder abuse and   196–8, 255–9,
      259–60
   frequency of contact with social
      workers   160–3
   gender issues   174–5
   health perspective   11–12, 127–48
   health services help   131–42;
      accident and emergency
      departments   140–1; GPs 12,
      133–7; health visitors   12,
      137–40; principles for
      intervention   145–7;
      psychotherapy   141–2;
      recommendations for good
      practice   144–5
   multi-agency approaches   169–72
   nature   111–13
   police responses   118–20
   politics of   102–7
   possible indicators   155
   prevalence and incidence
      109–11, 127–30, 152–3
   programmes for violent men
      172–4
   recipients and perpetrators   10,
      107–11, 154–9
   social perspective   12–15, 149–77
   social work practice and   152–4
   staying, leaving and surviving
      124–6
   training   14–15, 142–4, 167, 168,
      169–72
   understanding   154–60

victims' opinions of social work
   response   163
way ahead for social work   175–7
Women's Aid   168–9; housing
   and   163–5
Domestic Violence Intervention
   Project   109
Domestic Violence and Matrimonial
   Proceedings Act (1976)
   (DVMPA)   110, 120–1
Domestic Violence Units   119, 258
dominant disease model   51
Dr Barnardo's   42
Duluth model   174
Duncan, S.   35, 40

Eastman, M.   3, 181, 193, 223,
   228
Edinburgh 'Zero Tolerance'
   campaign   170–1, 257
Edleson, J.   173
education see training
effects of abuse   111–13, 130–1,
   246–7
Eisikovitz, Z.   173
elder abuse   2, 15–19, 181–261
   assessment   213–19
   characteristics of abused and
      abuser   3, 187–9, 254–5
   child abuse and   see child abuse
   definitions   184–6
   diagnosing   19, 206–8
   and domestic violence   196–8,
      255–9, 259–60
   extent of   16, 186–7
   health perspective   17–18, 204–21
   historical background   222–6
   indicators   17, 208–9
   institutional abuse   189–92
   intervention   200–2, 240–3,
      257–9; categories of abuse
      200–1
   legislation   16, 198–200, 219–20,
      241–2, 258–9
   marginalisation   237–40
   memory clinic   218–19
   mental state assessment   216–19
   raising awareness   208–10
   re-discovery   183–4
   screening instruments   215–16

information, professionals'
knowledge of 144–5, 163
injunctions 120–1, 198, 258–9
institutional abuse 16, 189–92, 201,
242
institutional care 197, 220, 241–2,
252, 258
integrated models of family violence
48
interactionist theory 46, 194–5
inter-agency coordination *see*
multi-agency approaches
inter-generational mediation 203
inter-generational transmission of
violence 11, 115–16, 156–7
reversed 248
International Society for the Study
and Prevention of Child Abuse
and Neglect 29
intervention 49, 247, 261
child abuse 60–1, 73; *see also*
child protection
domestic violence 146, 147,
257–9
elder abuse 200–2, 240–3,
257–9; principles 201–2
interviewing
children 89–91
older people 211–12, 213–16
women 161, 162
Irvine, R. 45
isolation 112–13, 192, 238, 246
Iwaniec, D. 43

Jackson, H. 31
Jaffe, P. 113, 131, 166
Jehu, D. 59–60
Jenkins, G. 236
Jezierski, M. 145–6
Johnson, J. M. 158
Johnson, T. F. 184
joint investigations 172
joint training 14–15, 72, 172
Jones, A. 154, 160
Joseph, Sir K. 26
judgement 220
Judicial Statistics 110
justice principle 65–6
juvenile offenders, persistent 94,
96

Kalmuss, D. S. 117
Kayser-Jones, J. 190
Kempe, C. H. 25, 53
Kempe, R. S. 53
Kingston, P. 189, 193, 240, 242,
243
Kitsuse, J. 103, 104
Koning, A. de 44
Kosberg, J. I. 17, 214
Kurz, D. 10

La Fontaine, J. 35
Large, S. 53
Lasch, C. 48
law/legislation
child abuse 61–3, 66–7;
discourse analysis 81–2,
87–8, 92–5, 97; *see also*
Children Act
domestic violence 258
elder abuse 16, 198–200,
219–20, 241–2, 258–9
Law Commission 121–2, 198, 216,
225, 241
'learned helplessness' 14, 115,
157–8
learning disabilities, people with 3,
16, 152, 257
leaving violent relationship 125,
158
legitimation of social problems
231–4
Leroux, T. G. 227–8, 228, 230, 235
lesbian women 152
Lloyd, S. 172
local authorities
child abuse 67
Children Act 79, 83; complaints
and representation procedures
95–6
Children's Departments 42
housing obligations 122–3, 168
multi-agency approaches to
domestic violence 169–72
local connection 122
London poster campaign 171
Loney, M. 54
Loseke, D. R. 3
Lynch, M. 24, 44
Lyon, C. 51–2, 53

294

male dominance   117, 141, 142, 148
Mama, A.   109, 117, 133, 151, 161,
    164
management of abuse   *see*
    intervention
managerialism   83–4, 97
mandatory reporting legislation
    241, 242
Mandt, A.   12, 143–4
Manning, N.   23
Manthorpe, J.   239
marginalisation   19, 195, 237–40,
    240
market economy discourse   83,
    93–4, 97
Marsden, D.   128
material abuse   185, 187, 189, 201,
    253
Matrimonial Homes Act (1983)
    (MHA)   120, 121, 198
Matrimonial Homes (Family
    Protection) (Scotland) Act
    (1981)   163–4
Matthews, S.   187, 195–6, 197–8
Maynard, M.   106, 153, 159, 161–2
McIlwaine, G.   12, 142
McLeer, S.   11–12, 128–9
media   233–4
medical model   51
memory clinic   214, 218–19
men
    intervention for violent   114,
        172–4
    possible indicators of domestic
        violence   155
Men's Centre, London   114
Mental Health Act (1983)   198
mental state assessment   214,
    216–19
'mental test score'   218–19
Metropolitan Police   119
Miller, D.   52
Millett, K.   102–3
'minimental state' test   219
mobilisation of action   19, 234–6
'moderate' physical injury   37, 38–9
money control/management   117
Moore, D.   192
Moore, J. G.   157
moral panic   229

Morgan, P. A.   106
multi-agency approaches
    child abuse   7, 49; Children Act
        68, 70–3
    domestic violence   14–15, 142–4,
        167, 168, 169–72
    elder abuse   221
    training   14–15, 72, 172
multi-infarct dementia   217–18
Munhall, P.L.   51
murder of partner   125–6, 128,
    158–9

Naish, J.   57
NALGO   150, 170
Narducci, T.   70
National Children's Bureau   167,
    168
National Health Service and
    Community Care Act (1990)
    15, 198, 233
National Inter-Agency Working
    Party on Domestic Violence
    117, 120, 121, 125
National Women's Aid Federation
    104, 105
needs-led intervention   92–6, 243
neglect
    child abuse   27, 28, 30, 36, 42–3
    elder abuse   185, 186–7, 188,
        200–1, 253
    gender of abuser   249
Nelson, B.   23–4
Nethercott, S.   57
'New Nursing'   56–7
New Zealand   35
Newberger, E.   30, 31–2
Newson, E.   34
Newson, J.   34
Nixon, J.   111, 130
'no-criming' domestic violence
    110, 118, 119
'no order' principle   79, 86
Noble, J.   33–4
'non-accidental injury syndrome'   45
non-consequentialist (deontological)
    theory   63–4
non-maleficence principle   65
non-molestation injunctions   120–1,
    122

Scottish Women's Aid   168, 169, 173
screening instruments   215–16
Seedhouse, D.   54–5, 65
Select Committee on Violence in Marriage   105, 109–10, 123
self-determination   *see* empowerment
self-help   107, 257
self-neglect   197–8
sexual abuse
    children   3, 44, 205; case study 58–61; definitions   27, 28, 30, 52–3; family systems model   26–7; nature 39–42; preconditions   60; prevalence   34–5, 36; professionals and identification   31; risk factors   60; sociological model   48
    domestic violence   111–12
    elders   3, 17, 205, 210–13; indicators   208, 209
    myths surrounding   212–13
    people with learning disabilities 3, 257
sexual abuse continuum   213
Shakti   153
shame   124
Shapiro, J.   115, 124
Shemmings, D.   88
Simnett, I.   54, 55
situational model   193
Skelton, R.   57
skin, ageing and   206–7
Smith, L.   101, 108–9, 109, 110, 128
    causes of domestic violence   116, 117
Smith, M.   34
Smith, S.   12
Snell, J.   115
social class   31–2, 109
social construction of child abuse 23–7
social construction of old age 195–6, 229–30, 238
social learning theory   11, 115–16, 156–7
    reversed   248

social movements   *see* battered-women's movement; pressure groups; women's movement
social perspective
    child abuse   8–9, 77–97; care proceedings   84–6; child protection case conferences 86–8; children's rights 91–6; interviewing children 89–91
    domestic violence   12–15, 149–77; children   165–8; frequency of contact between victims and social workers 160–3; gender issues   174–5; housing   163–5; individual social workers' good practice 176; multi-agency approaches 169–72; programmes for violent men   172–4; social work agencies' good practice 175–6; social work practice 152–4; understanding domestic violence   154–60; Women's Aid   163–5, 168–9; women's opinion of social work's response   163
    elder abuse   18–19, 222–44; intervention   240–3
social problems   103–4
    child abuse   23–7, 223
    domestic violence   153–4, 223
    elder abuse   226–37; critical juncture   243–4; emergence 228–31; legitimation 231–4; mobilisation of action 234–6; official action plan 236–7
    stages in development   226
social services department, prior contact with   33
Social Services Inspectorate (SSI) 85–6, 234, 235
Social Services Select Committee 78
Social Work Services Group   28
social work agencies   175–6
social workers
    good practice in domestic violence 176

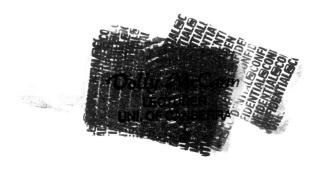